Congenital Adrenal Hyperplasia
A Comprehensive Guide

Congenital Adrenal Hyperplasia
A Comprehensive Guide

PETER C. HINDMARSH
University College London, London, United Kingdom

KATHY GEERTSMA
Dorset, United Kingdom

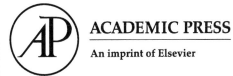

ACADEMIC PRESS
An imprint of Elsevier

Academic Press is an imprint of Elsevier
125 London Wall, London EC2Y 5AS, United Kingdom
525 B Street, Suite 1800, San Diego, CA 92101-4495, United States
50 Hampshire Street, 5th Floor, Cambridge, MA 02139, United States
The Boulevard, Langford Lane, Kidlington, Oxford OX5 1GB, United Kingdom

Notices

Knowledge and best practice in this field are constantly changing. As new research and experience broaden
our understanding, changes in research methods, professional practices, or medical treatment may become
necessary.

Practitioners and researchers must always rely on their own experience and knowledge in evaluating and using
any information, methods, compounds, or experiments described herein. In using such information or methods
they should be mindful of their own safety and the safety of others, including parties for whom they have a
professional responsibility.

To the fullest extent of the law, neither the Publisher nor the authors, contributors, or editors, assume any
liability for any injury and/or damage to persons or property as a matter of products liability, negligence or
otherwise, or from any use or operation of any methods, products, instructions, or ideas contained in the
material herein.

Library of Congress Cataloging-in-Publication Data
A catalog record for this book is available from the Library of Congress

British Library Cataloguing-in-Publication Data
A catalogue record for this book is available from the British Library

ISBN: 978-0-12-811483-4

For information on all Academic Press publications visit our website at
https://www.elsevier.com/books-and-journals

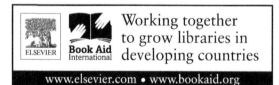

www.elsevier.com • www.bookaid.org

Publisher: Mica Haley
Acquisition Editor: Tari Broderick
Editorial Project Manager: Timothy Bennett
Production Project Manager: Karen East and Kirsty Halterman
Designer: Maria Ines Cruz

Typeset by Thomson Digital

CONTENTS

SECTION THREE: TREATMENT FOR CONGENITAL ADRENAL HYPERPLASIA

This book provides all the theoretical knowledge necessary to understand CAH in terms of pathophysiology, clinical presentation, diagnosis and management. It is extremely well written and very easy to follow and comprehend. It covers all aspects pertaining to the condition in great detail. There isn't another book available on the market like this one! Also, it is a wonderful book to read! The text covers all aspects of CAH in great detail and the figures are amazing and most informative. The book covers the topic extensively and teaches with great clarity about how to use the knowledge to make the most appropriate decisions for patients.

Evangelia Charmandari
Professor of Paediatric and Adolescent Endocrinology,
University of Athens Medical School

A MEDICAL VIEW

Over the last 10–15 years there have been many changes in the way that Congenital Adrenal Hyperplasia (CAH) is managed. These changes have come about by better understanding the way cortisol is naturally produced and how the body handles the synthetic form of cortisol, hydrocortisone. From knowledge of what happens with cortisol production during a 24 hour period, coupled with insights gained from working to mimic replacement therapy with a hydrocortisone pump, a greater depth of understanding of therapy in CAH has evolved.

My research in CAH focuses on improving cortisol replacement. The aim of replacement therapy is to mimic as closely as possible, the normal circadian rhythm of cortisol. To achieve this, knowledge of how the individual handles hydrocortisone (the synthetic form of cortisol) is necessary. Over the last 10 years we have studied the absorption and clearance of hydrocortisone in individuals with CAH and in other patients with a variety of disorders causing adrenal insufficiency. These studies use 24 hour blood cortisol profiles to help understand what happens in the circulation when a tablet of hydrocortisone is taken. This information is then processed with knowledge of the clearance of hydrocortisone from the circulation, obtained by intravenous studies of the fate of a bolus of hydrocortisone. From studies such as these, it is possible to define: fast, normal and slow absorbers and fast, normal and slow clearers. These data then inform how best to dose with hydrocortisone and how often the tablets should be taken.

24 hour blood cortisol profiles form the mainstay of my clinical practice. I make no apologies for using them extensively in this book, as they serve to illustrate and illuminate the many problems we face in treating people with this condition. This is evident when you look at the complexity of the dynamics of cortisol secretion in people without adrenal problems and even more so when tackling replacement therapy itself.

These 24 hour studies of the effect of therapy has been informed by the application of pump technology. What has been learned from pump therapy is that it is possible to mimic the normal cortisol circadian rhythm exactly without over or under exposure to hydrocortisone. If the cortisol is right then the other parameters often measured in

CAH such as 17-hydroxyprogesterone and androstenedione follow suit. This means if we get cortisol replacement right then everything else will fall into place.

None of this would have been possible without the inspiration provided by Kathy Geertsma, who encouraged and motivated me to write this book together. This book aims to bring all this knowledge into a single cover and is a tribute to the hard work that all families with the condition put in to keep their loved ones safe. Working with Kathy on this has opened my eyes to the wider impact of the condition on everyday living. I hope this has been conveyed in this book as well.

Peter C. Hindmarsh

INTRODUCTION

This book is about congenital adrenal hyperplasia and ways to manage it. It is written for a varied group of people but mainly patients, parents and families with the condition. It will also be valuable for health care professionals, as it deals with areas not usually covered by standard textbooks of endocrinology.

Medical practice has changed dramatically over the last 15 years with greater engagement of patients and families in care. This has come from the seminal work by the Institute of Medicine—Crossing the Quality Chasm published in 2001. One of the key components to improve quality in medicine is to put the patient at the centre of all endeavours.

Such a move needs a major change in the way health care professionals and patients and families interact. This is especially the case for long term conditions of which adrenal disorders and congenital adrenal hyperplasia, in particular, are examples. Health care professionals and particular doctors are great at getting the diagnosis right. That is what they are primarily trained to do. However, getting the diagnosis is only the first step in the journey which will involve the introduction of treatment, monitoring that treatment and watching out for long term problems, either associated with the condition and/or the treatment.

The traditional way to do this has been to attend clinics where treatments can be reviewed, as well as questions and concerns addressed. The problems people face may not be the ones that health care training can address. For example, what one needs to do with tablets while travelling to New Zealand. Fitting the condition into the life style and demands of the family is key to success and one solution will not fit all. Clinics are busy places and unless the patient and family have worked out beforehand what information they need the consultation may not be of value, as not everything is maximised for them and in essence, their time is wasted. This is important because the patient and family really understand how the condition affects them. If there are three to four clinics planned per year and each consult takes 30 minutes, then the health care involvement over a year might only amount to 2 hours at the most, whereas families live with this all the time. On the basis of the time spent to become an expert, it is the patients and families that know the condition and how its treatment affects them.

The book uses this depth of practical experience to create a guide for all those involved in congenital adrenal hyperplasia. At diagnosis there is a lot for a family to understand and learn about, in addition to all the practicalities which need to be considered to keep the child safe on the new medication. Section One covers the basics of the condition, what the adrenal glands do and the actual cause of the problem. It then progresses to two key aspects of paediatric endocrinology, namely growth and puberty. These two areas define the difference between adult and paediatric endocrinology and are referred to constantly in clinics. One additional aspect which we have added to this section, is on tests. Although there are numerous tests possible, we have covered most of the common ones.

Section Two discusses the problems which can occur in this condition. At the first read, it seems that numerous aspects can go wrong. In fact, the point about this section is to highlight why we need to carefully monitor and how we should go about monitoring to avoid problems. That is our satnav guide to the condition in Chapter 9! The important thing is to avoid problems in the first place. For various reasons this is not always possible, so should they occur we give an explanation on how they can be addressed.

Section Three is all about treatment and monitoring and how to deal with certain situations, such as sick days and travel. This section in particular, has drawn on the immense experience of families dealing with the condition and how they have tackled the practical issues. This is a rich resource and including these experiences within the chapters has been an education for us too. The main message we learnt was to always listen to the patient and family, as not only are they articulating the problem, but they also have a solution for most of the issues. Too often, health care professionals are quick to raise issues of compliance with therapies when things don't work out the way they should. Section Three shows just how complicated the whole system is and how much individual variation there is in absorption and clearance of a drug, thus making therapies effective is hard work. Everyone is different, so it pays to keep an open mind and recognise that it is more than just swallowing a tablet.

In Section Three, there is a chapter on pump therapy which is something we have pioneered for congenital adrenal hyperplasia and in fact anyone needing cortisol replacement. The chapter is of value, not only because we have been able to achieve perfect replacement of cortisol in several very difficult cases by using the pump method to continuously infuse cortisol with individualised infusion rates calculated to suit the individual's metabolism, but also such an approach has given greater understanding and in-depth knowledge on the hormones involved in CAH and how they interrelate. With the pump method, came the realisation of ways to fine tune and improve conventional therapy with the use of 24 hour cortisol and 17-hydroxyprogesterone profiles.

We use 24 hour cortisol and 17-hydroxyprogesterone profiles throughout the book to illustrate many of the points that are made. These are not available to all but we hope that by placing them in context within the chapters, people will see the immense value they bring to diagnosis and replacement therapy. Information is power and sharing this information with patients and families, especially in picture format, aids understanding and brings everyone into the decision making process. 'One picture is worth a thousand words', is never more true than in this situation. It all becomes obvious as one family said to us. Chapter 34 contains a quiz so you can sharpen up your interpretive skills. Sadly no prizes for getting the answers right!

The book represents a combined parent and health care professional approach in managing congenital adrenal hyperplasia. We have written, we hope, in a way which is easy to understand and have tried our best to avoid jargon, especially long medical words, where possible. Sharing information is the best way to promote better care which is what we all want. We hope that we have achieved this in these pages and that you enjoy reading it as much as we did when putting the chapters together.

PERSONAL STORY

I am a parent of a young adult with Salt-wasting Congenital Adrenal Hyperplasia and the Chair of the CAHisus Support Group.

When you are informed that your child has a rare life-threatening condition, it is extremely difficult to comprehend and absorb all the information you are told. Many of us parents could write a book on the emotional circumstances, fear and heartache that follow the diagnosis, as many males, like my own son, are on the brink of death before they are diagnosed. There is very little information on the condition and what is available is often difficult to understand. What becomes very evident when you begin to try to understand the treatment and monitoring is that most doctors have very different ideas on the condition which is not only confusing, but also leaves you wondering if you are doing the best for your child. I truly believed I was.

Throughout my son's younger years, he battled with his health, stamina and debilitating headaches. I was told there was no relationship between the condition and the symptoms he suffered and that his 17OHP levels were within normal range. Following my instincts and knowing my son, I sought several opinions from different endocrinologists, who either had no answers or suggested chronic fatigue syndrome. His condition was monitored by using blood spots to measure 17OHP, which seems to be the 'way' to treat this condition. The journey was very difficult and emotional for him.

It was only when we were introduced to Professor Hindmarsh did things change. He looked in great detail at the way my son metabolised cortisol (in fact during his younger years, no one ever once measured his cortisol levels). It became evident that not only did he metabolise cortisol very rapidly with a half-life of 40 minutes, but also had a problem with the cortisol shuttle where cortisol from hydrocortisone, which is metabolised to cortisone in the kidney occurred too quickly and the conversion back to cortisol too slowly! This meant not only did he not absorb cortisol well, but what he retained was metabolised very quickly.

Our very supportive GP, Dr Beth Davies, suggested the use of a syringe driver, and Professor Hindmarsh took up the idea and worked ways around the problems by introducing a new method of treatment, the 'pump method'. This focused on getting the cortisol levels optimal, by mimicking normal production, and from this we realised that if only my son's cortisol levels had been measured since birth, the problem would have been identified. He would have had a healthy childhood and it would have prevented the many short and long term side effects which he suffered. Professor Hindmarsh was the first person in the world to devise a formula that would mimic the circadian rhythm.

His health is so much better now compared to his younger years, when he was unable to partake in sports due to lack of stamina, not able to attend school regularly and had a poor quality of life. This was simply due to long periods of cortisol absence between doses and it was thought that taking higher doses would result in cortisol lasting longer, but this was not the case; it led to high peaks causing periods of over treatment, followed by many hours of under treatment where he had no measurable cortisol in the blood. As the high peaks suppressed the 17OHP, the doctors assured me that all was well. However, the more I researched the condition, the more it seemed that each centre varied in their approach and even had their own optimal 17OHP level.

Some people with the condition seemingly had no problems, seeing it only as a bit of a nuisance in having to take tablets, but many battle with it. This is probably due to variations in individual half-life and clearance of hydrocortisone which a study showed can range from 40–225 minutes.

With the dramatic change in my son's wellbeing, he went on further to University and now lives a very normal life, goes to the gym, surfs, swims and has a managerial position in a very stressful and demanding job, often having to work long hours. As well as seeing this incredible, positive difference to his health once his cortisol replacement was optimal, my son also gained good growth and no longer had weight issues. I feel it is very important that others are given the opportunity to have 24 hour profiles to ensure their cortisol levels checked. All other measures used only indicate problems once they have occured and looking carefully at cortisol, 17OHP and other important levels by 24 hour profiling, most problems can be prevented. I encouraged Professor Hindmarsh to give every patient who wanted one, a 24 hour profile. Our experience showed that relying on 17OHP blood spots taken before each dose, could give a false picture of what the aim of treatment in congenital adrenal hyperplasia which is, to replace what is missing - cortisol. It became very obvious with my son's detailed data, that it is important to measure the cortisol levels over 24 hours, as once the distribution and replacement amount is correct, all the other measures used as markers also normalise.

The severity of congenital adrenal hyperplasia varies among individuals and the treatment needs to be tailored for the person, and not a blanket formula used for all. This can only be done by tailoring the dose of hydrocortisone to suit the patient using 24 hour cortisol and 17OHP profiles. The data that Professor Hindmarsh has shown at our meetings, a lot of which are in this book, I hope will help everyone understand how hydrocortisone works as a replacement for cortisol. Realising the importance of the timing of taking doses, how long it lasts in the blood stream, as well as how much cortisol is attained from the dose, what can go wrong and what to do about it can only be beneficial to all those with CAH.

We began by writing leaflets which were put on our website, and over the years these have helped so many patients, as well as saved lives worldwide. We started a parent and patient group which is well supported and appreciated and even caters to people from Europe. It is incredibly important for parents, patients and medical professionals to have a book like this which we have co-authored, as the data are accredited, scientifically based and very easy to understand. Over the years the knowledge I have gained and my experience in dealing with this condition, especially my involvement with my son pioneering the pump method devised by Professor Hindmarsh, which he has been on for over 13 years, has enabled me to fully contribute to this project.

Kathy Geertsma
Co-author

SECTION ONE

Congenital Adrenal Hyperplasia—Introduction

The first section covers the basics of the condition, what the adrenal glands do and what the cause of the problem actually is. It then progresses covering two key aspects of paediatric endocrinology, namely growth and puberty. These two areas define the difference between adult and paediatric endocrinology and are referred to constantly in clinics. One additional aspect we have added to this section is on tests. Although there are numerous tests possible, we have covered most of the common ones.

Growth and development largely separates paediatric endocrinology from adult endocrinology. Virtually all childhood conditions have an impact on growth and development. So, in this section we look into how growth and puberty take place and how to assess whether it is progressing in a normal manner or not. Congenital adrenal hyperplasia is a complex condition because, as we show, both the condition itself and the treatment of the condition, impact growth and puberty. This is a complicated area and we expand on this by looking at the contributions made by the adrenal glands and the gonads.

What we are not going to consider in Section One, are aspects of congenital adrenal hyperplasia care involved in determining the gender rearing of a child born with ambiguous genitalia. This is an area that deserves a book in its own right and is not really suited to this book which is about practical issues of treatment.

CHAPTER 1

Physiology of the Adrenal Glands: How Does It Work?

GLOSSARY

Adrenal androgens Male like hormones with a structure similar to testosterone. The two main androgens are dehydroepiandrosterone and androstenedione.

Adrenal cortex Outer layer of the adrenal glands which has three layers known as zones that produce corticosteroids.

Adrenal medulla Centre of the adrenal glands producing epinephrine (adrenalin) and norepinephrine (noradrenalin).

Adrenocorticotropin hormone (ACTH) Polypeptide hormone secreted by the anterior lobe of the pituitary gland, which stimulates the cortex of the adrenal glands to produce cortisol.

Androstenedione One of the adrenal androgens which is made from dehydroepiandrosterone by the action of the enzyme 3 beta hydroxysteroid dehydrogenase type 2. Level rises in CAH when cortisol replacement is suboptimal.

Backdoor pathway An alternative pathway for the formation of androgens by the fetal adrenal glands.

Circadian rhythm Changes in a hormone in this case cortisol through the 24 hour period where values peak in the morning and reach low levels late evening.

Corticosteroids Class of steroid hormones produced in the adrenal cortex, these being mineralocorticoids, glucocorticoids and adrenal androgens.

Cortisol The major glucocorticoid in humans. Made in the adrenal glands. Cortisol regulates over two thirds of human genes. Cortisol regulates blood glucose, muscle function, the body's response to infection, fat distribution and brain thought processes.

Cortisol binding globulin (CBG) A protein made by the liver which attaches itself to cortisol and carries it around the body. This is known as bound cortisol. 90–95% of cortisol is bound in this way with 5% in the free state. The free cortisol is the biologically active cortisol. In blood tests we measure bound and free cortisol and this is called total cortisol.

Dehydroepiandrosterone (DHEA) One of the adrenal androgens which is made from 17-hydroxypregnenolone by the action of the enzyme CYP17.

Fetal adrenal glands Large structures present in the fetus which mainly produces dehydroepiandrosterone and helps maintain the pregnancy. The fetal adrenal glands disappear by the third month after birth.

Congenital Adrenal Hyperplasia. http://dx.doi.org/10.1016/B978-0-12-811483-4.00001-5

Glucocorticoids Group of steroid hormones (glucose + cortex + steroid) which regulate glucose metabolism and suppress inflammation.

Mineralocorticoids Hormones which regulate the balance of electrolytes such as sodium and potassium. A member of the steroid family which increases sodium uptake from the kidney and large bowel.

Physiology Structure and function.

Renin–angiotensin system Group of hormones which act together to regulate blood volume and blood pressure.

INTRODUCTION

We are going to start by looking at where the adrenal glands are situated in the body and how they are made up. Then we will look at the way the body makes cortisol and how it works out how much cortisol is needed. Then we will delve into what happens in congenital adrenal hyperplasia (CAH).

The two adrenal glands sit above the kidneys and are made up of two distinct parts (Fig. 1.1). In the middle is an area called the adrenal medulla which produces the stress hormones, adrenaline and noradrenaline. Outside of this is the adrenal cortex which is divided into three zones which make corticosteroids.

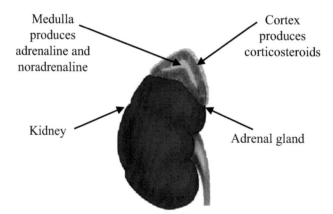

Figure 1.1 *Relation of the adrenal gland to the kidney showing the cortex and medulla of the adrenal gland.*

The corticosteroid family is made up of three groups: mineralocorticoids which are salt retaining hormones, of which aldosterone is the main one, glucose regulating hormones or glucocorticoids of which cortisol is the main one and adrenal androgens which are male like hormones and are produced by all males and all females.

Mineralocorticoids or aldosterone are regulated mainly by the renin-angiotensin system and to a lesser extent by adrenocorticotropin hormone (ACTH). Glucocorticoids are regulated by the pituitary gland through the hormone ACTH. Adrenal androgens are produced under the regulation of ACTH.

To understand how the adrenal glands work under the regulation of both the hypothalamus and the pituitary gland we need to look at each gland and learn a bit about their role.

THE HYPOTHALAMUS AND PITUITARY GLAND

The regulation of virtually all hormones produced by the body is undertaken by the pituitary gland. The pituitary gland sits at the base of the brain in a bony hollow called the pituitary fossa, this is behind the bridge of the nose and behind the eye socket, close to the nerves which come from the eyes. The pituitary produces six hormones: growth hormone (GH), adrenocorticotropin hormone (ACTH), thyrotropic hormone (TSH), prolactin (PRL), luteinising hormone (LH) and follicle-stimulating hormone (FSH) (Fig. 1.2). We will talk about several of these hormones as we go through this book.

The pituitary hormones are in turn regulated by a series of releasing factors produced by the hypothalamus. The hypothalamus acts as a coordinating centre bringing together information from various parts of the brain, the environment in terms of the day/night cycle and other inputs such as the levels of glucose and amino acids in the blood. Various parts of the hypothalamus are involved in the timing of hormone release.

Several genes which are known as 'clock genes' are important and are situated in the hypothalamus and the changes in the activity of these genes during the 24 hour period generate what we see with many hormones, namely a circadian rhythm. A circadian rhythm is something which changes through a 24 hour period, and these clock genes are sensitive to changes in light.

The hypothalamus produces a series of regulating factors which enter into a special blood stream connecting the hypothalamus to the pituitary, known as the portal venous system. This system proceeds down a very fine stalk which connects the hypothalamus to the pituitary. In the pituitary gland, these factors act on the various cells present and produce a specific hormone. The hormone then enters into the main blood stream travelling to the target glands, in our case the adrenal glands, to tell the glands to produce the target hormone. Once this hormone has been produced, it is also released into the blood stream and travels to the organs to carry out the various effects that are necessary. In addition, this target hormone feeds back onto the pituitary and hypothalamus to tell it that this job has been done and that no further hormone secretion is necessary.

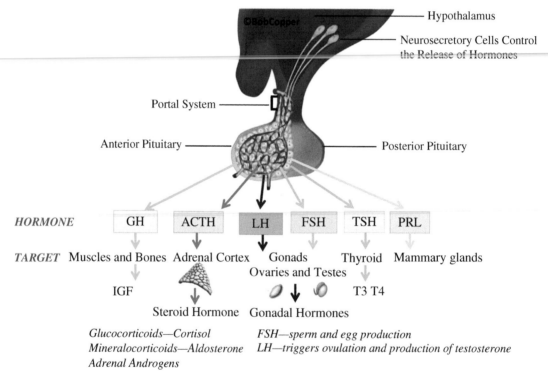

Figure 1.2 *The six major hormones that the anterior pituitary produces: growth hormone (GH), adrenocorticotropin hormone (ACTH), thyrotropic hormone (TSH), prolactin (PRL), luteinising hormone (LH) and follicle-stimulating hormone (FSH).*

In Fig. 1.3 we can see the complex control pathway from the pituitary gland leading to the formation of aldosterone, cortisol and adrenal androgens.

The adrenal glands are subdivided into the cortex and the medulla. The cortex is further divided into three zones and the adrenal steroid hormones are made in these different zones. Cells in the area called the zona glomerulosa make aldosterone whereas cells in the zona reticularis make androgens and the cells in the zona fasciculata make cortisol (Fig. 1.4).

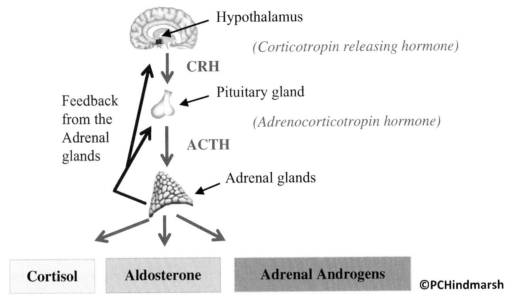

Figure 1.3 *Picture representation of the hypothalamo-pituitary-adrenal (HPA) axis.*

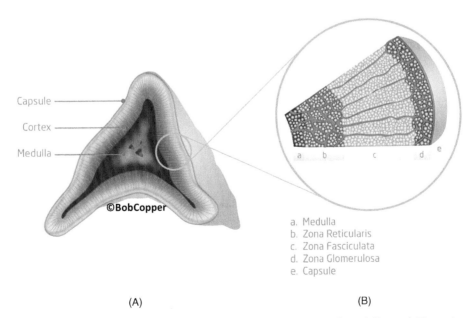

(A)   (B)

Figure 1.4 *(A) Sections of the adrenal gland to show the cortex and medulla and (B) a microscopic section of the cortex shows the three zones.*

WHAT ARE STEROIDS?

We have used this term already so it might be useful to consider what we mean. The name 'steroids' refers to a family of hormones which all share a similar structure based on cholesterol. The body takes cholesterol into the adrenal glands or the testes/ovaries and modifies it to make hormones called steroids.

There are branches of this steroid family, such as the adrenal steroids we have already mentioned, or the sex steroids such as the male hormone testosterone or the female hormone estrogen. Even Vitamin D is a part of the steroid family.

Steroids have received a bad name in the press because of the effect on making people gain weight or when athletes abuse them. However, steroids are vital hormones for the body in the right amounts. Too much as well as too little steroid can lead to illness and serious long term health issues as we shall see in Chapter 4 and Section Two.

REGULATION OF CORTISOL RELEASE

The amount of cortisol in the body is determined by the production of ACTH from the pituitary gland, which is in turn regulated by the corticotropin releasing hormone (CRH) produced by the hypothalamus. The process works rather like a thermostat in your oven. Just like the oven which keeps the temperature constant at a set value, the body will also always try to keep the cortisol concentration in the blood at certain preset values.

When cortisol concentrations fall below what is required, the body will increase the production of CRH and ACTH to make more cortisol. If cortisol values are higher than they should be at any particular point in time, then CRH and ACTH production will be switched off. Fig. 1.5 shows this in schematic form with cortisol acting back on the pituitary gland. Fig. 1.5 shows how CRH acts on the pituitary gland to release ACTH which travels in the blood stream to the adrenal glands to stimulate the release of cortisol. Cortisol then acts back on ACTH and CRH to reduce production.

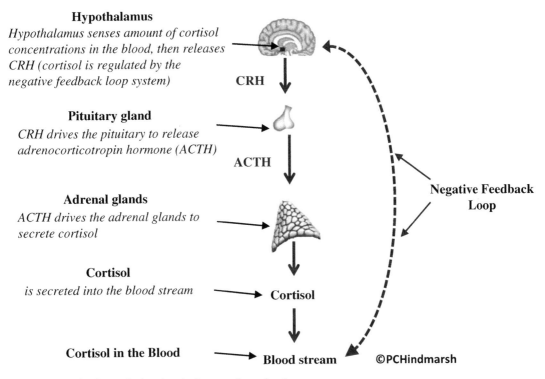

Hypothalamus
Hypothalamus senses amount of cortisol concentrations in the blood, then releases CRH (cortisol is regulated by the negative feedback loop system)

CRH

Pituitary gland
CRH drives the pituitary to release adrenocorticotropin hormone (ACTH)

ACTH

Adrenal glands
ACTH drives the adrenal glands to secrete cortisol

Negative Feedback Loop

Cortisol
is secreted into the blood stream

Cortisol

Cortisol in the Blood

Blood stream   ©PCHindmarsh

Figure 1.5 *The hypothalamic-pituitary-adrenal axis.*

THE CIRCADIAN RHYTHM OF CORTISOL—THE NATURAL PRODUCTION OF CORTISOL

The daily cortisol production rate is remarkably constant at all ages, but the amount of cortisol which can be measured in the blood, varies during the 24 hour period. This is called the circadian rhythm of cortisol and it reflects changes in the amount of CRH and ACTH produced during the 24 hour period. Circadian derives from the Latin words 'circa' meaning 'around, about or approximately' and 'diem' which is a Latin phrase for 'by the day' so simply means about a day and refers to the 24 hour period.

As you can see in Fig. 1.6, the highest concentrations of cortisol occur in the early hours of the morning so cortisol is really the 'get up and go hormone'. During the late afternoon and particularly in the evening, the amounts of cortisol present are very low but there is always some present which can be measured.

As we have already mentioned, the production of ACTH is also regulated by another hormone CRH, which comes from the hypothalamus which is the structure that occupies the base of the brain. CRH determines the amount of ACTH which in turn determines the amount of cortisol that can be produced so the whole system starts from a very small amount of CRH, an even greater amount of ACTH and a very high amount of cortisol. The whole system amplifies itself.

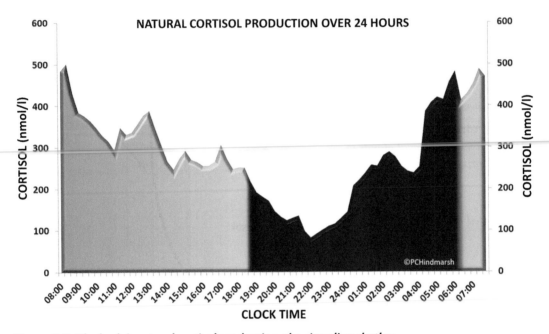

Figure 1.6 *The body's natural cortisol production, the circadian rhythm.*

It is important to remember this circadian rhythm of cortisol because it will determine how we go about replacing cortisol in CAH as part of our way of treating the condition. We will go into this in more detail in Section Three.

To make cortisol, the adrenal glands need to take up cholesterol from the blood stream. We often think of cholesterol as bad and that is true if there is too much of it present which can lead to problems with the blood vessels which become 'furred up' leading to heart problems. But we all need some cholesterol and it forms the basis of making all steroids.

ACTH tells the adrenal glands to pick up some cholesterol from the blood and it does this by using a series of proteins which help bring cholesterol into the adrenal glands. The main protein is called steroidogenic acute regulatory protein (StAR). Once cholesterol is in the adrenal glands, it starts to be used up in a series of steps converting cholesterol into the various steroids the adrenal glands make. Each conversion step is brought about by the action of an enzyme. Enzymes are proteins which speed up the process of the chemical reaction. You could think of them rather like baking powder in a cake recipe. Each of the steps requires a special enzyme and each of them has a different name for the different tasks that they perform.

We will be looking at this in more detail in the section on the different forms of CAH (Chapters 4 and 5). You will see that the pathway is built up with all the different enzymes needed to convert cholesterol. As this pathway is so complicated, it is easy to understand why things can go wrong in CAH.

Once the adrenal glands make cortisol, a small amount is stored but the majority is released immediately into the blood stream. As we said before, the amounts produced at different times of the day vary and Fig. 1.7 shows us the percentage of total amounts we find at different times of the day. These percentages differ because this is how the circadian rhythm changes. This represents the amount of cortisol produced by the adrenal glands between the time frames and not necessarily the times you need to take tablet replacement therapy (see Chapter 21).

Time Segment	Percentage of Total Cortisol Secretion during Time Segment	
	Children	**Adults**
06:00–12:00	38.4	26.4
12:00–18:00	21.2	21.2
18:00–24:00	10.7	7.2
24:00–06:00	29.7	45.2

Figure 1.7 *Percentage of the total cortisol produced by the adrenal glands at different times of the day in children and adults.*

Once cortisol is in the blood stream some of it goes around freely in the blood, i.e. not attached to anything, which is referred to as 'free' cortisol. 'Free' cortisol is cortisol which is ready to act in different cells in the body. However, a fair quantity of it becomes attached to different proteins present in the blood, in particular, one protein called cortisol binding globulin (CBG), takes up a fair amount of cortisol and acts as a little reservoir in the blood stream. We discuss this in more detail in Chapter 18.

This means as 'free' cortisol is removed from the blood stream there can be a top-up from the cortisol attached to the protein reservoir. 'Free' cortisol can be removed by the kidneys and passed out in the urine but the majority of the cortisol produced is broken down in the liver and is passed out of the body in various forms in the urine.

Cortisol is vital to life and is known as the stress hormone.

The diagram in Fig. 1.8 shows many of the effects of cortisol. For example, cortisol determines how much fat is laid down in various parts of the body as well as helping the body prevent blood glucose going low, by breaking down fat and protein into glucose. Cortisol also modulates how we fight infections and how much calcium we lay down in the bones. The effects of cortisol are numerous and about 60% of all our genes in the body are regulated by cortisol.

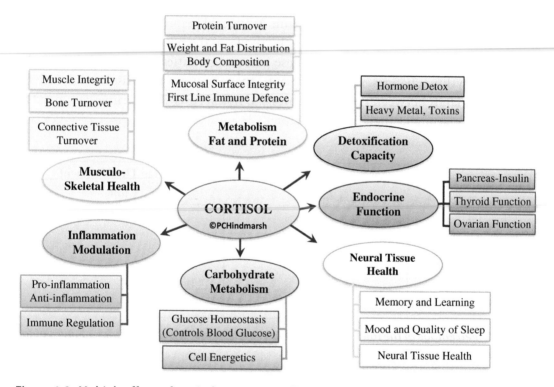

Figure 1.8 *Multiple effects of cortisol on a variety of body systems.*

RENIN-ANGIOTENSIN SYSTEM

The main function of the kidneys is to keep our blood clean and chemically balanced. They do this by removing salts and other water soluble waste which the body does not need, by making urine which is then excreted out of the body. The kidneys are also important in maintaining blood volume and blood pressure.

Sodium chloride is the most abundant salt in the body and it has many important roles in keeping the body healthy. There is a hormone which 'controls' the sodium keeping it at the correct level and this steroid hormone is called aldosterone and it is made in the adrenal glands. Aldosterone is responsible for how much sodium the kidneys keep (retain) and how much to pass out in the urine. As sodium retains water, it is very important to have the sodium level correct so the body can retain the correct amount of water, therefore maintaining the body's correct blood volume and blood pressure.

Just like the control of cortisol, aldosterone is regulated by a feedback system. Fig. 1.9 shows this system. So what are all these steps? Let's start by thinking about the main part which is blood pressure which is a measure of the force of blood moving around the body. A fall in blood pressure is detected by the kidneys which send a signal, renin, instructing the liver to make some angiotensin I from angiotensinogen. Angiotensinogen is a large molecule which is broken down by renin into angiotensin I.

Renin is a protein which conveys the message to the liver to make angiotensin I. Just like our oven thermostat, if blood volume changes or the amount of salt varies, renin levels will change. If the amount of salt decreases, then the amount of renin increases and similarly if the blood volume decreases, the renin also increases.

Angiotensin I is then converted in the lungs to angiotensin II which instructs the adrenal glands to make aldosterone. Aldosterone and angiotensin II instructs the blood vessels to narrow and the heart to pump harder, both of which increase blood pressure. In addition, aldosterone instructs the kidney to hold onto salt and water which increases the blood volume which also increases the blood pressure.

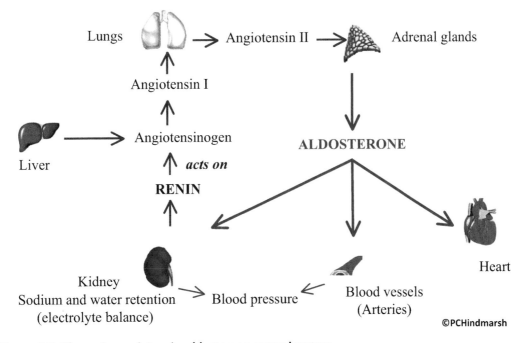

Figure 1.9 *The renin-angiotensin-aldosterone control system.*

The stimuli for renin release, angiotensin production and aldosterone synthesis, are decreasing sodium (salt) levels, low blood volume or blood pressure, high levels of potassium and adrenaline and low aldosterone levels. From these complex stimuli it is easy to see how serious the salt-wasting form of congenital adrenal hyperplasia (SWCAH) is. As aldosterone is missing, these people only get part of the response and so cannot hold onto sodium and maintain a good blood circulation.

Aldosterone is also controlled by ACTH but not to the same extent as renin.

ADRENAL ANDROGENS

Male hormones are called androgens and the body makes them in two places as shown in Fig. 1.10. In males, the testes make testosterone which is the strongest form of male hormone and a small amount of weak male hormones are made in the adrenal glands, namely dehydroepiandrosterone (DHEA) and androstenedione.

We say they are strong or weak depending on whether they alter the size of the penis and change body hair. In males, the testosterone from the testes is far stronger and produces greater effects than the adrenal androgens. The adrenal androgens can have testosterone like effects but you need to have very high levels of adrenal androgens (often 10 times those that are normally present) for a period of time in the blood to achieve the same effect.

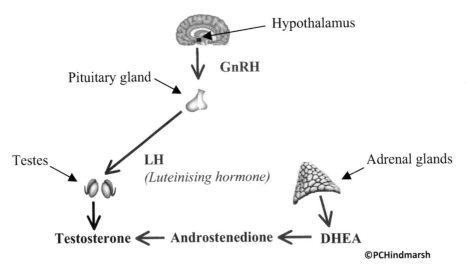

Figure 1.10 *Sources of male hormones in the male.*

One confusing element is that females also make small amounts of male like hormone but only from the adrenal glands as shown in Fig. 1.11 and this is androstenedione. This is a weak androgen which explains why axillary and pubic hair development in females are not to the same extent as in males.

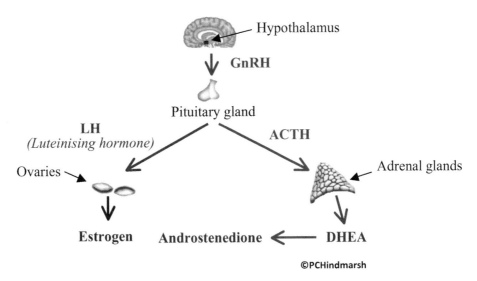

Figure 1.11 *Sources of male hormones in the female.*

In addition, the adrenal glands make another weak male like hormone called DHEA. DHEA and androstenedione are used in the testes to produce the strong male hormone testosterone, but the adrenal glands are very poor at making testosterone and even the amounts of androstenedione are quite low compared with the huge amounts of cortisol which are produced (about 300 times less).

DHEA is made in very large amounts but it is an extremely weak male like hormone. As a result, in males, although the adrenal glands do make these weak androgens, they have very little effect compared to the very powerful hormone testosterone made by the testes.

In females however, the appearance of pubic and axillary hair at puberty is dependent on the weak androgens, but the relatively finer and less dense distribution of pubic and axillary hair in females reflects the weakness of these androgens.

It is only when extremely high stimulation of the adrenal glands takes place that the weak androgens appear in any amounts which can influence the appearance of the individual. This is what we will see when we come to think about CAH and how it presents (Chapter 4).

THE BACKDOOR PATHWAY FOR ADRENAL ANDROGEN FORMATION

What we have described is the classic pathway for the production of 'male like' hormones in the adrenal glands. The production of 'male like' hormones from the adrenal glands are not very efficient and indeed the amounts of androstenedione and DHEA present in the blood, although comparable in total to testosterone, are not as potent.

Testosterone production from the adrenal glands is extremely difficult to achieve and can only occur when the adrenal glands are stimulated by extremely high amounts of ACTH for long periods of time. Although this can happen to a certain extent in the womb in babies who have CAH, it has always been difficult to understand how changes in the external genitalia in females can take place when it is so hard for the adrenal glands, at least in postnatal life, to make testosterone.

This has all seemed rather odd but more recently an alternative way of producing testosterone in the fetal adrenal glands has been identified. Rather than it going through DHEA and androstenedione, testosterone can also be formed from 17-hydroxypregnenolone and/or 17-hydroxyprogesterone through an alternative pathway involving androsterone (3alpha-hydroxy-5alpha-androstan-17-one) (Fig. 1.12).

This pathway involves quite a number of additional steps but it probably looks as though it is the more preferred pathway towards adrenal androgen production in the fetus.

This pathway ceases to work after birth as the fetal adrenal zone breaks down. In individuals who do not have any adrenal problems, this pathway is relatively underactive because 17-hydroxypregnenolone is preferentially converted to dehydroepiandrosterone (DHEA) and also down towards cortisol. However, when the conversion of 17-hydroxyprogesterone to 11-deoxycortisol is blocked as in CAH due to a deficiency of 21-hydroxylase, spillover from 17-hydroxypregnenolone into the alternative pathway takes place with the easier formation of testosterone.

It is probably this pathway which predominates in CAH and leads to the effects on the external genitalia in affected females.

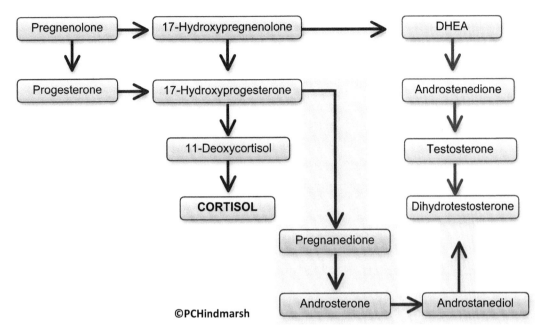

©PCHindmarsh

Figure 1.12 *The classic pathway to testosterone from 17-hydroxypregnenolone is shown in light blue. In the fetal adrenal glands there is an alternative pathway that allows the formation of dihydrotestosterone (the active form of testosterone) via androsterone shown in red.*

So what we see in Fig. 1.12 is a system which has many branching pathways and that changes with age. As we go through this book, we will be referring back to these pathways so it might be worth bookmarking them.

CONCLUSIONS

The adrenal glands are situated above the kidneys. Adrenalin is made in the middle of the gland and the cortisocosteroids, cortisol, aldosterone, DHEA and androstenedione are made in the outer area of the gland. Aldosterone production is regulated by the protein renin made by the kidneys and is involved in retaining salt in the body. Cortisol is regulated by the pituitary gland and has a circadian rhythm. Cortisol is a key hormone regulating many systems such as glucose, adipose (fat) tissue and the immune system. Dehydroepiandrosterone and androstenedione are weak, male like hormones produced in response to stimulation of the adrenal glands by the pituitary hormone ACTH.

FURTHER READING

Peters, C.J., Hill, N., Dattani, M.T., Charmandari, E., Matthews, D.R., Hindmarsh, P.C., 2013. Deconvolution analysis of 24 h serum cortisol profiles informs the amount and distribution of hydrocortisone replacement therapy. Clin. Endocrinol. (Oxf.) 78, 347–351.

CHAPTER 2

How Males and Females Develop

GLOSSARY

Anti-Müllerian hormone Hormone which is produced by the testes that causes resorption of tissues that would go on to form the womb and tubes.

Chromosomes Contain genetic information arranged on 22 pairs called autosomes and a pair called the sex chromosomes XY in males and XX in females.

Dihydrotestosterone Biologically active form of testosterone.

Primitive streak Part of the developing fetus that goes on to form the testes under instruction by SRY or in SRY absence, defaults to ovary formation.

SRY SRY (sex-determining region on the Y chromosome) gene on the Y chromosome which is critical in starting off the formation of the testes in males.

Testosterone Male sex hormone mainly produced by testes but can on occasion be produced by the adrenal glands when cortisol replacement is very poor.

GENERAL

The development of a human from a fertilised egg to the baby born after around 9 months of pregnancy is complex. To become either male or female requires a series of steps. The steps are rather similar to a cooking recipe in that different components have to be brought together at certain times in order for a male or female to develop. The gender or sex of an individual, depends on their genetic makeup and the hormones the testes or ovaries produce.

After birth, development is also influenced by the way in which parents and society view the person. Despite everything we try to do, there is an element of stereotyping which takes place. Parents tend to provide for a boy in a slightly different way to that of a girl. Society is conditioned to think of males doing certain tasks and females others. These are not conscious efforts but seem engrained in the way in which humans interact.

GENES MAKING MALES OR FEMALES

So let us start right at the beginning with the information which instructs us how to form a baby. The information which instructs how we develop is held in our genes and this is laid out on chromosomes. We have 23 pairs of chromosomes, 22 of the pairs are known as autosomes whereas the final pair is known as the sex chromosomes.

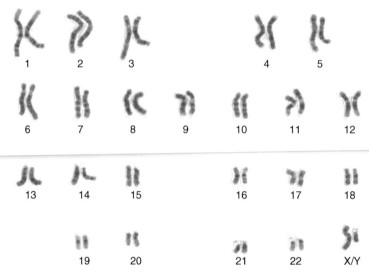

Figure 2.1 *Human chromosomes showing the 22 pairs and the X and Y indicating male.*

The picture (Fig. 2.1) shows what a male genetic makeup looks like. You can see the 22 chromosomes all nicely paired up and at the end the sex chromosomes called X and Y. Males have X and Y sex chromosomes (XY) whereas females have two X chromosomes (XX).

The Y chromosome carries a considerable amount of information which instructs the area (the primitive streak) which will develop into the gonad, to become a testicle. The most important of these is a gene called SRY which is the key piece of information instructing the gonad tissue to 'start becoming a testis'.

As we can see in Fig. 2.2 there are numerous complicated steps which go into making a testis. Each of the parts has to appear at a certain time and in a certain order. If any of the parts are missing or appear in the wrong order, the process stops and the gonad defaults to forming an ovary. In these situations, even though looking at the chromosomes they are XY, because small amounts of Y are missing, the individual will default and develop to look like a female.

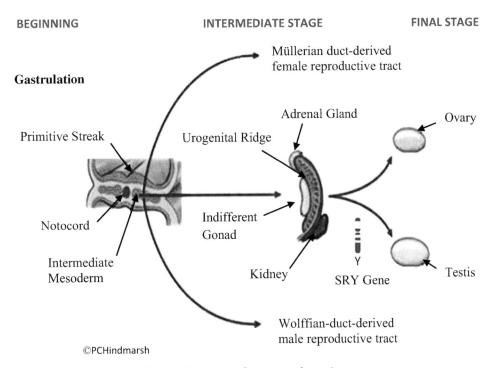

BEGINNING   INTERMEDIATE STAGE   FINAL STAGE

Gastrulation

Müllerian duct-derived
female reproductive tract

Primitive Streak

Urogenital Ridge

Adrenal Gland

Ovary

Notocord

Indifferent
Gonad

Intermediate
Mesoderm

Kidney

Y

SRY Gene

Testis

Wolffian-duct-derived
male reproductive tract

©PCHindmarsh

Figure 2.2 *Complex steps in the development of testes and ovaries.*

The diagram in Fig. 2.2 illustrates the complex developmental stages in both males and females. At about 5–6 weeks of development, germ cells migrate into the urogenital ridge; note that at this stage the gonads in the two sexes are identical and known as 'Indifferent'. The gonad development from thereon depends on the sex chromosome. As can be seen, if the Y chromosome SRY gene is present, this determines the fetus is male, however if there is no Y chromosome then an ovary develops.

Now let us assume that all goes to plan and the Y is intact and the testes develop properly. To look male and develop a penis, the testes have to produce the male hormone testosterone. This occurs quite early in development and by about 8–12 weeks after conception, the external genitalia, penis and scrotal area are formed. Testosterone not only forms the penis and scrotum, but also helps the tube that connects the testes to the penis to develop and it is along this tube that sperm are carried. In addition, the testes also make a special hormone called anti-Müllerian hormone which causes the primitive fallopian tubes and uterus to disappear.

In females, because there is no anti-Müllerian hormone, the primitive fallopian tubes and uterus do not disappear and continue to develop and form the womb.

We are now going to talk a bit more about testosterone. The reason for this, is that in congenital adrenal hyperplasia (CAH) the problem which arises with the appearance of external genitalia, relates to the presence of male like hormones produced by the adrenal glands. This means understanding what testosterone does is important.

It is very important to remember that in CAH in both males and females, the genetic plan to become a male or female is intact and sends the right messages to the gonad to become a testis or an ovary. There is nothing wrong with testis or ovary formation in CAH.

Equally, because the testes and ovaries form properly in males and females with CAH, there is nothing wrong with the internal structures in either males or females. In boys with CAH, the tube connecting the testes to the penis along which sperm travel is formed properly and sperm will be produced and move as they should. In girls with CAH, the tubes and womb form normally so eggs from the ovary can reach the womb.

What causes problems in CAH, is the development in the external appearances and we are now going to think about how these develop in boys and girls without CAH and how this can be altered in those with CAH.

EXTERNAL APPEARANCES—THE ROLE OF MALE HORMONES

As we have already said, the male hormone testosterone plays an important role in determining the appearance of the male. Testosterone is a member of the steroid family. To be a member of the steroid family, you have to have a structure which looks something like the structures in Fig. 2.3.

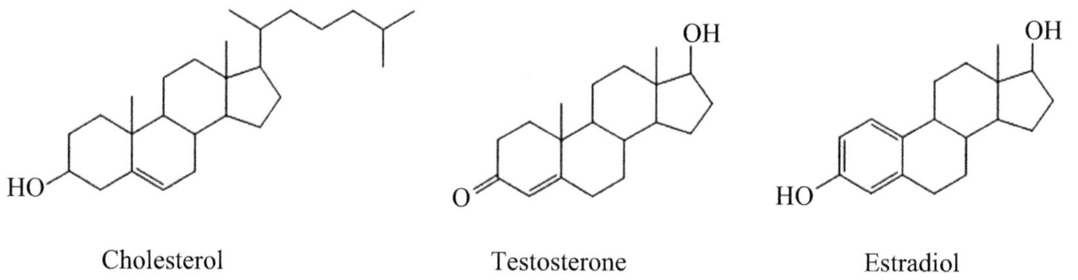

Cholesterol   Testosterone   Estradiol

Figure 2.3 *The structure of testosterone the male hormone and estradiol the female hormone. Both are made from cholesterol.*

On the left of Fig. 2.3 is cholesterol, from which all steroids in the body are made. We will look at this in more detail in the next chapter. The family characteristic is they have this ring structure with several open branches. Essentially, which branches are open determines what action the structure has as a hormone. The extra parallel lines are called double carbon bonds. These are also important for the steroid structure and action. We will show lots of steroid diagrams in the book so watch how the double bonds change.

In the next few chapters we will think about the male hormones, but at this stage we should remember that in males and females the adrenal glands make small amounts of weak male hormones or androgens. These adrenal androgens are called dehydroepiandrosterone (or DHEA for short!) and androstenedione (Fig. 2.4). In males the testes also produce the more powerful hormone, testosterone.

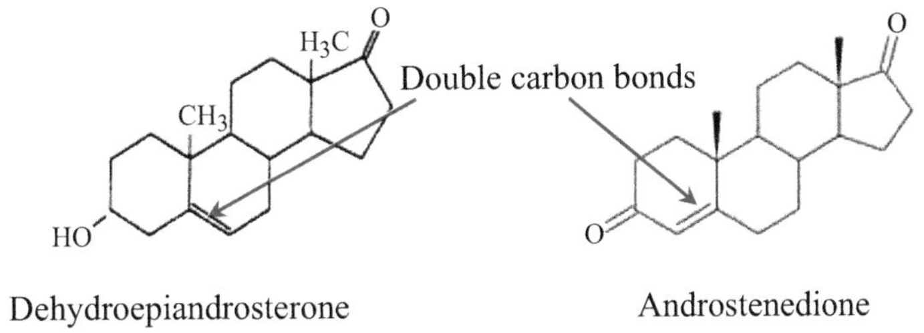

Figure 2.4 *Structures of dehydroepiandrosterone and androstenedione, two weak male like hormones made by the adrenal glands.*

To be fully active, testosterone has to be converted to dihydrotestosterone and it is this which causes the penis to develop in the male along with changes to the skin near the penis that form the scrotal sacs in which the testes sit.

As already said, testosterone is formed from cholesterol in the testes and it shares some of the formation steps with cortisol which is formed in the adrenal glands. Fig. 2.5 shows the common steps and also those steps which are different.

Don't worry about all the names as we will explain them in the next chapters. The important part for now is in the red box. This shows us how testosterone is formed in the testes. As the testes cannot make cortisol, everything is directed towards making testosterone.

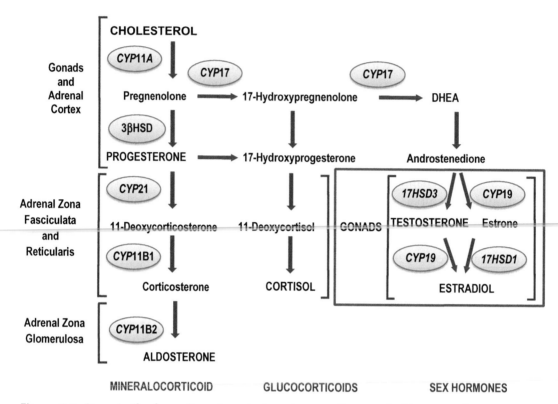

Figure 2.5 *Steps in the formation of cortisol, androstenedione and aldosterone by the adrenal glands and testosterone and/or estradiol by the gonads. The names in the ovals are enzymes.*

In addition, you can see there are a number of steps shared with the adrenal glands, namely up to the formation of androstenedione which both the adrenal glands and the testes can make. In CAH, because you cannot make cortisol, everything shifts towards making DHEA and androstenedione in the adrenal glands. This is the situation which results from a defect in the enzyme 21-hydroxylase (CYP21 in Fig. 2.5). Defects in this enzyme stop the formation of cortisol and for that matter, aldosterone. As the amount of cortisol falls or is very low, there is a marked increase in ACTH production from the pituitary gland (remember the thermostat in Chapter 1) which instructs the adrenal glands to make more cortisol. Due to the block, no further cortisol can be produced, so the pituitary keeps trying harder and harder to make cortisol, but to no effect. Unfortunately, the side effect of this is a shunting process takes place in which more of the steroids being built up before the block, are transferred down into the adrenal androgen pathway, making more DHEA and androstenedione.

If the developing baby is male (XY), these increasing amounts of DHEA and androstenedione do not make any appreciable difference to the external appearances. The external appearances were male anyway and having a bit more androstenedione from the adrenal glands makes no real difference.

In a female, however, the situation is more of a problem. As the female fetus does not receive any male hormone whatsoever, an increase in adrenal androgen production, as occurs with 21-hydroxylase deficiency CAH, will have effects on the external appearances. Remember that these babies have the genetic makeup XX so genetically are female. They have also formed ovaries, fallopian tubes and a uterus, so internally they are essentially normal females. The only difference comes from the effect of the male like hormones on the normal female external genitalia. What happens here is the structure which is going to form the clitoris enlarges, so in some situations it can look like a mini penis. In addition, the two tubes, the urethra and the vagina, do not separate well from each other so instead of there being two openings, there is often one.

The vagina is often merged into the back of the urethra at varying levels. In addition, sometimes the area where the urethra and vagina open out, can often be closed across looking a bit like a male scrotum in appearance. These effects all come about because of an increased amount of the weak adrenal androgens DHEA and androstenedione. The effects may vary from being a mild enlargement of the clitoris, right through to a mini penis with an overall appearance which is perhaps more male looking, than female. Sometimes this can be quite confusing and unless the baby is carefully examined, mistakes can be made in assigning them as males when in fact they are females.

Finally, there are forms of CAH where the block is right at the start of the pathway, e.g. CYP11A. What would happen in these cases? Looking at the pathway in Fig. 2.5 we can see that neither the adrenal glands nor the testes could make any of the hormones.

There would be no cortisol or aldosterone from the adrenal glands so an adrenal crisis would occur. In the testes, no testosterone would form and in the ovaries no estrogen (the female hormone).

So now in a male (XY), as testosterone cannot be formed in the developing testes even though the baby carries the Y chromosome and is genetically male, the external appearances will be female. However, because the testes are present and can make anti-Müllerian hormone, any early development of fallopian tubes and uterus will be suppressed. These individuals will have a genetic male makeup with female appearances, but they will not have internal female structures.

In the female, in these situations the genetic makeup is female and as the external appearances do not need estrogen to form, the appearance will also be female. The womb and tubes will also form normally.

ASSESSING THESE CHANGES

When babies are born with CAH the external appearances may be altered. To be able to make an estimate of how affected by hyperandrogenism a female baby with CAH is, a series of stages have been constructed. These are called Prader Stages named after a Swiss Paediatric Endocrinologist (Andrea Prader) who described the various points.

The staging ranges between a score of Stage 1 which is essentially the normal female external genital appearance, to Stage 5 which describes an appearance which is identical to that of normal male external genitalia. The accompanying table (Fig. 2.6) and illustration (Fig. 2.7) show the various stages described.

PRADER STAGE	APPEARANCE
STAGE 1	Appears normal but has a very slightly enlarged clitoris and no labial fusion. There may be a slightly reduced vaginal opening size. Virilisation is so mild, to such a slight degree, that it may go unnoticed.
STAGE 2	There is an increase to the degree of virilisation. The genitalia are abnormal to the eye, the clitoris is enlarged and the labia fused towards the back (posterior labial fusion). The vaginal opening is small.
STAGE 3	There is a greater enlargement of the clitoris, the labia are almost completely fused and there is a single perineal urogenital opening.
STAGE 4	The clitoris looks more phallic, there is a urethra like urogenital sinus at the base of the clitoris and the labia are almost completely fused, giving the appearance of an empty scrotum.
STAGE 5	This is the severest form of virilisation and results in male looking like genitalia. The clitoris looks like a penis with the urethral opening at the tip or near the tip. The scrotum appears to be normally formed but is empty.

Figure 2.6 *Table describing the changes in the external genital that can be seen in congenital adrenal hyperplasia (CAH).*

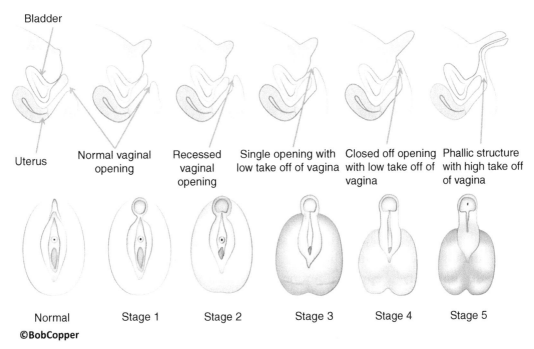

Bladder

Uterus   Normal vaginal   Recessed   Single opening with   Closed off opening   Phallic structure
          opening   vaginal   low take off of vagina with low take off of with high take off
                            opening   vagina   of vagina

Normal   Stage 1   Stage 2   Stage 3   Stage 4   Stage 5
©BobCopper

Figure 2.7 *Pictorial representations of the Prader Stages. Upper panel: the internal arrangement of the bladder, womb and vagina with the normal relationship on the left. Lower panel: appearance of the external female genitalia illustrating the 5 Prader Stages with the normal appearance on the left. Fig. 2.6 gives the actual description of the 5 Prader Stages.*

The overall appearance of the genitalia in Stage 4, the single small urethral/vaginal opening at the base or on the shaft of the phallus could be diagnosed as hypospadias in a baby boy. However, when examined by X-ray after an injection of dye into the opening, the X-ray shows the internal connection with the upper vagina and uterus (Fig. 2.7). The connection of the vagina to the tube leading out of the bladder can be high up in this situation, which makes surgery more complex. This opening can predispose the baby to urinary obstruction and recurrent urinary infections.

In Stage 5, the genitalia appears to be that of a normally formed penis with the urethral opening at or near the tip, with a normal looking scrotum; however, the scrotum has no palpable gonads. These babies are not visibly ambiguous and often are assumed to be ordinary boys with undescended testes; however, the internal pelvic organs include normal ovaries and uterus, the vagina connects internally with the urethra as in Stage 4.

The various losses of enzyme function seen in 21–hydroxylase deficiency, produce varying appearances. Where the defect is relatively mild the appearance is more towards Stage 1 or Stage 2. Where the defect is complete then it is possible the appearance may be more Stage 4 or Stage 5. In fact, for the majority of individuals affected by 21-hydroxylase deficiency in the United Kingdom, the appearance is more like Stage 3.

What is of interest is that within the same family, two girls affected by CAH may have different external genital appearances despite the fact they have exactly the same genetic abnormality. There are several reasons for this:

1. The drive to the adrenal glands in terms of ACTH formation may be variable resulting in varying amounts of adrenal androgen production.

2. The pathway to adrenal androgen production is quite complex as we have already discussed in Chapter 1. The presence of both the classic pathway through dehydroepiandrosterone (DHEA) and androstenedione to testosterone, has several steps within it, all regulated by different enzymes. The backdoor pathway is even more complex with many more steps involved. Variations in the strengths of the various enzymes, will lead to variable amounts of androgen production which might ultimately affect the appearance of external genitalia.

3. The situation becomes more complicated because in order for testosterone to have its affects, it has to be converted into a biologically active form called dihydrotestosterone. This step is also highly variable between individuals.

4. The final component is that all the 'male like' hormones have to affect the cells of the body involved. To do this, all steroids bind to a special protein within the cells called a receptor. Receptors are like docking stations where the steroid latches on and then the docking station, plus the steroid, has the effect on whatever component of the cell they are supposed to act on. Receptors are extremely important and with respect to the one that binds the 'male like' hormones, androgen receptors, are highly variable. Within the androgen receptor gene is a number of what are called 'repeats'. These repeats vary in length and depending on the length of the repeat within the gene, the function of the receptor is either better than average or less than average. So this adds an additional complication to the whole story in terms of what the external genitalia of the individual might look like. All these enzyme steps are different between individuals and in particular, the androgen receptor function will vary between individuals so it perhaps isn't too surprising that no two individuals with CAH, even though they might have the same gene abnormality in the 21-hydroxylase gene, have necessarily the same external appearances.

So now that we have covered how a male or female baby is formed, let's look in more detail in what goes wrong in someone with CAH. We will look at all the different types of CAH, some in more detail than others.

FURTHER READING

Achermann, J.C., Domenice, S., Bachega, T.A., Nishi, M.Y., Mendonca, B.B., 2015. Disorders of sex development: effect of molecular diagnostics. Nat. Rev. Endocrinol. 11, 478–488.

CHAPTER 3

Genetics of Congenital Adrenal Hyperplasia

GLOSSARY

Autosomal recessive This means both parents carry one abnormal gene copy each so that when the sperm fertilises the egg there is a 1 in 4 chance the two abnormal genes will be present (affected individual), a 1 in 4 chance both normal genes will come together and a 1 in 2 chance an abnormal will meet a normal (carrier state).

Heterozygote Name given to a person where one of the pairs of chromosomes carries an abnormality of a gene. When both pairs carry the same abnormal gene this is known as homozygote.

21-Hydroxylase Sometimes called CYP21, 21-hydroxylase is the enzyme which converts 17-hydroxyprogesterone to 11-deoxycortisol and also progesterone to deoxycorticosterone. This is the most common enzyme deficiency in CAH.

GENERAL

When we talk about congenital adrenal hyperplasia (CAH) we are referring to a number of conditions in which the adrenal glands have problems making cortisol. As we have already said cortisol is the most important hormone the adrenal glands make and the body will do anything to maintain normal production.

In CAH, blocks can occur at various levels leading to a lack of formation of cortisol. The commonest level of block is 21-hydroxylase or CYP21 and we will be looking at this in a bit more detail in the next chapter.

Wherever the block occurs however, the system reacts in a particular way. The reduction in cortisol leads the brain to detect it needs to produce more cortisol and the amount of ACTH produced in the pituitary (see Chapter 1) increases. ACTH not only tries to make cortisol, but in doing so it also increases the size of the adrenal glands and this helps us understand what the term CAH means:

- 'Congenital' refers to a condition that the person is born with and we will be thinking a little bit more about the genetics of this condition further on.

- The 'adrenal' is self-explanatory and is talking about a condition which affects the adrenal glands!

- The 'hyperplasia' is a little harder to understand but all it means is an increase in the size of a particular structure.

So if we put the whole story together, what CAH means is, a condition affecting the adrenal glands which leads to an increase in size of the adrenal glands and you are born with the condition.

We will be talking about 21-hydroxylase and 11-hydroxylase in the next chapter and the other forms in Chapter 5. You might be tempted to skip this chapter but please do not as we cover a fair amount about how this condition is inherited. So read on.

UNDERSTANDING THE GENETICS OF CONGENITAL ADRENAL HYPERPLASIA

CAH is a genetic condition. In other words we know that part of the DNA structure we all have is not quite right in people who have this condition. There are estimated to be about 25,000–30,000 genes in us. Each of them is tasked with a certain job, making proteins. The enzymes in the system which go towards making cortisol are proteins and as we said before, they are like baking powder in a cooking recipe in that they speed up the chemical reactions.

CAH occurs when there is an error in the coding of part of the genes which control the production of adrenal enzymes. This error which is a change to the structure of the gene is known as a 'mutation'. Mutations can be caused by several different types of changes such as:

- Deletion—part of the DNA structure is missing.

- Insertions—a bit of extra DNA is added to the structure.

- Point mutations—a small part of the DNA is altered leading to an error in the amino acid produced.

- Recombination—a part of the DNA structure is swapped with other different genes.

Each form of CAH is caused by a different mutation on a different chromosome as shown in Fig. 3.1. The mutation in each gene causes the deficiency of a different enzyme.

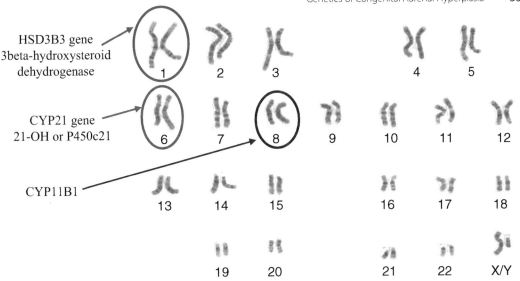

HSD3B3 gene
3beta-hydroxysteroid
dehydrogenase

CYP21 gene
21-OH or P450c21

CYP11B1

Figure 3.1 *Our chromosome map with the chromosomes involved in three forms of congenital adrenal hyperplasia shown, e.g. CYP21 gene is situated on Chromosome 6.*

Let us now think about the genetics of the condition and we are going to use 21-hydroxylase deficiency partly to explain this.

21-Hydroxylase is an enzyme and it plays a very special role converting 17-hydroxyprogesterone to 11–deoxycortisol. Do not worry about the names at this stage as all will become clear in the next chapter. This is a very key step in cortisol synthesis (production). The coding information for producing 21-hydroxylase is carried on one of the chromosomes, Chromosome 6. We talked a little about the chromosomes in previous chapters when we were talking about how we decide whether someone would become male or female. That information we said, is carried on the sex chromosomes. The genetic information to instruct you to make 21-hydroxylase is coded on part of Chromosome 6 (Fig. 3.2).

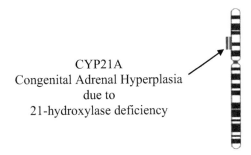

CYP21A
Congenital Adrenal Hyperplasia
due to
21-hydroxylase deficiency

Figure 3.2 *Map of Chromosome 6 showing where the CYP21A gene can be found.*

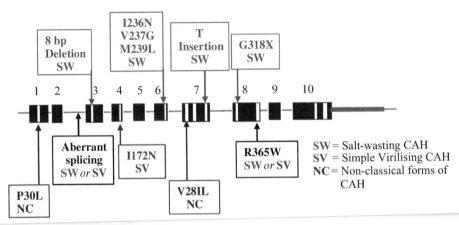

Figure 3.3 *Problems in the CYP21A gene which can cause congenital adrenal hyperplasia.*

In Fig. 3.3 we can see the gene in more detail with the codes for the abnormalities (mutations) often found. On this part of Chromosome 6, because the chromosomes come in pairs, it means there are two copies of the gene for 21-hydroxylase, one copy comes from the mother and one copy comes from the father. This is quite useful, because if one of the copies became damaged or did not work properly, then you would still have the other one and you would have about 50% of the activity of 21-hydroxylase, which is enough to maintain normal cortisol production, so you would be well. This is a situation which happens in those individuals who are called carriers of the 21-hydroxylase deficiency.

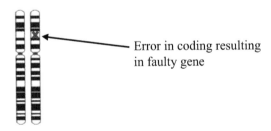

Figure 3.4 *Map of Chromosome 6 showing normal gene on left paired with abnormal gene on right. Overall result would be normal function. This is known as carrier state.*

To understand this a bit further, we need to think about how this genetic information is passed on to the next generation (Fig. 3.4). This diagram shows the two Chromosome 6's in the mother and father. As you can see, on one of the chromosomes we put a cross, to indicate that the 21-hydroxylase gene is not working properly on that particular chromosome, but is working perfectly well on the other one. The mother and father in this situation are called carriers of 21-hydroxylase deficiency because they have one chromosome which has the right information and the second chromosome contains the wrong information. As the system can still produce cortisol, the parents are well and suffer no untoward problems.

If we now look at Fig. 3.5, we can see what happens when the genetic information from the father meets that of the mother when the sperm fertilizes the egg. In this situation there are four possibilities. The normal chromosome from the father could join with the normal chromosome from the mother so the offspring inherits two normal chromosomes and would not have any problems with 21-hydroxylase.

Alternatively, one normal chromosome from the mother could join with the abnormal chromosome from the father, or the abnormal chromosome from the mother could join with the normal chromosome from the father and this would produce offspring who are carriers of the 21-hydroxylase deficiency, but again would be otherwise well, just like their parents. The situation which is more of a problem is when the abnormal chromosome of the mother meets the abnormal chromosome of the father. In this situation, the child inherits two non-functioning 21-hydroxylase enzymes and this means they cannot make cortisol. In this case, we get all the problems associated with 21-hydroxylase deficiency which we will talk about in the next chapter.

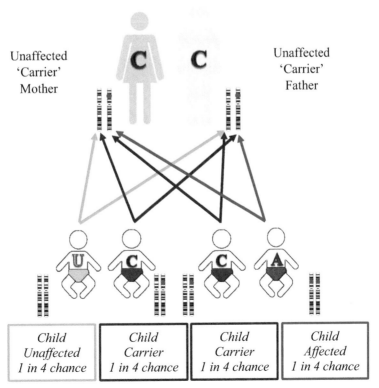

Figure 3.5 *Inheritance pattern when both parents are carries of a recessive (faulty) gene.*

What this diagram also tells us is that every time mothers and fathers who are carriers of 21-hydroxylase deficiency try to make a baby, there is a 1 in 4 risk the child will inherit both the abnormal copies and have the condition. Although carriers of 21-hydroxylase deficiency are quite common and there are probably 1 in every 80 individuals who are carriers, it is a very rare event two people come together to produce a child with 21-hydroxylase deficiency and this occurs probably only in 1 in every 18,000 live births.

So, as a recap if both parents are carriers of the faulty gene there is:

- 1 in 4 chance (25%) of having an unaffected child.
- 2 in 4 chance (50%) of having a child who will carry the defective gene.
- 1 in 4 chance (25%) of having child who will inherit both affected genes and therefore have the condition.

In Fig. 3.6 we can see when the affected parent (who has two defective genes) and the other parent who is a carrier have children, the children will be either carriers or affected.

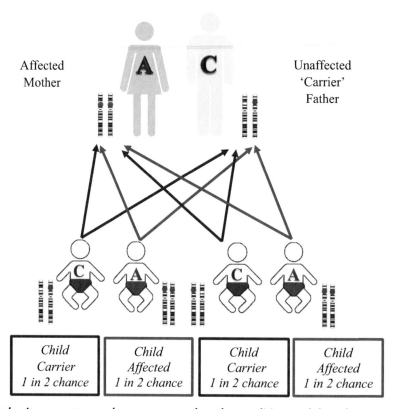

Figure 3.6 *Inheritance pattern when one parent has the condition and the other parent carries the recessive (faulty) gene.*

To recap if one parent is affected and the other a carrier:

- 2 in 4 chance (50%) of having a child who will carry the defective gene.
- 2 in 4 chance (50%) of having a child who will inherit both affected genes and will have the condition.

If both parents are affected (have the condition) as illustrated in Fig. 3.7, this will mean both the parents will have the two defective genes. This means each child they have together will inherit one faulty gene from the mother and one faulty gene from the father, resulting in each child having two faulty genes, so they will have the condition (affected).

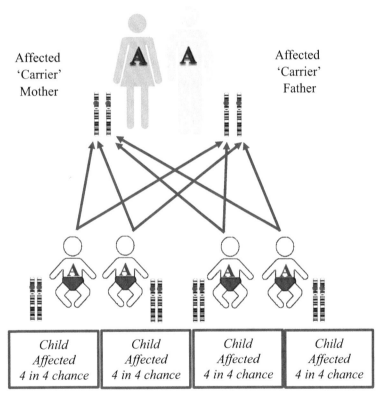

Figure 3.7 *Inheritance pattern when both parents are 'affected' and have two defective genes and therefore have the condition.*

As a recap if both parents have two defective genes there is:

- 4 in 4 chance (100%) of being affected, i.e. inherit the condition.

Although we have focused on 21-hydroxylase deficiency, this inheritance pattern is the same for any recessive disorder and true of the other variations of CAH.

ANTENATAL DIAGNOSIS AND TREATMENT

All this information means it is now possible to diagnose the condition whilst the baby is in the womb. This requires the genetic problem is known before the pregnancy and the carrier status of the parents is known along with the genetic problem in the affected child.

What is done is to take a small part of the forming placenta (the placenta is made by the baby not the mother!) and check the CAH gene for the abnormality. This is not an easy procedure and is done by experts in Fetal Medicine. Even so, there is a risk of miscarriage of about 1–2%.

This is not usually done just to get this kind of information but has been coupled with treatments given to the mother to try and prevent the virilisation of female babies. What happens is the mother is given dexamethasone to switch off the baby's adrenal glands. The dexamethasone is given as soon as the mother knows she is pregnant as the adrenal glands in the baby are active from 6 weeks of the pregnancy. Dexamethasone is a synthetic form of cortisol which can cross from the mother to the baby. Dexamethasone because it is like cortisol, switches off ACTH production from the baby's pituitary gland. This reduces the drive to the adrenal glands and the amounts of adrenal androgens fall. This means there are less androgens available in the affected female baby to change the external genitalia.

Then at 8 weeks of pregnancy, a blood test is taken from the mother. Baby cells can be detected in the mother's blood stream all through pregnancy and these cells are used to tell whether the baby is male or female. If the baby is male, dexamethasone is stopped irrespective of whether the baby might have CAH or not, as having extra adrenal androgen production as a male is not a significant issue as far as we know at present. If the baby is female, then the special placenta test (chorionic villus biopsy) is carried out and if the baby is not affected by CAH, dexamethasone is stopped. If the baby is affected, then treatment is continued until birth.

The problem with this is the baby is exposed to dexamethasone which is not good for many reasons, including future risks of diabetes and hypertension in adulthood. In addition, there are concerns about how well the brain develops when exposed to dexamethasone. Also, all babies whether they have CAH or not (see Fig. 3.3), will be exposed to dexamethasone at some point with all the potential risks and no benefit. For these reasons, the Endocrine Society in the USA has said this should not be viewed as standard treatment and should be thought of as experimental. Antenatal treatment with dexamethasone is not permitted any more in Germany and Sweden. We agree and urge caution if thinking about this approach.

FURTHER READING

Miller, W.L., 2015. Fetal endocrine therapy for congenital adrenal hyperplasia should not be done. Best Pract. Res. Clin. Endocrinol. Metab. 29, 469–483.

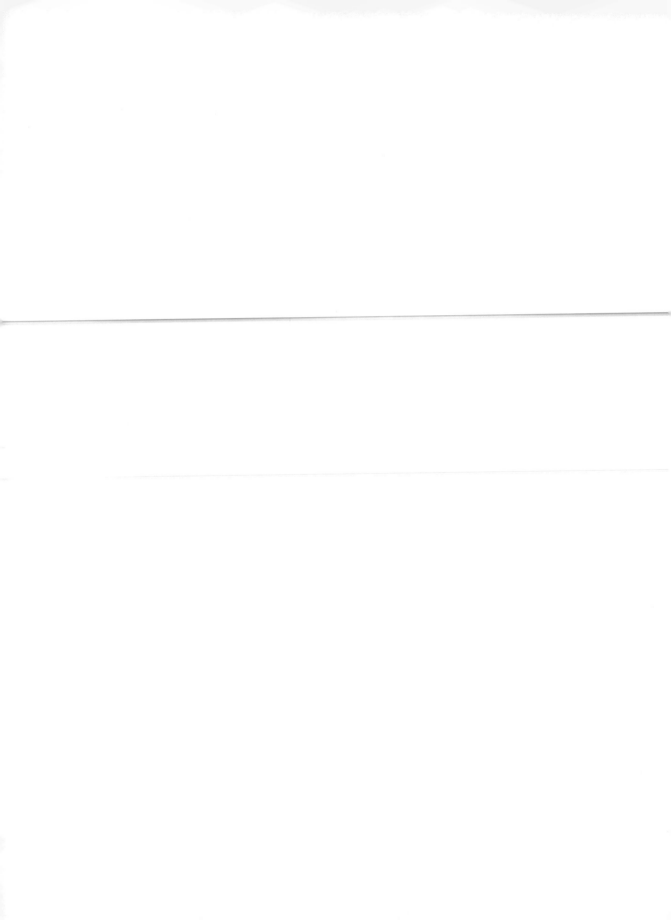

CHAPTER 4

Common Forms of Congenital Adrenal Hyperplasia

GLOSSARY

11-Hydroxylase Sometimes called CYP11B1, 11-hydroxylase is the enzyme which converts 11-deoxycortisol to cortisol and 11-deoxycortisocosterone to corticosterone.

21-Hydroxylase Sometimes called CYP21, 21-hydroxylase is the enzyme which converts 17-hydroxyprogesterone to 11-deoxycortisol and also progesterone to deoxycorticosterone. This is the most common enzyme deficiency in CAH.

Non-classical CAH (NCCAH) Also known as late-onset CAH (LOCAH) Mildest form of CAH and often not detected until adolescence or sometimes as late as adulthood.

Salt-wasting CAH (SWCAH) This is when there is loss of cortisol and aldosterone formation, so the individual often presents with an adrenal crisis. Cortisol is replaced with a glucocorticoid (hydrocortisone) and a mineralocorticoid (fludrocortisone) is needed to replace aldosterone. In infancy, salt (sodium) supplements are often required.

Simple virilising CAH (SVCAH) Presents in childhood with rapid growth, body hair development and body odour. Cortisol production is maintained by high ACTH drive.

GENERAL

When we talk about congenital adrenal hyperplasia (CAH) we are referring to a number of conditions in which the adrenal glands have problems making cortisol. As we have already said, cortisol is the most important hormone which the adrenal glands make and the body will do anything to maintain normal production.

In CAH, blocks in enzyme activity can occur at various levels leading to a lack of formation of cortisol. We will be talking about 21-hydroxylase (CYP21) and 11-hydroxylase (CYP11B1) in this chapter and the other forms in the next chapter. You might, if you have one of the other forms, be tempted to skip this chapter but please do not as we cover a fair amount about what being deficient in cortisol and aldosterone means. So read on.

CLASSICAL CAH - 21-HYDROXYLASE DEFICIENCY OR CYP21 DEFICIENCY

Salt-wasting Congenital Adrenal Hyperplasia (SWCAH)

This is the most common form of CAH. The gene lies on Chromosome 6 and the incidence of this condition is 1 in 18,000 live births. This means that in the United

Congenital Adrenal Hyperplasia. http://dx.doi.org/10.1016/B978-0-12-811483-4.00004-0

Kingdom, there would be approximately 35 new individuals diagnosed each year with the condition presenting at various ages, but mainly at birth.

The 21-hydroxylase gene is quite complicated but essentially problems arise if large parts of it are deleted or if small changes take place within the gene, at critical points. These are known as point mutations. When a large chunk of the gene is lost, then a lot of enzyme activity is absent and it becomes very difficult to make the steps to cortisol synthesis. If only a little point of the gene is altered, there will still be some enzyme activity enabling some cortisol production. The gene codes for the protein that makes the enzyme 21-hydroxylase. There are various classification schemes in use, so it is also known as CYP21 or P450c21. This means that the enzyme is a part of the cytochrome P450 enzyme family.

Now let's have a look at what the lack of 21-hydroxylase or CYP21 will do.

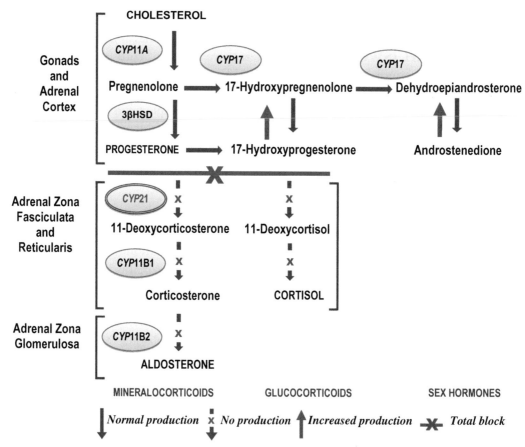

Figure 4.1 *Pathway for cortisol, aldosterone and adrenal androgen formation. Block at CYP21 (solid red line) leads to lack of formation of cortisol and aldosterone and an increase (red arrows) in 17-hydroxyprogesterone and androstenedione.*

Fig. 4.1 shows the position of the block in the pathway. As you can see, the enzyme is present in both the glucocorticoid pathway making cortisol and the mineralocorticoid pathway that makes aldosterone. So if there is no activity we can predict what might happen. Initially, with no cortisol present, there is a significant chance of becoming very unwell with poor feeding, vomiting and low blood glucose. Fig. 4.2 tells us the symptoms we might expect. This is going to happen from quite early on, from about 7 days after birth (Fig. 4.3). If we lose the ability to make aldosterone the person will not be able to retain salt and this leads to a salt-wasting crisis around 7–10 days of life as salt is lost in the urine and stool. The person becomes very dehydrated and can collapse. The rise in potassium which takes place in the blood at the same time can be dangerous, as it can produce irregular heartbeats. The combination of these features is known as an 'adrenal crisis' or a 'salt-wasting crisis'. Urgent treatment is required in terms of a vital bolus injection of hydrocortisone, intravenous fluids containing salt and glucose as well as the start of treatment with regular amounts of hydrocortisone. Once the individual can take feeds again, oral 9 alpha-fludrocortisone should be introduced to replace the aldosterone which is missing. We will be talking about these treatments in later chapters in more detail.

We will now go back to Fig. 4.1 to see what else might happen as a result of the loss of cortisol. As we said the body will do anything to keep cortisol production normal and it does this by increasing the amount of ACTH the pituitary gland produces. We have said that ACTH will stimulate the adrenal glands to try to produce more cortisol but because of the block, (shown by the solid red line with a cross) what starts to happen is the steroids start to accumulate before the block (shown by the red arrows pointing upwards). This is why the 17-hydroxyprogesterone (17OHP) is a marker for 21-hydroxylase (CYP21) deficiency.

When we want to work out where a block happens, we measure the hormones before the block, in this case 17OHP which will be elevated and after the block, where we have a choice, we could measure either 11-deoxycortisol or cortisol as both will be absent. We tend to use cortisol because it is easier and quicker to measure but we could also measure 11-deoxycortisol for completeness if we wanted to. As the block will cause the 17OHP to accumulate, there will also be a buildup of the steroid 17-hydroxypregnenolone which allows the adrenal glands to shunt all this extra production into the formation of androgen, particularly via the backdoor pathway (Fig. 1.12).

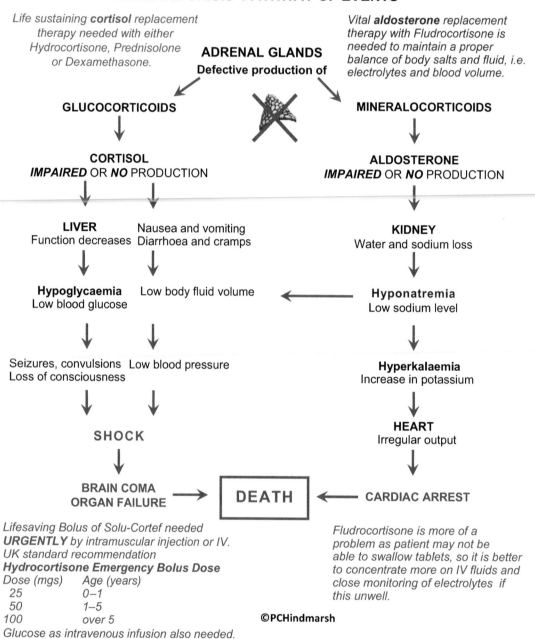

ADRENAL CRISIS–PATHWAY OF EVENTS

*Life sustaining **cortisol** replacement therapy needed with either Hydrocortisone, Prednisolone or Dexamethasone.*

ADRENAL GLANDS
Defective production of

*Vital **aldosterone** replacement therapy with Fludrocortisone is needed to maintain a proper balance of body salts and fluid, i.e. electrolytes and blood volume.*

GLUCOCORTICOIDS   **MINERALOCORTICOIDS**

CORTISOL
***IMPAIRED* OR *NO* PRODUCTION**

ALDOSTERONE
***IMPAIRED* OR *NO* PRODUCTION**

LIVER   Nausea and vomiting
Function decreases Diarrhoea and cramps

KIDNEY
Water and sodium loss

Hypoglycaemia   Low body fluid volume
Low blood glucose

Hyponatremia
Low sodium level

Seizures, convulsions   Low blood pressure
Loss of consciousness

Hyperkalaemia
Increase in potassium

SHOCK

HEART
Irregular output

BRAIN COMA
ORGAN FAILURE   →   **DEATH**   ←   **CARDIAC ARREST**

Lifesaving Bolus of Solu-Cortef needed
***URGENTLY** by intramuscular injection or IV.*
UK standard recommendation
Hydrocortisone Emergency Bolus Dose
Dose (mgs)   Age (years)
25   0–1
50   1–5
100   over 5
Glucose as intravenous infusion also needed.

Fludrocortisone is more of a problem as patient may not be able to swallow tablets, so it is better to concentrate more on IV fluids and close monitoring of electrolytes if this unwell.

©PCHindmarsh

Figure 4.2 *Components of an adrenal crisis that results from lack of cortisol and aldosterone. An adrenal crisis is a medical emergency.*

The adrenal glands cannot really make much testosterone, but do make quite a lot of DHEA and to a certain extent androstenedione. In the fetus, there is another alternative pathway for testosterone formation so that in the womb, additional testosterone can be made by the high levels of ACTH. In male babies this does not matter too much as all that will happen, will be that the penis will grow a little bigger. In females, all the extra male hormones will cause changes to take place in the external genitalia (Fig. 2.6). The clitoris will enlarge and will look a little more like a male penis and in extreme situations, the separation of the tube from the bladder and the vagina may merge into a single tube low down.

Finally the gap where the vagina should be, sometimes closes over. These changes are very variable in individuals, but the general principle is the same as they all reflect an increase in the production of male like hormones from the adrenal glands.

The aim of treatment is not only to replace the hormones which are missing and get the circulation back to full health, but also to reduce the amount of male hormone that can be produced in both females and males. In females, this is to prevent any further changes in the external appearances and in both sexes we like to keep the adrenal androgens low, because we know they will affect the speed at which the skeleton matures. If you want to know more about bone maturation, we talk about it in more detail in Chapter 6.

Classical CAH—Salt-wasting Congenital Adrenal Hyperplasia (SWCAH): Summary

- Females: Present at birth with ambiguous genitalia; virilisation of external genitalia from clitoromegaly to a mini penis due to excess androgens whilst in the womb. The ambiguous appearance can be mild to severe.
- Males: The excess androgens do not affect the proper formation of male genitalia and usually present with a salt–wasting crisis within the first 2–3 weeks of life.
- Salt–wasting crises in both boys and girls.

Physical Symptoms	Biochemical Findings
Salt-wasting	Low sodium
Adrenal crisis	High potassium
Failure to thrive	High plasma renin activity
Poor feeding	Low aldosterone
Poor weight gain	High 17OHP level
Weight loss	High androgens
Vomiting/reflux	Low cortisol
Lethargy	Low blood glucose
Low urine output—(very few wet nappies when dehydrated)	High ACTH
Low body temperature	
Prolonged jaundice	

Figure 4.3 *Physical symptoms and biochemical findings of salt-wasting congenital adrenal hyperplasia.*

There are other forms of 21-hydroxylase (CYP21) deficiency which arise because of differences in the enzyme activity. We have just described when the enzyme activity is absent. However, some of the point mutations decrease activity to about 10–15%. This means that these cases are less likely to present early on in the newborn period with either a salt-wasting crisis or changes to their external genitalia, if they are female.

Simple Virilising Congenital Adreanl Hyperplasia (SVCAH)

The components of this section are slightly complicated. There are patients that present with early virilisation but no salt loss and those that present around 5–6 years old with virilisation and no salt loss. These patients are referred to as simple virilising CAH or SVCAH. The only difference between SVCAH and salt-wasting congenital adrenal hyperplasia (SWCAH) is the degree of loss of CYP21. In SWCAH, loss is complete whereas in SVCAH there is some CYP21 activity which leads to increased ACTH drive and an increase in the adrenal androgens (Fig. 4.4). As the block is not complete, cortisol can still be produced in sufficient quantities to keep the person reasonably well, but at the expense of a high ACTH drive and increased adrenal androgen production.

So although the enzyme which is affected is the same (CYP21), the reason that we have these differences in timing and ways of presenting, is due to the amount of activity of the enzyme which remains.

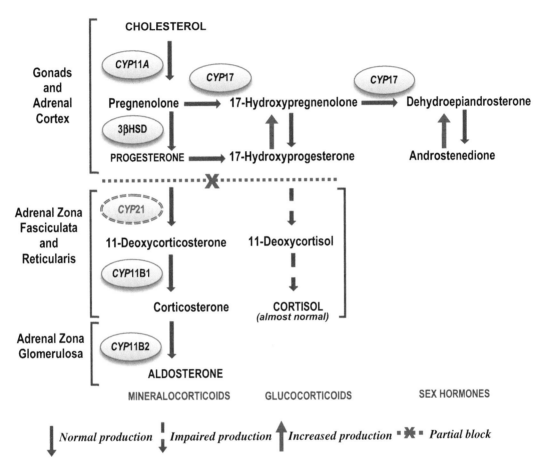

Figure 4.4 *Pathway for cortisol, aldosterone and adrenal androgens formation. A less severe block at CPY21 (dashed red line) leads to normal or slightly reduced formation of cortisol and aldosterone and an increase (red arrows) in 17-hydroxyprogesterone and androstenedione.*

In SVCAH, individuals usually present around 5 or 6 years of age. They do not usually present with a salt–wasting crisis, but are often noticed to be growing a bit faster than their friends; they may have an increase in body hair, body odour, acne. Boys may have an increase in the size of the penis and increase of pubic hair, but the testes do not increase in size. In girls, there may be a slight increase in the size of the clitoris and appearance of pubic and axillary hair (Fig. 4.5).

In this situation the diagnosis is made by measuring 17OHP and of course cortisol to define the block. The treatment, as with the salt-wasting form, is with hydrocortisone. Once hydrocortisone is started, the adrenal production of cortisol is switched off, so the person needs full cortisol replacement and monitoring. Many of these individuals if tested by measurement of plasma renin activity and aldosterone, are on the borderline of needing fludrocortisone replacement. Many endocrinologists prescribe fludrocortisone for these individuals.

One of the problems with the SVCAH, is that the parts of the brain involved in regulating the timing of puberty will have been exposed to adrenal androgens in the run up to diagnosis. This seems to prime the system to start an earlier puberty once hydrocortisone treatment is introduced. It is not unusual for an individual to have presented originally with the appearance of pubic and axillary hair and not to be in true puberty, because that system has not switched on. However, at a later date once hydrocortisone treatment has been introduced, the whole puberty system switches into action. This is often a bit confusing to everyone and we talk about this in more detail in our section on 'Puberty' (Chapter 7).

Understanding this however, is important. The reason for this is that the adrenal androgens will start to mature the skeleton a bit faster, which means there is less time available to grow and so the height of the individual might be less than it was destined to be. If you then add in real puberty with all the hormone changes that take place, which include effects of the sex hormones on maturing the skeleton even further, then a very serious situation can arise in which the adult height of the individual can be very seriously compromised (Fig. 4.5).

It is important when treating SVCAH, not only to get the hydrocortisone treatment correct, but also to carefully monitor the individual from the puberty and bone age perspective once treatment has been started with hydrocortisone, because early puberty might follow on.

Simple Virilising Congenital Adrenal Hyperplasia: Summary

- Females: May present at birth with ambiguous genitalia; virilisation of external genitalia from clitoromegaly to mini penis due to excess androgens whilst in the womb. The ambiguous appearance can be mild to severe.
- Males: Normal external genitalia with hyperpigmentation of scrotum and postnatal virilisation.

If there is no genitalia ambiguity, SVCAH is diagnosed when the physical symptoms appear as listed in chart Fig. 4.5.

Physical Symptoms	Biochemical Findings
Accelerated growth	Usually normal sodium and potassium
Acne	Normal or slightly high plasma renin activity
Pubic and axillary hair growth	
Body odour	Normal or slightly low aldosterone
Very oily/greasy hair	High 17OHP
Signs of early puberty	Normal or low cortisol
Advanced bone age	Slightly high ACTH

Figure 4.5 *Physical symptoms and biochemical findings of simple virilising congenital adrenal hyperplasia.*

Non-Classical Congenital Adrenal Hyperplasia (NCCAH) also known as Late-Onset Congenital Adrenal Hyperplasia (LOCAH)

Non-classical CAH (NCCAH) also known as late-onset CAH (LOCAH), refers to a series of features which present much later in adolescents or early adulthood (Fig. 4.6). The features here are more of an increase in body hair known as hirsutism, acne and irregular periods and again reflect the loss of 21-hydroxylase (CYP21) activity, which is far less than seen in the salt-wasting form. In females hirsutism develops in a male like pattern, i.e. facial hair, hair growth on the back, chest and abdomen.

Many of the symptoms that occur in NCCAH, are similar to those that occur in the simple virilising form, but because the loss of CYP21 function is less than in SVCAH, the changes are milder and present in adolescence or early adulthood.

Non-Classical Congenital Adrenal Hyperplasia: Summary
- Usually not diagnosed until adolescence or as a young adult.
- Symptoms typical of high androgens rather than salt–wasting.

Physical Symptoms	Biochemical Findings
Genital virilisation is not usually a problem	Normal cortisol
Hirsutism	High androgen production
Irregular menstrual periods	High 17OHP
Infertility in both males and females	Normal plasma renin activity
Acne	Normal aldosterone
Amenorrhea (no menstrual period)	Normal sodium and potassium
Body odour	
Muscular build in females	
Deepened voice in females	
Premature balding in males	
Accelerated growth	
Early puberty with advanced bone age	

Figure 4.6 *Physical symptoms and biochemical findings non-classical, also known as late-onset congenital adrenal hyperplasia.*

11-HYDROXYLASE OR CYP11B1 DEFICIENCY

11–Hydroxylase (CYP11B1) deficiency is the next most common form of CAH. If you look at Fig. 4.7 you will see that the block is now further down than 21–hydroxylase (CYP21). In the cortisol pathway, it is the final step from 11–deoxycortisol to cortisol. In the aldosterone pathway, it is the next step from 11–deoxycorticosterone into the final steps towards aldosterone formation.

Knowing this, we can then start to think about how this condition might present. Again, we would expect a buildup of the steroids before the block, so you would be right to think that in both males and females, an increase in adrenal androgens would take place.

This is exactly what happens and the presentation can be very similar in terms of the appearance of external genitalia, to that observed in a salt-wasting 21-hydroxylase (CYP21) individual. Usually, these individuals present at birth, however they can often present a bit later at 3–5 years of age.

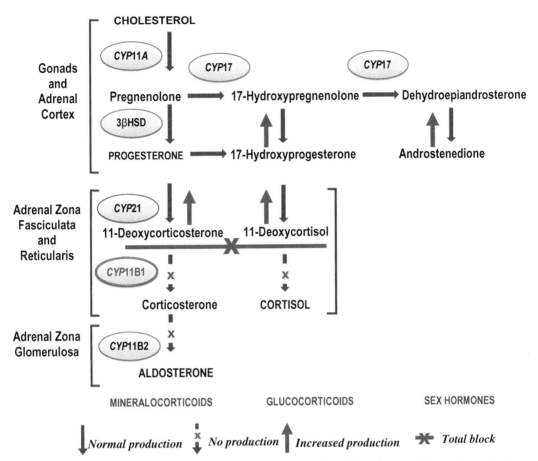

Figure 4.7 Pathway for cortisol, aldosterone and adrenal androgen formation. *Block at CYP11B1 (solid red line) leads to lack of formation of cortisol and aldosterone and an increase (red arrows) in 11-deoxycortisol, 11-deoxycorticosterone and androstenedione as well as an increase in 17-hydroxyprogesterone.*

Again, like the individuals with 21-hydroxylase (CYP21) deficiency, these patients with 11-hydroxylase (CYP11B1) deficiency, will not be able to make cortisol properly. Unlike the individuals with 21-hydroxylase (CYP21) deficiency, they do not get experience as many problems early on, as salt-wasters. The reason for this is not clear, but it is likely that the increased amount of deoxycorticosterone probably acts to some extent like cortisol and helps them get through the first few years of life.

Now we think about the mineralocorticoid pathway. You might think at first that because the individual cannot make aldosterone, these people will have salt-wasting problems. In fact, this does not occur because deoxycorticosterone is an extremely potent mineralocorticoid and is much more potent than aldosterone. So, in this situation where we get lots and lots of deoxycorticosterone built up, what we get is salt retention, water retention and a rise in blood pressure, often to very serious and dangerous levels. Indeed, some of these individuals can present with mini strokes because of the severity of the high blood pressure (Fig. 4.8). So, in contrast to 21-hydroxylase (CYP21) deficiency, the main aspect that differentiates 11-hydroxylase (CYP11B1) deficiency from 21-hydroxylase (CYP21) deficiency, is that in 21-hydroxylase (CYP21) there is salt loss, whereas in 11-hydroxylase (CYP11B1) there is salt retention.

Physical Symptoms	Biochemical Findings
(Classical)	Low/normal cortisol
High blood pressure *(sometimes)*	High androgen production
Mini strokes	High 17OHP
Rapid growth	High 11-deoxycortisol
Girls virilisation	Low/normal plasma renin activity
Male increase in pubic and axillary hair and penile enlargement	Low/normal aldosterone
	Normal sodium
Acne and increase in body hair in milder forms	Low/normal potassium
	High ACTH

Figure 4.8 *Physical symptoms and biochemical findings of congenital adrenal hyperplasia due to classical 11-hydroxylase (CYP11B1) deficiency.*

The treatment for 11-hydroxylase (CYP11B1) deficiency is as you would expect, to give hydrocortisone to replace the cortisol which is missing. However, we have to remember, that the defects in the system operate in both pathways that make glucocorticoids and mineralocorticoids which occupy different parts of the adrenal glands. When we introduce hydrocortisone, what happens is ACTH is switched off. As ACTH production is switched off, the drive down the system lessens and initially the amount of deoxycorticosterone which is made from the cells which also make cortisol, is reduced. In this situation we find that the plasma renin activity (Chapter 1) is very low because the deoxycorticosterone is being made off the ACTH pathway. For a short while, we get actual salt loss until the renin system wakes up and gets into action. When it does, it goes into overdrive because it cannot make aldosterone due to the block. It can make deoxycorticosterone in the zona glomerulosa and this is what leads to the high blood pressure in 11-hydroxylase deficiency when treated with hydrocortisone alone. In this situation, it is best to switch off the renin system using fludrocortisone. So you end up in an odd situation, where you treat a salt retaining condition with a salt retaining hormone.

Just as there are milder forms of 21-hydroxylase deficiency, there are classical and non-classical forms of 11-hydroxylase deficiency (Figs 4.9 and 4.10).

Physical Symptoms	Biochemical Findings
(Non-classical)	Low/normal cortisol
High blood pressure	High 11-deoxycortisol
Premature adrenarche	Normal/high 17OHP
Growth acceleration	High ACTH
Bone age advancement	High androgens
Polycystic ovarian disease	Low/normal potassium
Irregular menses	High sodium
Acne	Low plasma renin activity
Hirsutism	Low aldosterone
Infertility	
Body odour	

Figure 4.9 *Physical symptoms and biochemical findings of congenital adrenal hyperplasia due to non-classical 11-hydroxylase (CPY11B1) deficiency.*

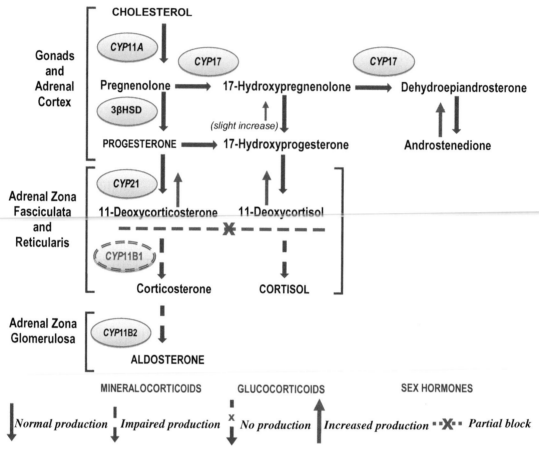

Figure 4.10 *Pathway for cortisol, aldosterone and adrenal androgen formation. A partial block at CYP11B1 (dashed red line) leads to a reduced formation of cortisol and aldosterone production and an increase (red arrows) in 11-deoxycorticosterone, 11-deoxycortisol and androstenedione 17-hydroxyprogesterone is only slightly increased.*

11-Hydroxylase (CYP11B1) Deficiency: Classical summary

- Females: Present at birth with ambiguous genitalia; virilisation of external genitalia from clitoromegaly to mini penis due to excess androgens whilst in the womb. The ambiguous appearance can be mild to severe.
- Males: The excess androgens do not affect the proper formation of male genitalia. However, there may be hyperpigmentation of scrotum and postnatal virilisation.
- Males usually present between the ages 3 and 5 years.

11-Hydroxylase (CYP11B1) Deficiency: Non-classical summary

- Usually presents in mid–childhood with premature adrenarche (early pubic and armpit hair).

As there are many steps to cortisol formation, there are other forms of CAH that can occur. These are rarer than the two conditions we have just described, so in the next chapter for completeness we will consider them.

FURTHER READING

White, P.C., Speiser, P.W., 2000. Congenital adrenal hyperplasia due to 21-hydroxylase deficiency. Endocr. Rev. 21, 245–291.

CHAPTER 5

Other Blocks in the Pathway Causing Congenital Adrenal Hyperplasia

GLOSSARY

Cytochrome P450 oxidoreductase This is part of a system that facilitates the enzymes CYP 17, 19 and 21. Deficiency means that the classic formation of cortisol, aldosterone and adrenal androgens (and testicular androgens) is not possible, but the backdoor alternative pathway to testosterone is not affected.

21-Hydroxylase Sometimes called CYP21, 21-hydroxylase is the enzyme which converts 17-hydroxyprogesterone to 11-deoxycortisol and also progesterone to deoxycorticosterone. This is the most common enzyme deficiency in CAH.

StAR Steroidogenic acute regulatory protein. After cholesterol is taken up by adrenal cells, it is transported in the cell by this protein. When this protein is not present, not only can other steroids not be made, but the accumulating cholesterol destroys the adrenal cells, as well as the testes and ovaries.

GENERAL

In this chapter we are going to look at other blocks which can happen in the pathway to making cortisol. Many of these causes of CAH are rare, so if you have the common ones talked about in Chapter 4, you might want to skip this section. If you do want to read on, make sure you have the cortisol pathway handy so that you can see where the block is and what will happen to the steroids made.

17α-HYDROXYLASE/17, 20-LYASE (P450C17) OR CYP17 DEFICIENCY

In this situation, the block stops the production of cortisol and sex steroids but allows an increased synthesis of mineralocorticoids. This is not a very common form of CAH, but because the enzyme is present in both the adrenal glands and gonads, the effects are quite dramatic.

Patients with P450c17 deficiency (partial or complete), have reduced or absent levels of both gonadal and adrenal sex hormones. This means they will be cortisol deficient

Congenital Adrenal Hyperplasia. http://dx.doi.org/10.1016/B978-0-12-811483-4.00005-2

but will not lose salt as the mineralocorticoid pathway is intact. If anything, they may retain salt and develop hypertension (Fig. 5.1). These patients do not develop adrenal crises as the 11-deoxycorticosterone acts like cortisol. This is similar to the situation in 11-hydroxylase deficiency described in Chapter 4.

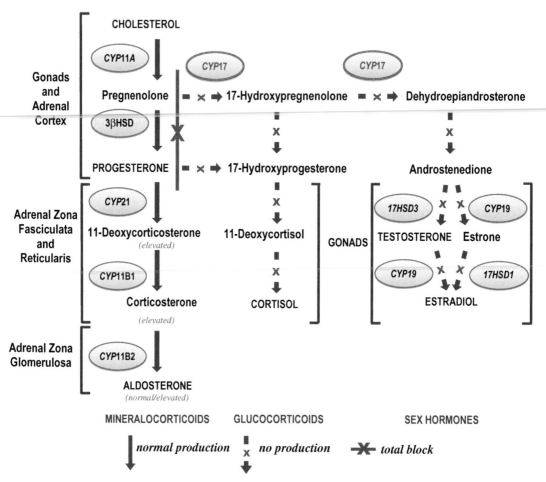

Figure 5.1 *Complete block in the enzyme 17 α-hydroxylase (CYP17 or P450c17) deficiency (solid red line) leads to loss of production of all steroids to the right side of the diagram.*

In females (46XX), in addition to the cortisol loss, puberty is unlikely to take place as the ovaries cannot make estrogen. In males (46XY), the problem is that the testes cannot make testosterone, so the normal external genitalia development either does not take place, or is less than normal. However, the testes can still instruct the body not to make a womb, so the overall appearance is female, but there is no womb.

If the cortisol production is not totally compromised, 46XY males or 46XX affected females, may go undetected until puberty, at which time they present as an apparent female patient with a hernia, or lack of periods and lack of secondary sex development, (including pubic and axillary hair) (Fig. 5.2).

Physical symptoms	Biochemical findings
Females:	High pregnenolone
Normal external genitalia	High progesterone
Males:	Low/normal potassium
Ambiguous genitalia with most presenting looking female	Normal sodium
	High 11-deoxycorticosterone
Hypertension present in 85–90% of patients	Low cortisol
	High LH and FSH
No periods and lack of secondary sex characteristics	Low sex steroids
	Low plasma renin activity
46XY males may present as females with hernia	Normal/high aldosterone
	High ACTH

Figure 5.2 *Physical symptoms and biochemical findings in the enzyme 17α-hydroxylase (CYP17) deficiency.*

Partial combined P450c17 (CYP17) deficiency in females may present with irregular periods and subsequently, loss of periods, hypertension, hypokalaemia (low potassium in the blood) with under developed or absent breast development and no axillary or pubic hair. Again, as with the total block, adrenal crises are unusual due to the increased production of 11-deoxycorticosterone which have a similar action to cortisol.

The goal of treatment for patients with P450c17 (CYP17) deficiency is to suppress ACTH secretion, decrease 11-deoxycorticosterone levels in particular and normalise serum potassium and blood pressure.

Patients who remain hypertensive on glucocorticoid replacement therapy require the addition of a mineralocorticoid antagonist (e.g. spironolactone) or calcium channel blocker to control their blood pressure.

Dietary control of sodium intake is recommended.

Sex steroid replacement therapy appropriate for the gender of the child, is started at the expected time of puberty to induce secondary sexual characteristic development, cyclic menstrual bleeding in 46XX females and to promote bone mass accrual.

3BETA-HYDROXYSTEROID DEHYDROGENASE TYPE-2 (3β-HSD 2) DEFICIENCY

In severely affected individuals, decreased mineralocorticoid secretion results in varying degrees of salt-wasting in both males and females and the deficiency of androgen production results in ambiguous genitalia in 46 XY males. This condition is due to defects in 3beta-hydroxysteroid dehydrogenase type 2 (3β-HSD 2), an enzyme that occurs almost exclusively in the gonads and adrenal glands. Just as with CYP21 deficiency, the deficiency of 3β-HSD 2 occurs in varying degrees and subsequently the severity in the loss of the function of this enzyme, results in different presentations and physical symptoms. This is due to a variety of mutations in the HSD3B2 gene. As this enzyme is involved in sex steroid formation as well, it behaves in a similar way to P450c17 deficiency but because mineralocorticoids are not formed, the patient does not develop hypertension.

With severe deficiency, the most common presentation is that of a newborn infant with an adrenal crisis due to both glucocorticoid and mineralocorticoid deficiency and ambiguous genitalia in 46XY patients (Fig. 5.3). 46XY infants present with varying degrees of under virilisation ranging from a small penis to a poorly formed penis (known as penoscrotal hypospadias). Conversely, 46XX infants may present with normal genitalia or mild to moderate enlargement of the clitoris and/or partial labial fusion (Figs. 2.6 and 2.7, Prader Stages) due to peripheral conversion of elevated DHEA to testosterone by the isozyme 3β-HSD type 1 in the liver and the conversion of 17-hydroxypregnenolone by the alternative backdoor pathway (Fig. 1.12).

Infants with less severe (non salt-wasting) forms may be relatively asymptomatic. There are also some non salt-wasting forms of 3β-HSD 2 deficiency, which can be diagnosed in infancy in the presence of perineal hypospadias in males and mild enlargement of the clitoris in female newborns, especially in the presence of other factors, such as a family history of death in early infancy (Fig. 5.4).

Some patients may present at a later age with the early development of pubic hair, growth acceleration and bone age advance (Fig. 5.5).

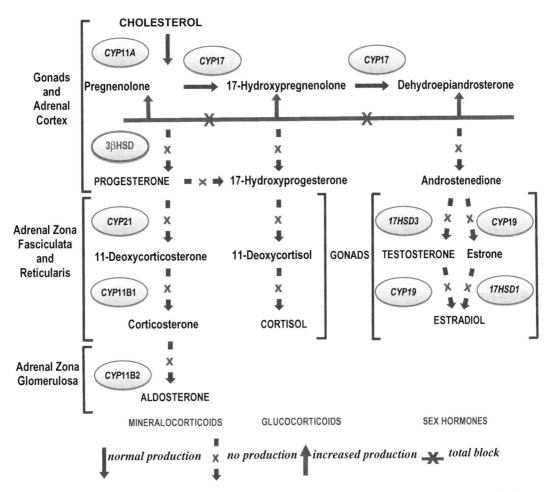

Figure 5.3 *Effect of the block in the enzyme 3Beta-hydroxysteroid dehydrogenase type-2 leads to lack of formation of any steroids below the block (solid red line) with increase in pregnenolone, 17-hydroxypregnenolone and dehydroepiandrosterone.*

Older patients with mild defects in 3β-HSD 2 activity (late-onset or non-classical variant), may present with premature pubic hair development, hirsutism, irregular menstrual cycles or primary amenorrhea.

Glucocorticoid replacement and mineralocorticoid therapy are indicated in patients with the salt-wasting form. Sex steroid replacement therapy is started in patients who fail to develop secondary sex characteristics.

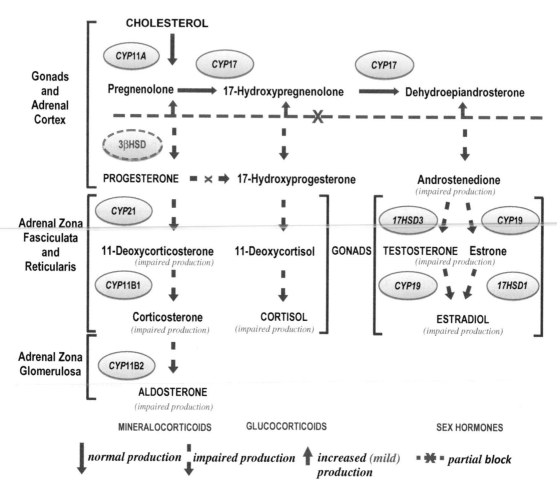

Figure 5.4 *Effect of a partial block (dashed red line) in the enzyme 3Beta-hydroxysteroid dehydrogenase type-2 produces a non salt-wasting situation with milder elevations of pregnenolone, 17-hydroxypregnenolone and dehydroepiandrosterone (red arrows).*

3Beta-hydroxysteroid dehydrogenase type-2: Summary

- Usually presents in early infancy with adrenal insufficiency and salt–wasting.
- Some cases of non salt-wasting are diagnosed due to:
  - Perineal hypospadias in males.
  - Mild enlargement of the clitoris in newborn girls.

Physical symptoms	Biochemical findings
Severe Deficiency Salt-wasting (Figure 5:3)	***Severe Deficiency***
Birth	High potassium
Failure to thrive	Low sodium
Salt-wasting crisis	No cortisol
Hypoglycaemia and adrenal crisis	Low blood glucose
Males: underdevelopment of external genitalia from small penis, severe hypospadias to appearance of female genitalia.	No sex hormones
	High plasma renin activity
	Low aldosterone
Females: Near normal to enlarged clitoris.	***(Severe and Mild Deficiencies)***
Milder defects (Figure 5:4) ***(Non salt-wasting and non-classical)***	High ACTH
	High 17a-pregnenolone
Early pubic and axillary hair development	High DHEA
Premature puberty	High LH and FSH
Growth acceleration	Low cortisol
Bone age advancement	Low androstenedione
Acne	Low testosterone
Excess body hair (hirsutism)	Occasionally elevated 17OHP
Polycystic ovaries	
Irregular/no periods	
Gynecomastia common in pubertal males	
Fertility problems in males and females	

Figure 5.5 *Physical symptoms and biochemical findings in the enzyme 3Beta-hydroxysteroid dehydrogenase type-2 deficiency.*

CONGENITAL LIPOID ADRENAL HYPERPLASIA (LIPOID CAH) (StAR DEFICIENCY)

Congenital lipoid adrenal hyperplasia (lipoid CAH) is the most severe form of CAH, in which adrenal and gonadal steroidogenic cells are unable to convert cholesterol to pregnenolone, effecting the synthesis of virtually all adrenal and gonadal steroids (Fig. 5.6).

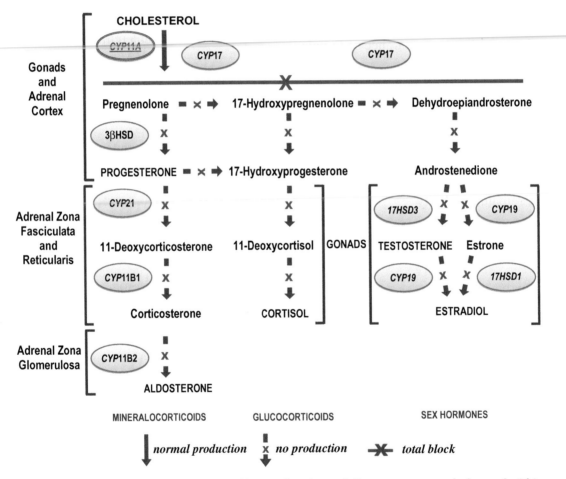

Figure 5.6 *Block in the pathway (solid red line) either due to failure to transport cholesterol within the adrenal cells (StAR deficiency) or to loss of function of CYP11A1 or side-chain cleavage enzyme (in red) leading in either situation to loss of all steroid production.*

The defect in lipoid CAH is primarily in the steroidogenic acute regulatory protein (StAR), which shuttles cholesterol into the mitochondria, where the P450scc enzyme catalyses the conversion of cholesterol to pregnenolone. A few patients so far, have been reported with lipoid CAH due to mutations of the CYP11A1 gene that result in P450scc enzyme deficiency. StAR loss leads to accumulation of cholesterol which destroys the adrenal glands, as well as the testes and ovaries.

The majority of affected patients with lipoid CAH present during the first month of life with salt-wasting and adrenal crisis as well as female appearance, irrespective of the genetic makeup. In 46XY patients the testes can be in the abdomen or groin.

Most affected patients present with hypoglycaemia and generalised pigmentation at birth due to intrauterine glucocorticoid deficiency which results in elevated ACTH. Affected 46XX patients, unlike the 46XY patients, may experience spontaneous puberty, normal periods and an early menopause because their ovaries are able to produce estrogen through StAR-independent pathways, but in the long term the ovaries will fail.

As in other forms of CAH, a non-classical form can occur where there is 10–25% of normal StAR activity. Presentation in males is often with salt loss, whereas in females early menopause may occur after a normal onset and progression through puberty. In both classic and non-classical forms the adrenal glands are large and filled with cholesterol. Similarly, the gonads accumulate cholesterol which in the classic form, takes place in males in the womb leading to complete loss of testicular function. In females, the ovaries continue to function as the cholesterol accumulation does not become a major problem until the pubertal years. The main feature which distinguishes this condition from adrenal hypoplasia congenital, is that in the latter the adrenal glands cannot be visualised whereas in StAR deficiency, the adrenal glands on ultrasound are very large. (Fig. 5.7).

StAR Deficiency: Summary
Most severe form of CAH

- Usually presents within the first month of life.
- High mortality in infancy.

Milder form

- Usually presents in childhood or adolescence.

Physical symptoms	Biochemical findings
Severe Deficiency	***Severe Deficiency***
Failure to thrive	All adrenal steroids absent
Salt-wasting crisis	Low blood glucose
Hypoglycaemia and adrenal crisis	High potassium
Generalized hyperpigmentation	Low sodium
Males: Look female externally	High LH and FSH
Females: Normal genitalia	High plasma renin activity
Milder defects (non-classical)	***Milder defects (non-classical)***
Females	Low cortisol
Spontaneous puberty	Low aldosterone
Periods start normally	***Severe and Milder defects***
Premature menopause	High ACTH
Males	
Late-onset adrenal insufficiency with reduced cortisol and aldosterone	
Enlarged adrenal glands	

Figure 5.7 *Physical symptoms and biochemical findings in steroidogenic acute regulatory protein (StAR) deficiency.*

P450 OXIDOREDUCTASE DEFICIENCY

This is a new condition which has been identified (see Fig. 5.8 and Chapter 1).

Rather than there being a problem in the classic enzymes in P450 oxidoreductase (POR), there is a problem in one of the systems that help the enzyme to work. The problem is this helper system is involved in many enzymes like CYP21 (P450c21) and CYP17 (P450c17) as well as the conversion of testosterone to estradiol by aromatase (CYP19).

The diagnosis is usually made in the newborn period. This condition is a bit mixed with features of mild 21-hydroxylase (CYP21) and mild CYP17 deficiencies as well as low androgens and in females no estradiol at puberty.

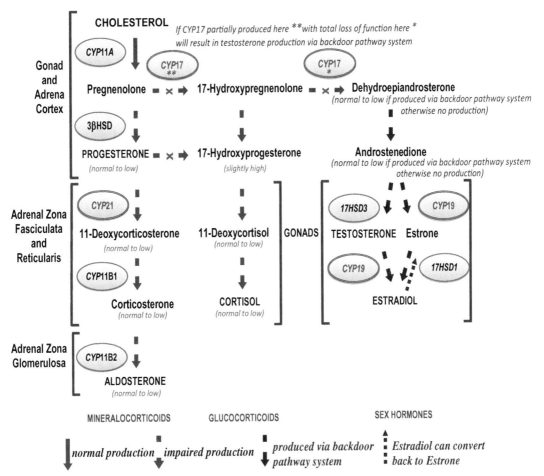

Figure 5.8 *Loss of activity of P450 oxidoreductase (POR) deficiency leads to loss of function of the enzymes CYP21, CYP17, CYP19 (in red). It is important to realise that the manifestations of this defect are very variable and the degree of block differs between individuals. This can range from a reduction in enzyme activity to total loss of function.*

The majority of patients with POR have some skeletal abnormalities characteristic of Antley–Bixler syndrome as the helper system is also involved in bone formation.

Affected girls are born with ambiguous genitalia but in contrast to what is occurring in other virilising forms of CAH, there is no progression of virilisation because circulating adrenal androgens after birth are low or normal.

To explain the antenatal androgen excess and postnatal androgen deficiency in patients with POR, an alternative pathway in androgen synthesis which is present only during fetal life, ceases after birth has been identified.

Conversely, affected boys are born with a range of appearances ranging from just a small penis to poor formation of the penis with the tube that passes urine coming out at the base of the penis, a condition known as penoscrotal hypospadias.

This is due to an impairment of the CYP17 enzyme in the testes (Fig. 5.9). Some women who are pregnant with fetuses affected by POR, can experience mild symptoms of the disorder even though they themselves do not have the disorder. They may develop excessive body hair growth (hirsutism), acne, and a deep voice. These changes go away soon after delivery.

Physical symptoms	Biochemical findings
Birth	*(Dependent on block)*
Males:	Normal to low cortisol
Undervirilised	Cortisol may not increase as expected following ACTH stimulation.
Females:	
Ambiguous genitalia	Slightly high 17OHP
Post Birth	Normal to high plasma renin activity
Skeletal malformations similar to Antley–Bixler including cramped facial appearance, narrowing of nasal passage, poor growth of skull bones, incurved little finger, poor formation of bones in the arms.	Normal to low aldosterone
	Normal to high potassium
	Normal to low sodium
	High 17-OH pregnenolone
No progression of virilisation in females.	Normal DOC
Mothers may experience virilisation during pregnancy, which resolves after birth.	Normal to low androgens
	Androgens unresponsive to ACTH or HCG stimulation
	High LH and FSH

Figure 5.9 *Physical symptoms and biochemical findings in P450 oxidoreductase (POR) deficiency.*

P450 Oxidoreductase Deficiency: Summary

Diagnosis usually made in newborn period.

Depending on the degree of CYP21 and CYP17 deficiencies, treatment can include:

1. Glucocorticoid replacement therapy in patients with low ACTH stimulated cortisol.
2. Testosterone treatment in infancy in males with a small penis at birth.
3. Sex steroid replacement for induction of secondary sex characteristics in individuals with decreased CYP17 activity.

FURTHER READING

Frindik, J.P., 2016. 3-beta-hydroxysteroid dehydrogenase deficiency. Medscape. Available from http://emedicine.medscape.com/article/920621-overview#a4.

White, P.C., Speiser, P.W., 2000. Congenital adrenal hyperplasia due to 21-hydroxylase deficiency. Endocr. Rev. 21, 245–291.

CHAPTER 6

Growth

GLOSSARY

Bone age An estimate from an X-ray of the hand on how much growth has taken place to date. This can then be used to work out what the adult height is likely to be.

Growth hormone A protein made by the pituitary gland, which is secreted in bursts particularly overnight. It causes cartilage to divide and expand in size under the influence of its target protein insulin-like growth factor-1.

Parental height 70% of height is explained by the heights of the parents. On average, people come out somewhere midway between their parents' heights. To work this out for girls, MINUS 5.08 cm (2 inches) from the average parental height which gives you her estimated height, whereas for boys, ADD on 7.62 cm (3 inches) which will give you his estimated height.

GENERAL

We are all familiar with children growing and it is an area which parents are often concerned about, too little, too much or too early or will it be too late. When we are thinking about any condition in children, we have to include growth assessment as part of the way in which we handle the condition. We all want the condition and/or its treatment to impact as little on growth as possible, so we monitor growth at regular intervals in the clinic.

When we talk about growth, what we mean is height and weight and the combination of the two, which gives you the body mass index or BMI. BMI is a way of deciding if the current weight is appropriate for the height and generally can be used as a marker of body fat, although this is not always the case.

In this chapter we are going to consider growth from birth to adulthood and look at the ways to assess growth. We will concentrate particularly on height.

THE PROCESS

Postnatal growth can be considered to consist of at least three distinct phases:

1. Infancy

2. Childhood

3. Puberty

The infancy component is largely a continuation of the growth process observed in the womb. This displays a peak speed of growth at around 27–28 weeks of gestation with a decline in growth rate during the last trimester of pregnancy.

In fact, you will never grow as fast as during this period again. Even the pubertal growth spurt is small compared to this.

The picture in Fig. 6.1 illustrates this and tells us the different factors which make you grow at different stages of life.

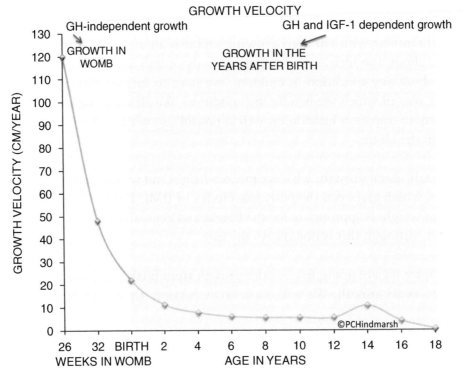

Figure 6.1 *Growth velocity chart showing where growth hormone (GH) and insulin-like growth factor 1 (IGF-I) act in the growth process.*

Birth, in a sense, is incidental to this declining growth rate which continues during the first 3 years of life reaching a plateau at or around the fourth year of life, remaining at this level until the commencement of the pubertal growth spurt. The factors influencing these distinct growth periods are different. We know little of the factors influencing fetal and early infant growth. At around 6 months of age, growth becomes dependent on how much growth hormone (GH) you make. The final step in the growth process, the pubertal growth spurt, comprises a 50% contribution from sex steroids and 50% contribution from GH.

GH, like ACTH, is produced in the pituitary gland and acts on the growth plates, which are made up of cartilage in the bone causing them to expand. GH is produced in bursts with most GH produced during the night. This might mean that grandma was right about going to sleep early to grow better.

Generally speaking, height and weight go hand in hand especially over the first 2 years of life. Thereafter, weight gain is quite slow at only 2 kg/year whereas height is 5–6 cm/year. So that we can better understand the growth of a child we plot data on standard growth charts.

GROWTH

At each clinic visit you will notice that your child's growth is measured. The measurements we take are usually height and weight. We plot these measurements on a standard growth chart so we can keep track of how your child is growing. In childhood, growth normally follows a regular pattern, which is depicted by a set of curves on the growth chart; each curve represents a different percentile line of growth, which differs in girls and boys, so a different chart is used for each gender (Figs 6.2 and 6.3).

To plot height, we first take the age of the child and then make a dot for the height at that age. This tells us what centile they are on. So if the child is on the 50th centile, then their height is average. If the child is on the 10th centile, then the child is on the shorter end of the height range, as only 10 out of every 100 children of that age would have the same height or less.

This tells us where we might expect the child to be with respect to the general population, but what is more important is where the child should be in relation to the height of their parents. This is known as the genetic height potential or target height. The reason this is more important is that if you have tall parents you might expect them to have tall children. So if they have a small child it might mean that there is something wrong with the child, as you would have expected them to be taller than they actually are, so they may not be growing normally.

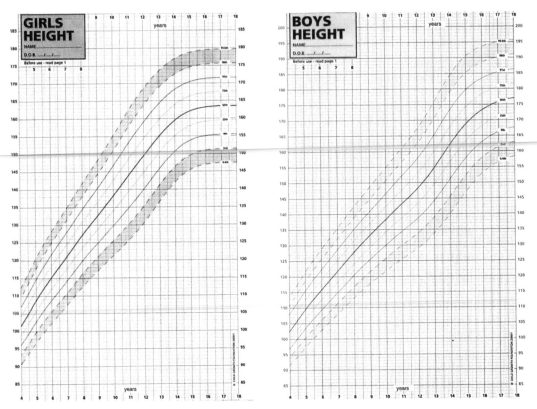

Figure 6.2 *Girls growth chart.* *(All height, weight and body mass index charts reproduced in this chapter are with permission from the Child Growth Foundation).*

Figure 6.3 *Boys growth chart.* *(All height, weight and body mass index charts reproduced in this chapter are with permission from the Child Growth Foundation).*

How to estimate genetic height potential

Genetic height potential can be roughly estimated by taking the height of each parent, adding these heights together and dividing this by two, to get an average parental height.

- For girls MINUS 5.08 cm (2 inches) from the average parental height which gives you her estimated height.

- For boys ADD on 7.62 cm (3 inches) to the average parental height which will give you his estimated height.

Please note that this is an estimated height.

Growth in childhood

From birth to 2 years old is the period when the most rapid growth takes place:

- In the first year of life a baby grows on average 25.4 cm (10 inches) and in the second year an average of 12.7 cm (5 inches).

- From 2 years old until a child starts puberty, growth averages approximately 5–6 cm/year (2–2½ inches/year) for boys and girls.

These are the numbers we think of when looking at growth in height. As long as you are averaging these numbers, you are growing normally no matter what centile line you are on.

People hold onto their centile line/channel very tightly. They rarely move off it either upwards or downwards to any great extent. Children do have mini bursts of growth especially around 7–8 years of age, but they tend to track back to the centile that they were on.

Growth in puberty

Growth accelerates again in puberty:

- In girls, puberty usually begins between the ages of 8 and 11 years, which is when their ovaries become active. Girls usually have the biggest part of their growth 'spurt' at the beginning of puberty. By the time they have their first menstrual period, only about 5 cm of growth is left to come.

- In boys, puberty usually begins between the ages of 10 and 13 years which is when their testes become active. Boys usually have their biggest growth spurt in the second part of puberty.

The growth spurt in boys occurs a bit later and is more intense than in girls and this is what leads to the difference in adult height between men and women, which is about 12.5 cm.

Growth slows down towards the end of puberty and then stops. In girls this usually happens at the age of 15 years and in boys around 17 years of age, as shown in the graph in Fig. 6.4.

In both sexes growth comes to an end due to the effect of estrogens on the growth plate. This is easy to understand in girls but what is happening in boys? Well boys can make a small amount of the female sex hormone and the small amount they make is important, as it matures the skeleton and plays an important role in preventing osteoporosis just as it does in females.

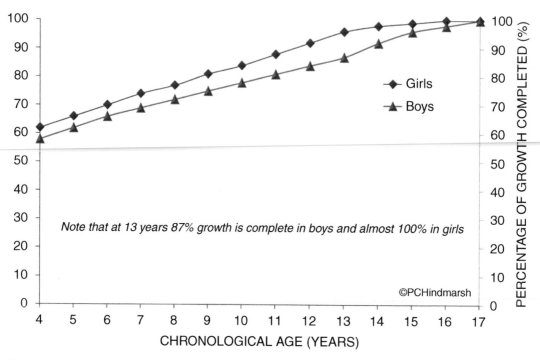

Figure 6.4 *Percentage of growth completed at a particular age.*

WEIGHT

The weight charts (Figs 6.5 and 6.6) look very similar to the height charts and are used in a similar way. Since weight does not change that much year on year in children (only about 2 kg/year), it is not as useful as height for monitoring growth overall.

However, it is quite useful as part of our assessment of the effects of hydrocortisone treatment, because if you give too much hydrocortisone this will result in weight gain and if too little is given, weight loss will occur.

BODY MASS INDEX

The problem with using weight alone is that a change in weight can take place simply because you increase your height. After all, to increase your height several things have to increase as well, e.g. bone, which is heavy. So what we do is to adjust the weight for the actual height.

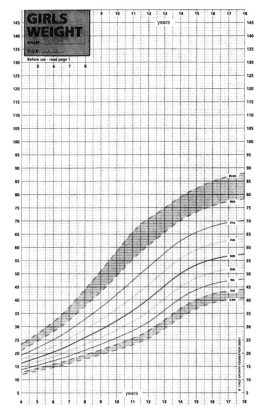

Figure 6.5 Girls weight chart. (All height, weight and body mass index charts reproduced in this chapter are with permission from the Child Growth Foundation).

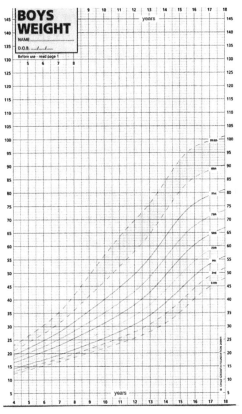

Figure 6.6 Boys weight chart. (All height, weight and body mass index charts reproduced in this chapter are with permission from the Child Growth Foundation).

We do this by calculating Body Mass Index or BMI. You can do this yourself as all you do is multiply the current height by itself and divide it into the current weight.

Or:

$$BMI = Weight(kilograms)/Height(metres) \times Height(metres).$$

There are charts for BMI just like there are for height and weight as shown in Figs 6.7 and 6.8.

The chart has the same style with centiles. On this chart we are concerned about becoming overweight, which is when you are above the 90th centile.

BMI is quite useful but can be a problem at times. For example, if you look at the England Rugby team, their BMI is in the obese range. The reason is not that they are obese but they have a much greater muscle mass contributing to their weight.

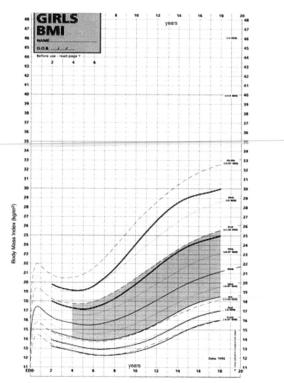

Figure 6.7 *Girls body mass index chart.* *(All height, weight and body mass index charts reproduced in this chapter are with permission from the Child Growth Foundation).*

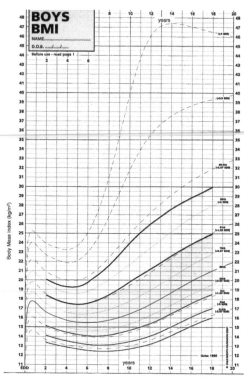

Figure 6.8 *Boys body mass index chart.* *(All height, weight and body mass index charts reproduced in this chapter are with permission from the Child Growth Foundation).*

We can refine this a little more by thinking about another factor that helps determine how tall you will be, namely the maturity of the skeleton, i.e. bone age. This is particularly important in CAH so we will think about how we measure it and what it means.

BONE AGE

Using X-rays which show us the bone age is another valuable tool we use to keep track of growth. We use the growth charts to show the growth in relation to the chronological age (birth age); however, the bone age shows us the skeletal development.

In normal growth these ages usually do not vary too much, although sometimes there may be a difference of 1–2 years. In childhood, growth and development targets are more often linked to bone age rather than chronological age, so this measurement is a good marker for long term growth.

We can plot the bone age on the growth chart alongside the actual physical growth as shown in Fig. 6.9, which gives us a very clear picture of how both of these measurements correlate.

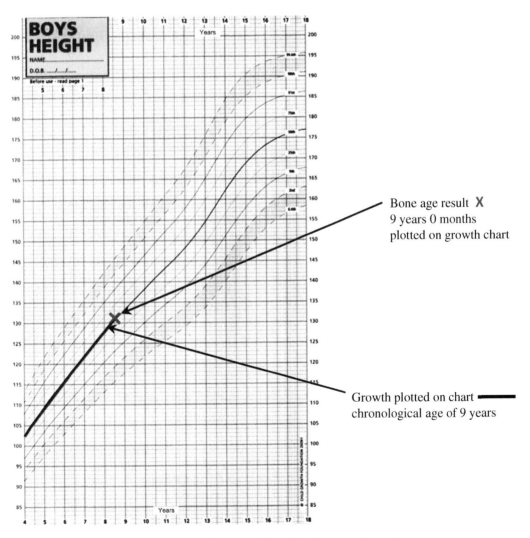

Bone age result **X**
9 years 0 months
plotted on growth chart

Growth plotted on chart ▬▬
chronological age of 9 years

Figure 6.9 *Bone age and chronological age on chart showing equal match.*

How bone age is done

The bone age measures the maturity of the growth plates in the skeleton (Fig. 6.10).

An X-ray of the hand is taken; the hand is used because it has lots of growth centres which can be scored. Various scoring systems are available, but all give a score for the shape and size of the growth plate area. The total of these scores give a maturity score, which can be translated into a bone 'age'.

These values tell us how much growth has taken place, so from this the estimated adult height can be predicted. However, it is important to know that because the bone age reading involves interpreting a visual picture, the results can be variable so it is a good idea to get the same doctor (preferably your endocrinologist) to read it each time.

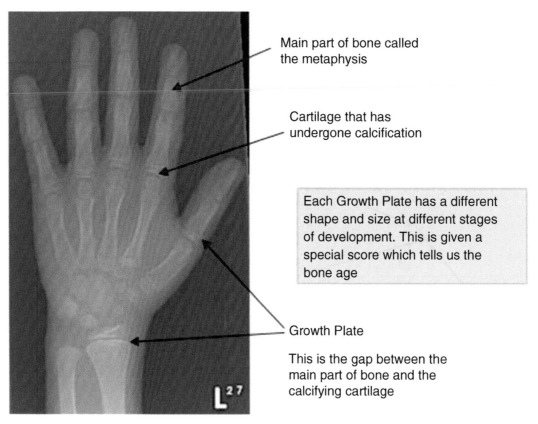

Main part of bone called the metaphysis

Cartilage that has undergone calcification

Each Growth Plate has a different shape and size at different stages of development. This is given a special score which tells us the bone age

Growth Plate

This is the gap between the main part of bone and the calcifying cartilage

Figure 6.10 *Bone age X-ray.*

When should the first bone age X-ray be taken?

The first bone age X-ray is usually taken at 3 years of age and then repeated once a year. As you can see from the hand X-ray picture, there are a lot of bones in the hand. Each of them has a special score attached to them depending on shape and size. Before the age of 3 years, there are not that many bones to assess and giving a score is not very accurate, so we use 3 years as the time point to start bone age measurements.

Growth is quite a slow process and changes in bone maturity take time to show. There is also a slight error in scoring the X-ray, so that if you repeat the same assessment it may differ from the first one by about 3 months. This means that doing X-rays every 6 months is not helpful because the changes are slow.

CONCLUSIONS

This chapter has looked at growth and how it is measured. We can see that it is a very useful measure for monitoring how well we are doing from the point of view of managing CAH. A normal height, weight and body mass index for parents is one of the key goals for doctors managing CAH. Before we look more at the practical treatment side, we need to finish our story on growth by considering the puberty process in more detail.

FURTHER READING

Tanner, J.M., 1989. Foetus Into Man, second ed. Castlemead Publications, Hertfordshire.

CHAPTER 7

Puberty

GLOSSARY

Follicle-stimulating hormone (FSH) Hormone produced by the pituitary gland which is involved in sperm formation from the testes in males. In females, along with luteinising hormone, it is involved in egg selection and production of estradiol.

Luteinising hormone (LH) Hormone produced by the pituitary gland which generates testosterone from the testes in males. In females, along with follicle-stimulating hormone, it is involved in egg selection and production of estradiol.

Pituitary gland A small gland divided into anterior and posterior parts which sits below the hypothalamus at the base of the brain. It produces six hormones from the anterior part and two from the posterior.

Pubertal growth spurt The final component of human growth which adds on approximately 30 cm to the final height in males and 20-25 cm in females.

GENERAL

Puberty is defined as the acquisition of reproductive capability and is attained through a series of physical changes, which have their onset in more than 50% of boys and girls by their 12th birthday. The appearances of puberty are brought about by a number of mechanisms.

In girls, these consist of changes in the breast tissue and the appearance of pubic hair. In boys, these are the change of the size of the testes and penis along with the appearance of pubic and axillary hair.

In association with these changes, the pubertal growth spurt contributes about 30 cm in boys and 20–25 cm in girls to the adult height of the individual. Between the sexes there is a slight difference of the timing of the pubertal growth spurt, occurring quite early on in puberty around the age of 11 years in girls and later in boys, around the age of 13–13.5.

HORMONAL CONTROL OF PUBERTY

The system regulating puberty is known as the hypothalamo-pituitary-gonadal axis. The hypothalamus is an area of the brain which produces hormones and is situated at the centre of the base of the brain. You can read more about this in Chapter 1 where we talk about the pituitary gland.

Congenital Adrenal Hyperplasia. http://dx.doi.org/10.1016/B978-0-12-811483-4.00007-6

In this system, the hypothalamus secretes a hormone called gonadotropin releasing hormone (GnRH), in little bursts every 90 minutes, which stimulates the production of luteinising hormone (LH) and follicle-stimulating hormone (FSH) from the pituitary (Fig. 7.1). These bursts of GnRH are extremely important, because if GnRH is introduced as a constant amount which does not pulse, the system will not work.

We will see how this phenomenon is used to switch puberty off when we look at various treatments used in CAH in Chapter 11.

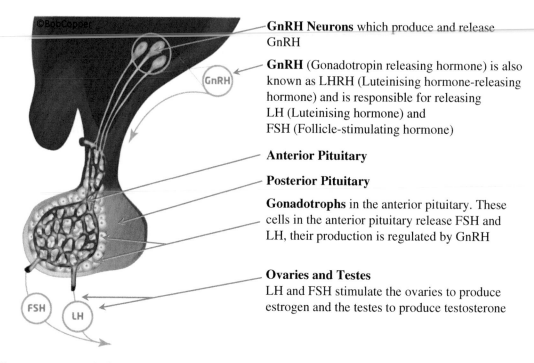

GnRH Neurons which produce and release GnRH

GnRH (Gonadotropin releasing hormone) is also known as LHRH (Luteinising hormone-releasing hormone) and is responsible for releasing LH (Luteinising hormone) and FSH (Follicle-stimulating hormone)

Anterior Pituitary

Posterior Pituitary

Gonadotrophs in the anterior pituitary. These cells in the anterior pituitary release FSH and LH, their production is regulated by GnRH

Ovaries and Testes
LH and FSH stimulate the ovaries to produce estrogen and the testes to produce testosterone

Figure 7.1 *Hypothalamo-pituitary-gonadal axis.*

LH and FSH appear in the blood as bursts or pulses as shown in the graphs in Figs 7.2–7.4 and are sometimes called the sex hormones. Before 8–9 years of age, the system is switched off but thereafter becomes more active at night initially and then during the day and night once puberty is established. This can be seen in Figs 7.2 and 7.3, which show the system becoming more active as we can see LH and FSH activity at night but not during the day. This happens when a child has entered the first stage of puberty. Fig. 7.4 shows the adult situation with LH and FSH activity present during the day and night.

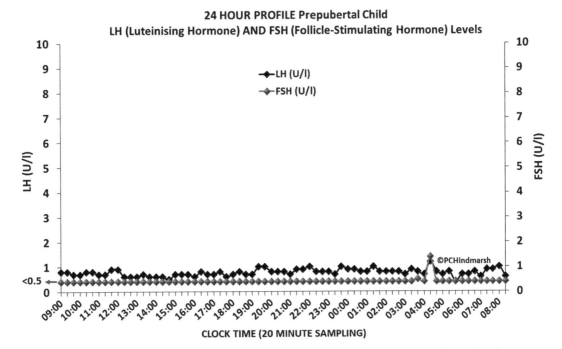

Figure 7.2 *LH and FSH over a 24 hour period in a prepubertal child. The data show that there is no activity.*

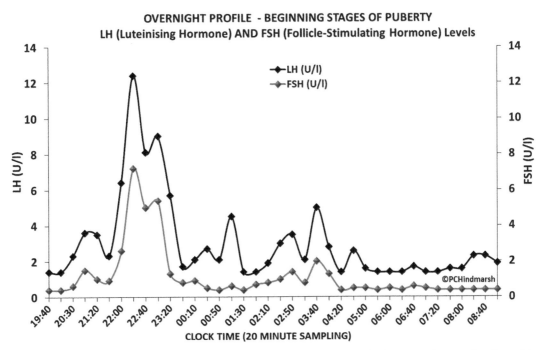

Figure 7.3 *LH and FSH activity have become more active at night but not during the day, this happens when a child has entered the first stage of puberty.*

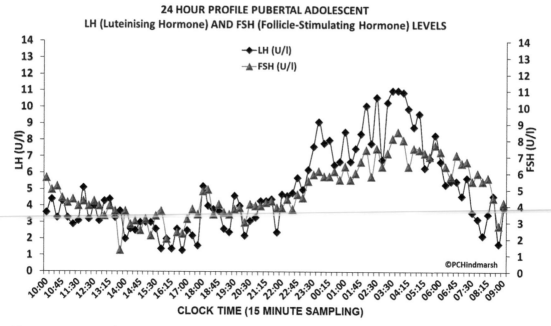

Figure 7.4 *LH and FSH production are very pulsatile throughout the full 24 hour period in late puberty and adulthood.*

HOW WE MEASURE THE STAGES OF PUBERTY

LH and FSH then impact on either the testes or the ovaries to produce an increase in size of the testes in boys and the development of ovarian follicles in girls. We can measure this in boys, by comparing changes in size with a special set of beads known as an Orchidometer or Prader's balls, as can be seen in Fig. 7.5. The string of 12 different sized beads increases in size from 1 to 25 ml and are compared with the size of the testicles and the volume is matched as closely as possible to the size of the bead.

- Prepubertal sizes are 1–3 ml.
- Pubertal sizes are considered 4–12 ml.
- Adult sizes are 15–25 ml.

In girls, by using ultrasound, we can measure change in the appearance of the ovary to a multicystic appearance as shown in Fig. 7.6.

We can also ultrasound the testes, this procedure is known as a sonogram, to determine their size but we tend to reserve testes ultrasound to check for the presence of adrenal rests. We talk about this in more detail in Chapter 14. Fig. 7.7 shows what a normal testes ultrasound looks like.

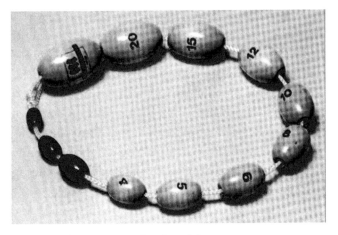

Figure 7.5 *Orchidometer used to measure the size of the testes.*

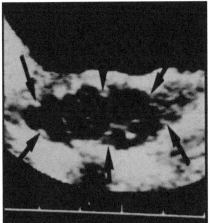

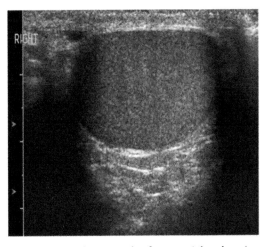

Figure 7.6 *Ultrasound showing a multi-cystic ovary.*

Figure 7.7 *Ultrasound of a testicle showing uniform grey colouring.*

SEX STEROID PRODUCTION

The testes and ovaries produce the sex steroids testosterone and estradiol, respectively. These hormones also have a pulsatile pattern, but the more important rhythm is a circadian rhythm with respect to testosterone, with higher values in the early hours of the morning and low values in the late afternoon.

The situation with the ovaries is more complex because of the presence of the menstrual cycle, which requires a close interaction between LH and FSH as well as the generation of estradiol and progesterone from the ovary leading to ovulation and menstruation.

Fig. 7.8 shows the hypothalamo-pituitary-ovarian axis as a girl goes through the menstrual cycle. This cycle occurs on average once every 28 days with a range between 23 and 35 days. The bleeding part of the cycle lasts between 5 and 8 days. GnRH from the hypothalamus tells the pituitary to release LH and FSH into the blood stream. In the ovaries, LH and FSH set about the maturation of the immature egg/follicle, growth of the follicle, as well as estradiol production. This increase in estradiol production leads to a thickening of the lining of the womb and at day 14 of the cycle (14 days after the end of the last period), a massive surge in LH. You might have expected the estradiol to have suppressed LH but in this early part of the cycle it has the opposite effect.

This surge of LH causes release of the mature egg from the follicle. If the egg is fertilised by sperm then the residual material called the corpus luteum, continues to make estradiol and progesterone until the fertilised egg is embedded in the lining of the womb.

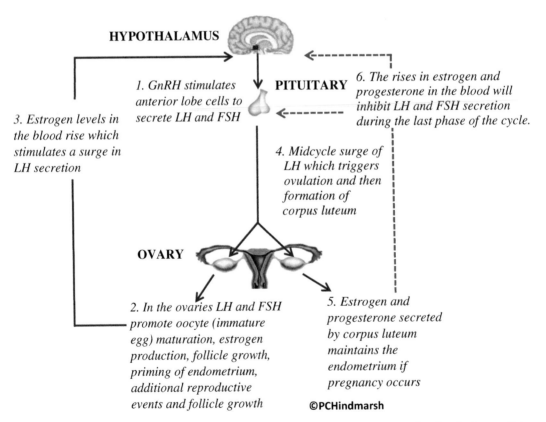

Figure 7.8 *The menstrual cycle.* On the left for up to 14 days there is positive feedback of estradiol on the hypothalamus and pituitary leading to a surge in LH which starts egg release. Once this has occurred if the egg is not fertilised, then estradiol and progesterone have negative feedback (right side) effects on LH and FSH leading to the menstrual period.

If the egg is not fertilised then the estradiol and progesterone now have a negative effect on LH and FSH, switching off production and with that comes the period which is when the lining of the womb is shed.

The pathway of testosterone and estradiol production uses several of the steps used in the formation of cortisol in the adrenal glands. Like the adrenal glands, the gonads use cholesterol as the starting point. However, the gonads do not contain 21-hydroxylase (CYP21) so they cannot form cortisol and instead there is a shift in the pathway towards the formation of testosterone and estradiol.

In the male, the hypothalamic-pituitary-gonadal axis is predominant because of its ability to produce testosterone. This gives all the secondary appearances which we associate with puberty. In girls, however, estradiol is the predominant hormone produced during puberty from the ovary and the male like hormones which are required for pubic hair development, do not come predominately from the ovary but from the adrenal glands. This difference leads to a number of problems and potential confusion as to what system is regulating what in the appearances we see. However, it is important to realise that these two systems do operate independently, particularly in females and they need to be considered separately.

As such, when we come to start thinking about puberty (Fig. 7.9) in congenital adrenal hyperplasia, it is extremely important for us to remember this additional role adrenal glands play in females in particular.

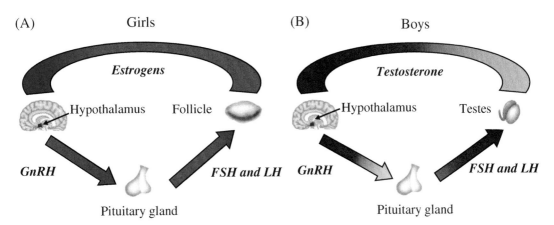

Figure 7.9 *Gonadal control in girls (A) and boys (B).*

We then add, as can be seen in Fig. 7.10, the hypothalamo-pituitary-adrenal axis making cortisol and androgen and to a certain extent, aldosterone.

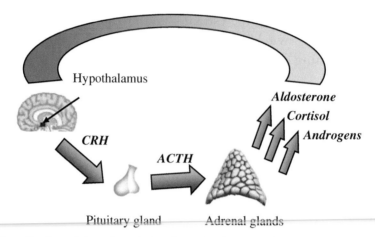

Figure 7.10 *Contribution of the adrenal glands to circulating androgens.*

ORDER OF PUBERTY

The pubertal changes in boys and girls take place in a sequence which reflects the increased production of LH and FSH from the pituitary gland. In the early stages of puberty in both sexes, the production of LH and FSH is at night only and this is associated with a small but significant increase in the circulating concentrations of the sex steroids. These only produce early changes of puberty, but in order to progress to full menstrual cycles and to develop an adult size testes in boys, the LH and FSH production has to switch from being predominantly at night, to taking place during both the day and night time. This is also associated with an increase in the sex steroid production and the completion of the changes which take place in puberty.

Fig. 7.11 shows the actual sequence of events which take place. As illustrated, in boys the predominant factor is the production of testosterone from the testes and this leads to the changes. In girls, however, the adrenal glands produce the androgens which are necessary to give pubic and axillary hair changes, but it is the ovary in its production of estradiol which leads to breast changes and the associated growth spurt.

You can see therefore, that it is possible for someone to display some pubic and axillary hair as they are able to make some androgen, but as they have an ovarian problem, they have no breast development. Equally, we know that in people with pituitary problems where only hydrocortisone is given and estrogen replaced, the girls do not develop adequate pubic and axillary hair because they are lacking in adrenal androgens due to the pituitary problem.

Boys—development of external genitalia

Stage 1:   Prepubertal.

Stage 2:   Enlargement of scrotum and testes; scrotum skin reddens and changes in texture.

Stage 3:   Enlargement of penis (length at first); further growth of testes.

Stage 4:   Increased size of penis with growth in breadth and development of glans; testes and scrotum larger, scrotum skin darker.

Stage 5:   Adult genitalia.

Girls—breast development

Stage 1:   Prepubertal.

Stage 2:   Breast bud stage with elevation of breast and papilla; enlargement of areola.

Stage 3:   Further enlargement of breast and areola; no separation of their contour.

Stage 4:   Areola and papilla form a secondary mound above level of breast.

Stage 5:   Mature stage: projection of papilla only, related to recession of areola.

Boys and Girls—pubic hair

Stage 1:   Prepubertal (can see vellus hair similar to abdominal wall).

Stage 2:   Sparse growth of long, slightly pigmented hair, straight or curled, at base of penis or along labia.

Stage 3:   Darker, coarser and more curled hair, spreading sparsely over junction of pubes.

Stage 4:   Hair adult in type, but covering smaller area than in adult; no spread to medial surface of thighs.

Stage 5:   Adult in type and quantity, with horizontal distribution ('feminine').

Figure 7.11 *Stages of pubertal development in boys and girls.*

WHAT HAPPENS IN CAH WHEN THE ADRENALS MAKE TOO MANY ADRENAL ANDROGENS

In CAH, the situation becomes quite complicated because of the additional adrenal androgen production from the adrenals in both males and females, especially when there is poor suppression of the androgens.

For males, when androgens are high, this will lead to a situation which looks rather similar to puberty and is known as precocious sexual development and this starts earlier than normal puberty because of the increase in adrenal androgens. These are relatively weak androgens compared to testosterone, but would be sufficient to produce an increase in growth rate, appearance of pubic and axillary hair and also an enlargement of the penis. However, because there is feedback of the adrenal androgen on the pituitary gland, the production of LH and FSH will be switched off so that there is no increase in the size of the testes and testosterone production from the testes will be low (see Fig. 7.12). So, from a simple examination using the beads (Fig. 7.5), we can tell that the androgens are from the adrenal glands because the testes are not enlarged.

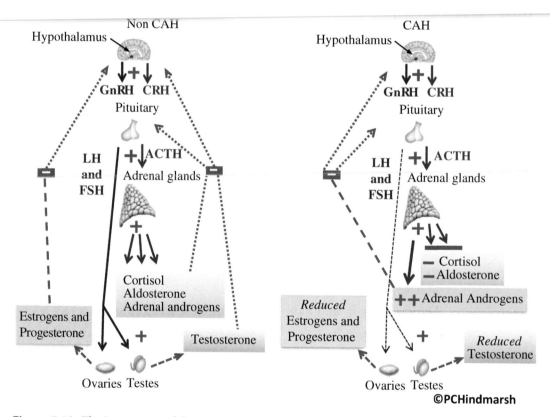

©PCHindmarsh

Figure 7.12 *The interaction of the gonadal and adrenal systems showing on the right that adrenal androgens act like gonadal testosterone, switching off LH and FSH production thereby reducing testicular testosterone production and ovarian estrogen and progesterone production.*

In girls, what would happen is adrenal androgen production would lead to an increase of body hair and sometimes an enlargement of the clitoris. Again because LH and FSH are suppressed by the adrenal androgens, there would be no estradiol production and there would be no breast development (Fig. 7.12).

Although people often refer to these changes as puberty, strictly speaking they are not, because the LH and FSH are suppressed and the drive to the change is not from the changes in LH and FSH production, but from the over production of adrenal androgens. Fig. 7.13 summarises all of this. Normal puberty would see the pituitary gland make LH and FSH, which would instruct the testes or ovaries to make testosterone or estrogen. These would then modulate the activity of the pituitary, but would not suppress LH and FSH production.

If however, cortisol was poorly replaced, the adrenal glands would start to enlarge, generating a lot of adrenal androgens, such as androstenedione and testosterone which would feedback on the pituitary and suppress the LH and FSH production and suppress gonad activity.

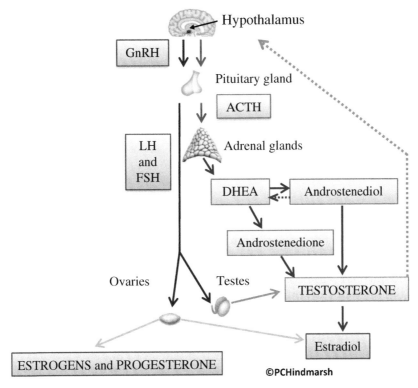

Figure 7.13 *Overall cascade with interaction of adrenal and gonads in sex steroid production.*

SYMPTOMS AND SIGNS OF PRECOCIOUS PUBERTY

Let's just go through that again, but in relation to the findings we would expect in true early puberty. The reason we need to consider this is because excess androgen due to under treatment in CAH, or in someone who is just diagnosed with SVCAH or NCCAH or LOCAH, can lead to precocious puberty. If the following signs and symptoms develop before the age of 9 years in boys and 8 years in girls, the endocrine team needs to look into this very carefully:

Both genders

- Fast growth—rapid increase in height.
- Body odour.
- Appearance of pubic or axillary hair.
- Acne.

Boys

- Facial hair (usually on the upper lip).
- Deepening voice.
- Enlarged penis or testicles.

Girls

- Breast growth.
- Menstruation (first period).

CONCLUSIONS

Puberty is a complex process and often doctors do not really understand it fully. The most important point to understand is that two systems are involved. The hypothalamo-pituitary-gonadal axis drives puberty making the puberty hormones testosterone in boys and estradiol in girls. These produce the external appearances, with the exception in girls where pubic and under arm hair comes from adrenal hormone production of weak male like hormones and not estradiol.

FURTHER READING

Tanner, J.M., 1989. Foetus Into Man, second ed. Castlemead Publications, Hertfordshire.

CHAPTER 8

Biochemical Tests Used for Diagnosis

GLOSSARY

Adrenocorticotrophic hormone (ACTH) Polypeptide hormone secreted by the anterior lobe of the pituitary gland, which stimulates the cortex of the adrenal glands to produce cortisol.

Bioavailability The amount of drug which is available for the target cells when administered either by oral, intramuscular injection or intravenous routes.

Clearance How fast or slow the body removes a drug from the circulation.

Immunoassay A technique where antibodies are raised to the steroid which is to be measured and then labelled with a marker, so that the amount which attaches to the steroid in the blood, can be determined.

Tandem mass spectroscopy A method for separating steroids based on their mass, which is unique to each steroid.

GENERAL

In previous chapters we have outlined how people with CAH either present at birth or at later stages in their lives. In this chapter, we are going to consider how that diagnosis is made and what we use tests for, in managing the condition. Tests fall into these two broad categories of diagnosis and monitoring of treatment. When we think about diagnosis, it is useful to have the pathways which are shown in Chapter 4, handy for reference. We need to refer to these because in this chapter we will be considering 21-hydroxylase (CYP21) deficiency. This is the most common form of CAH and we are going to use this as the model for how you go about making a diagnosis. The principles we will be talking about are similar to those of the other forms of CAH.

When we think about making a diagnosis of CAH, we need to remember one important principle. This principle states that we need to measure the steroids on either side of the block in the pathway which we are looking for. So, if we look at our diagram (Fig. 8.1) of how we form cortisol, we can see when we are considering 21-hydroxylase (CYP21) deficiency, we would want to measure the steroids before the block, 17-hydroxyprogesterone and then also the steroids after the block,

Congenital Adrenal Hyperplasia. http://dx.doi.org/10.1016/B978-0-12-811483-4.00008-8

11-deoxycortisol or cortisol itself. We usually measure cortisol because it is easier to do than 11-deoxycortisol but you could measure both and many clinical services do this.

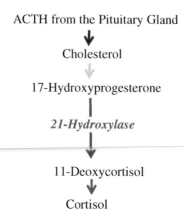

Figure 8.1 *Simplified Cortisol Synthesis Pathway shown in italics (red) the enzyme 21-hydroxylase (CYP21) which is blocked.*

BLOOD MEASUREMENTS

Steroids can be measured in blood samples. The blood samples are generally taken at the time the person presents, usually with a salt-wasting crisis. Blood samples taken at that stage would show a very high ACTH and 17-hydroxyprogesterone (17OHP) whilst the level of 11-deoxycortisol and cortisol would be low. That would of course pinpoint the block to 21-hydroxylase (CYP21) deficiency. If we were talking about a diagnosis of 11-hydroxylase (CYP11B1) deficiency, then we would expect 11-deoxycortisol to be high, ACTH to be high but cortisol to be low. It is by comparing these particular ratios of steroid before and after the block that we arrive at the diagnosis.

As said, we measure steroids in the blood using a very specific analysis called immunoassay. This process allows us to measure very small amounts of hormones in the blood. This technique was developed in the 1960's and has been refined further so that we can measure extremely small quantities of virtually any hormone that we want to.

Considerable care has to be taken with the steroids in the newborn period because the fetal adrenal zone is still active at this time and does not stop working until about 3 months of age. The hormones which the fetal adrenal glands make, sometimes upset the steroid hormones we wish to measure and because of this, we need to use laboratories that can carefully assess the difference between these steroid hormones. There are not many laboratories that do this, because most are geared to measuring steroid hormones in adults who do not have a fetal adrenal zone. As a result, we are always very careful in interpreting results when we receive information from laboratories we are not familiar with. In our laboratory at University College London Hospitals, we measure the steroid hormones by a process called liquid chromatography/tandem mass spectroscopy, which is a very specific method for identifying the steroid hormones based on their molecular size. A bit like a sieve with different size holes in it. This particular process overcomes the problems associated with the fetal adrenal zone (Fig. 8.2) and gives us a very accurate specific measure.

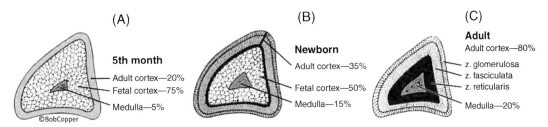

Figure 8.2 *Changes in the adrenal glands with age. (A) The fetal adrenal zone with a small amount of adult cortex. (B) The newborn with increased adult cortex. (C) Adult adrenal glands with loss of the fetal zone.*

The other thing which is important about blood measurements, is that we take them as a proper blood sample. Many people collect steroid hormone measurements on filter paper using blood spots (Fig. 8.3). This is a quick method for assessing the level of the steroid hormone, but there are considerable problems associated with it and we prefer not to make important clinical decisions based solely on this measurement.

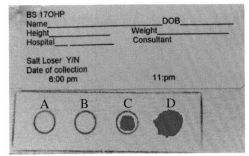

- Two circles must be completely soaked with blood for each time from the same bleed.
- A and B should be filled from the same finger prick.
- C Example of an insufficient sample.
- D Example of a correct sample.

Note centres may vary in instructions and the timings, some ask for pre morning dose only, whereas some centres ask for four specific times which may not coincide with dosing and many ask for both circles to be filled pre dose. NOTE only 17OHP is measured.

Figure 8.3 *Blood spot samples showing how they should be collected.*

URINE SAMPLES

Virtually all the steroid hormones are metabolised in the liver and excreted, in solution, in the urine. In the urine there are specific patterns of the metabolites of all the steroid hormones which we see in the adrenal pathway. These hormones do not have the same names, but we can easily identify them using chromatography in the same way that we can do on blood.

The advantage of doing the test on urine is that we can get very large volumes from which to undertake tests. In the newborn we rely very heavily on this technique. From a single processed urine test we can get an idea of every single steroid hormone above and below a certain block. This is a very efficient and effective way of making a diagnosis and is the one which we prefer in the initial phases, to blood testing.

SALIVA SAMPLING

These seem like a good way of measuring steroid hormones because no blood sample is required. In fact, because they measure the free cortisol level, they are not so good. The reason is that the amount of steroid hormone has to be high in the blood to appear in the saliva and the whole point is that cortisol is likely to be low. Saliva samples are helpful in diagnosing conditions where there are high levels of cortisol in the saliva, such as in Cushing's syndrome; however, they should not be used to measure cortisol in any condition where cortisol is being replaced because you cannot measure low cortisol levels in saliva. Measuring 17OHP in saliva is not a good way to estimate what is happening to blood 17OHP, because 17OHP is also influenced by the effect of the binding proteins like cortisol. We will look at the later in Chapter 18.

Measuring saliva is also measuring cortisol at a distance because it has been through the blood system first, so there will be a delay between what is happening in the blood and what is measured in the saliva. When measuring cortisol to assess the correct level in the body, you need to measure the amount of cortisol in the blood which is being taken to the organs.

There are also many factors which can influence the saliva sample and cause inaccurate readings, such as too much acid in the mouth, food and drink. In illness, not only could the samples be contaminated, but it would be difficult to obtain enough saliva in which to measure the cortisol level.

STIMULATION TESTS

In the newborn period the major presentation is with either ambiguous genitalia or an adrenal crisis. In both situations the ACTH drive to the adrenal is extremely high and it is usually very easy to determine the level of the block in the pathway.

In individuals with simple virilising or non-classical CAH the level of ACTH is sometimes not that high and cortisol concentrations in the blood may at first sight appear to be normal. They are usually normal, but are only achieved by a slightly higher ACTH drive which still could be within the normal range.

Assessing this situation can be quite difficult and what we do then is to undertake a synacthen stimulation test (Fig. 8.4). In this test we give some synthetic ACTH (synacthen) to stimulate the adrenal glands. We give a fairly large amount to mimic the very high levels of ACTH which are often seen in untreated CAH. This high level of ACTH maximally stimulates the adrenal glands and will then drive the adrenal glands and unmask the block. For example, if 17OHP is only slightly elevated and cortisol concentrations are normal, giving a large amount of synacthen will stimulate the system and magnify the discrepancy between 17OHP production and cortisol.

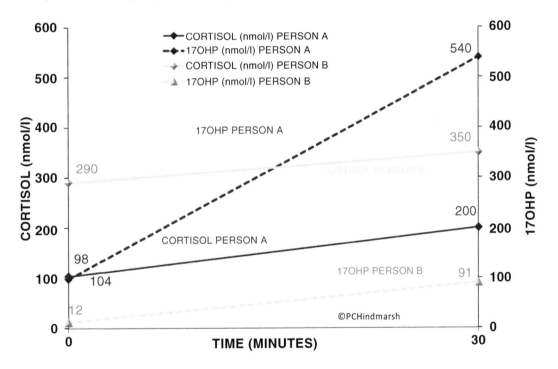

Figure 8.4 *Examples of response to synacthen.*

The graph, Fig. 8.4, shows how the synacthen test produces information which helps us to evaluate the extent of the block.

Person A has a high 17OHP at baseline of 98 nmol/l. Normal values are usually less than 10 nmol/l. Note, despite massive stimulation with synacthen, how the cortisol level hardly changes, moving from 104 to 200 nmol/l and does not get over the threshold value for a normal response of 500 nmol/l. In contrast, 17OHP is high at 98 nmol/l before the ACTH is given and then rises even higher to 540 nmol/l.

Person B has a cortisol level of 290 nmol/l before stimulation and after the ACTH is given, the cortisol rises to 350 nmol/l whereas 17OHP is only slightly high at 12 nmol/l before stimulation but rises to 91 nmol/l once stimulated. This suggests that the block in Person B is not as complete as the block in Person A.

We tend to reserve the synacthen test for situations where we want to be absolutely sure of the diagnosis, such as simple virilising CAH or non-classical forms. The slight difficulty with the ACTH test is that if you are a carrier of CAH you will also, when given ACTH, have a small rise in 17OHP. This can be a slight problem but we do have some normal ranges which we use to help overcome this, as they help separate those who are carriers from those with very mild CAH. These ranges can be seen in Fig. 8.5; however, we would always confirm these findings with genetic testing of the 21-hydroxylase gene.

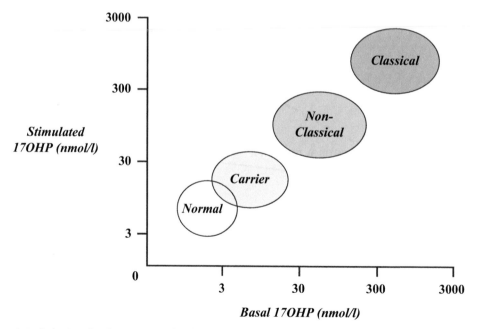

Figure 8.5 *Relationship between 17-hydroxyprogesterone before and after synacthen stimulation.* Definitions for the 17-hydroxyprogesterone levels for the various forms of 21-hydroxylase are: salt-wasting disease, up to 3000 nmol/l; simple-virilising disease, 30–300 nmol/l. Note the overlap that can occur. (Data derived from White, P.C., Speiser, P.W., 2000. Congenital adrenal hyperplasia due to 21-hydroxylase deficiency. Endocr. Rev. 21, 245–291).

In Fig. 8.5 we can see how the test separates the different groups. If we put Patient 'A' values on this, they come out in the non-classical area. Patient B is more difficult as they come out as a possible carrier or possible non-classical, although the poor cortisol response would be in favour of the latter. In this situation we would need additional help from genetic analysis.

GENETIC CONFIRMATION OF THE DIAGNOSIS

Once a biochemical diagnosis has been made, this can be confirmed by undertaking genetic testing of the gene responsible. Have a quick look back at Chapter 3 to see where the 21-hydroxylase gene is. When we do a genetic test, we usually use a blood sample and look at the gene directly with a series of special probes. These probes are designed to pick up the common mutations or deletions which are missing in the 21-hydroxylase gene. This is a very efficient way to screen for abnormalities and covers about 90% of cases in the United Kingdom. You can also use another technique called gene sequencing where each building block of the gene (called the bases), are analysed one by one. This can be quite a task, especially for a large gene like 21-hydroxylase, so this technique is reserved for situations where the common mutations/deletions are not identified.

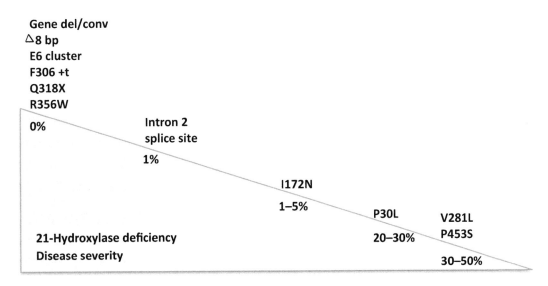

Figure 8.6 *Severity of congenital adrenal hyperplasia ranging from 0% to 30–50% enzyme activity and the various mutation codes.*

Fig. 8.6 shows how the different deletions or point mutations associate with the different forms of CAH. Once we know the actual genetic make up for the person who is affected, we then can offer antenatal diagnosis. Nowadays we do not offer antenatal treatment because of a variety of problems which are discussed in Chapter 2.

Before we embark on antenatal diagnosis, we need to know the genetic make up of the parents. We will see why this is important shortly.

The first step in antenatal diagnosis is to determine whether the baby is going to be male or female. This can be easily done by taking a blood sample from the mother at about 6–8 weeks of pregnancy. As this is a sample from the mother, it works because in the mother's blood are cells from the baby.

The test identifies these cells then tests whether the make up is XX (female) or XY (male). If we want to then define whether the baby is affected with CAH, or is carrier, or not affected, then we need to take a piece of tissue from the baby. This procedure is done under ultrasound guidance by taking a biopsy of the placenta and is known as a chorionic villous biopsy. The tissue we get is then analysed for the 21-hydroxylase genetic make up just as the blood sample was.

We use the information from the child who was affected to pin point the part of the gene to look at. We also use the parental genetic information to help us locate the genetic area as well, which is why we like to have parents' gene analysis.

TESTS TO WORK OUT ABSORPTION AND CLEARANCE

Clearance studies

Clearance studies are undertaken to work out the half-life of a drug, in our case hydrocortisone. In the study, two cannulas are inserted into veins. One cannula is used to give the hydrocortisone by a bolus injection and the other to sample blood for cortisol which appears in the circulation as a result.

A blood sample for cortisol is taken, we then immediately administer 30 mg hydrocortisone intravenously, then sample very frequently every 5 minutes for the first 45 minutes, every 15 minutes for the next 45 minutes and then half hourly for the next 90 minutes. The picture you get is shown in Fig. 8.7. We use 30 mg IV hydrocortisone, because the cortisol peak is so high that the laboratories have to dilute the higher values to get accurate cortisol readings.

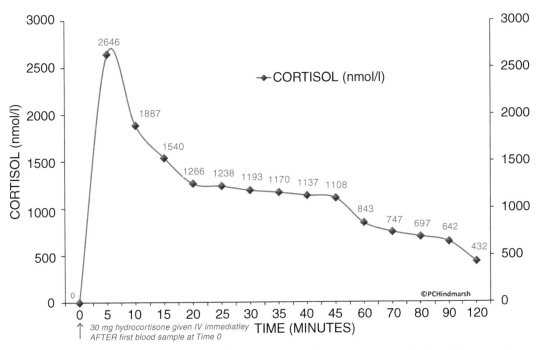

Figure 8.7 *Intravenous hydrocortisone clearance test.* A 30 mg intravenous bolus of hydrocortisone is given at time zero and frequent samples taken for the next 120 minutes.

From the data derived from the frequent sampling we measure various parameters such as the maximum concentration achieved, time to maximum concentration and of course, half-life.

From this we use mathematical formulae to derive the clearance.

Bioavailability

If we have the data from an intravenous study, we can go a step further and work out the bioavailability of hydrocortisone from either intramuscular or oral administration. In this we give the same amount of drug, usually 30 mg intravenously and then intramuscularly and/or orally. Fig. 8.8 shows the level of cortisol in the blood that is achieved via the three routes of administration.

We then work out how much cortisol is in the blood as a result and for this we sample over a 4–6 hour period. We then compare the area under the blood profile in the three cases using the intravenous route as the standard at 100%. Usually what we find is there is less hydrocortisone available over the total period by the other two routes, but not by much. For hydrocortisone, it is approximately 98% by the intramuscular route and 94% by the oral route. This is quite good compared to some medications.

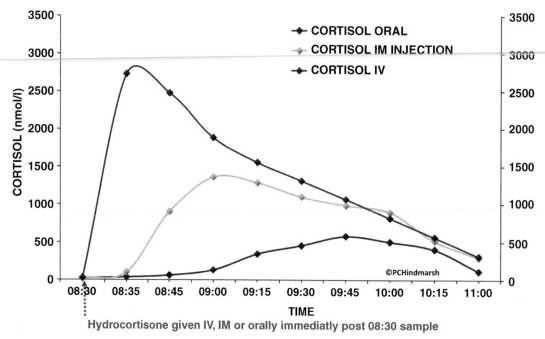

Figure 8.8 *Blood cortisol levels achieved after administration of 30 mg of hydrocortisone by the intravenous (purple line), intramuscular (green line) or oral (blue line) routes.*

TESTING FOR EARLY PUBERTY

The most important test for establishing whether puberty has started is the gonadotropin releasing hormone (GnRH) stimulation test.

In this test, blood is taken before an intravenous bolus of GnRH is given for the measurement of the sex hormones, luteinising hormone (LH) and follicle-stimulating hormone (FSH). Further samples are then taken at 20 and 60 minutes to measure the sex hormone response. Fig. 8.9 shows a typical pubertal response of LH and FSH to GnRH.

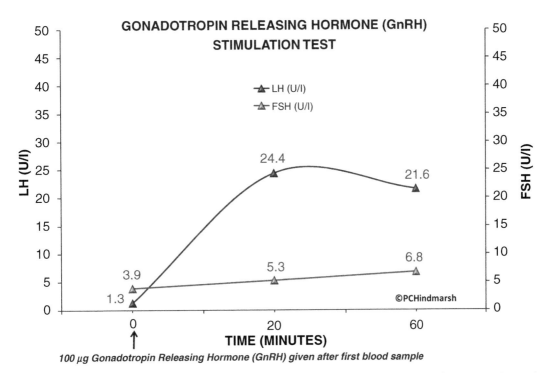

Figure 8.9 *Pubertal sex hormone response to gonadotropin releasing hormone (GnRH). Luteinising hormone in dark blue rises to a peak value of 24.4 U/l 20 minutes after administration of GnRH. Follicle stimulating hormone rises more slowly. This dominance of LH over FSH is very typical of puberty.*

Sometimes, in males, a further test is done where human chorionic gonadotropin (HCG) is given to stimulate testosterone production from the testes.

HCG is chemically similar to LH. This test is often done in cases where puberty is delayed to check whether the testes are working properly or not. The test involves three intramuscular injections of HCG on alternate days with a measurement of testosterone at the start and finish. Another way to look at this is to undertake testosterone measurements over 24 hours.

Fig. 8.10 shows the rhythm of testosterone with high values in the early hours of the morning. A short course of HCG amplifies testosterone.

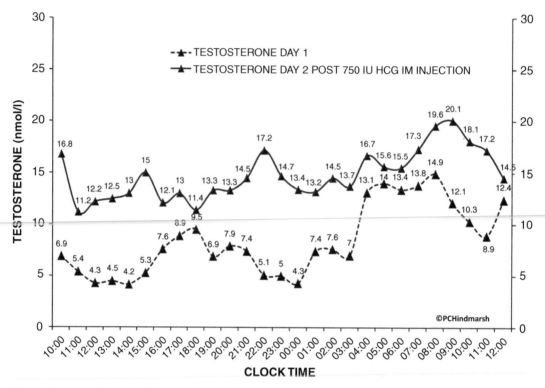

Figure 8.10 *24 hour profile of testosterone with amplification by HCG.*

TESTING THE FEEDBACK FROM ADRENAL TO PITUITARY

Quite often it is important to know how the feedback from the adrenal glands to the pituitary gland works. You might want to quickly refresh yourself on this by looking at Chapter 1 again. What we are interested in this test is whether the pituitary is producing ACTH that can be switched off by cortisol. Sometimes, when CAH has been difficult to manage and ACTH levels have been high, the pituitary gland can end up producing ACTH in an uncontrolled way.

We can test this by giving the individual dexamethasone rather than hydrocortisone. The reason we use dexamethasone rather than hydrocortisone is because it lasts longer, making blood testing easier. ACTH is measured along with 17OHP and androstenedione (A4). This is done every day at 09:00. Fig. 8.11 shows this over the study period of 4 days. After the 09:00 sample has been taken, dexamethasone is given as total daily dose of 2 mg for the next 2 days and then at 8 mg/day for the subsequent 2 days. What happens in Fig. 8.11 is that the pituitary gland takes a bit of time to respond, with the ACTH starting to fall which in turn brings the 17OHP and A4 down. Notice that this is not instantaneous and takes some days. Nonetheless it comes down. If it does not, this suggests the pituitary gland is producing ACTH in an uncontrolled way and this would need attention and possibly surgery, to remove the source of ACTH production. This is often called Nelson's disease and is a major problem in adult endocrinology. It is a rare issue in paediatrics.

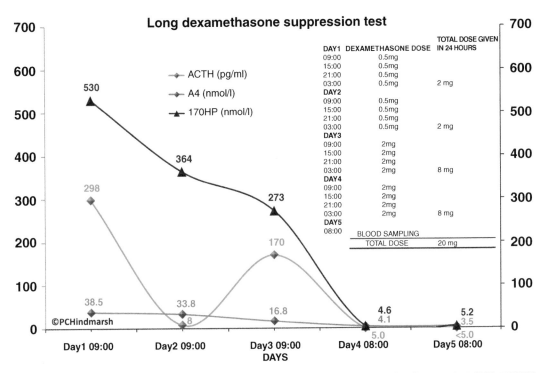

Figure 8.11 *Long dexamethasone suppression test showing the gradual reduction in ACTH, 17OHP and androstenedione (A4) over the study period.*

MONITORING THERAPY

Testing hydrocortisone replacement

We use blood tests to help us alter hydrocortisone and fludrocortisone replacement therapy. This is a complex area and Section Three of this book looks at the way to measure hydrocortisone replacement using 24 hour profiles. This area needs a book in itself.

Testing the mineralocorticoid axis

As we have outlined in previous chapters, many individuals with 21-hydroxylase (CYP21) deficiency present in the newborn period with either ambiguous genitalia or, in the case of the males, with a salt–wasting crisis. In this situation the plasma sodium concentration falls due to sodium loss through the kidney. The result of this is to increase the amount of renin produced by the kidney, which drives the pathway in the adrenal glands to produce aldosterone as discussed in Chapter 1 (renin–angiotensin system).

So, for diagnosis, what we would do in this situation is to measure the plasma sodium concentration along with the plasma renin activity.

If plasma sodium concentrations are low, then plasma renin activity will be very high and this will indicate there is reduced production of aldosterone. We can also measure aldosterone in the blood, so the combination of plasma renin activity, plasma sodium and aldosterone helps us to identify a loss of the salt retaining hormone aldosterone. Fig. 8.12 summarises the block. This combination, taken with the results from the blood or urine steroid analysis, supports the diagnosis of a salt–wasting crisis, due to 21-hydroxylase (CYP21) deficiency. Another clue is that before the sodium actually falls to low levels we see the potassium levels in the blood start to rise.

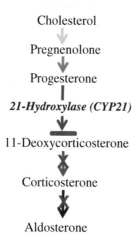

Figure 8.12 *Block in the enzyme 21-hydroxylase (CYP21) in the mineralocorticoid pathway leads to reduced production of aldosterone.*

In both simple virilising and non–classical CAH, the plasma renin activity may be normal or at least at the top end of the normal range and the plasma sodium concentration normal. In this situation it is of interest that if the individual is placed in an environment of increasing sodium loss, e.g. a very hot climate where they sweat a lot or if they are challenged with a very low sodium diet, then the plasma renin activity will rise quite markedly, plasma sodium may fall but more importantly the plasma aldosterone concentration does not rise in response to the increase in plasma renin activity.

This combination would imply there is a block in the formation of aldosterone, but the block is not complete and can be overcome with a slightly increased drive to the system through an increase in plasma renin. Whether this requires some treatment with fludrocortisone is a debatable point and is not resolved as yet. In fact, because hydrocortisone also retains sodium, we often find that simply using hydrocortisone keeps the sodium system stable in individuals with either simple virilising CAH or non-classical CAH. Another good reason to always use hydrocortisone!

ELECTROLYTE MEASUREMENT

Throughout the book we refer to the measurement of electrolytes. These measurements refer to several chemicals in the blood namely sodium, potassium, chloride and bicarbonate. Sodium and potassium have an overall positive charge associated with them, whereas chloride and bicarbonate have negative charges. This means the positives and negatives can combine to maintain electrical neutrality. One example is sodium chloride also known as common salt.

Sodium and potassium balance each other so that when one goes up the other goes down. The electrolytes are filtered by the kidneys but only a small proportion is excreted in the urine. The kidneys for example, reabsorb lots of sodium and the key factor in absorbing sodium is aldosterone. This is why loss of aldosterone has such profound effects leading to sodium loss. As sodium is lost in the urine, it takes with it water so that severe dehydration ensues. The way aldosterone works is to swap sodium for potassium, which also explains why in an adrenal crisis the potassium rises as this swap cannot take place.

We refer to high and low amounts of electrolytes as hyper and hypo. Low sodium is called hyponatraemia and high potassium as hyperkalaemia. The actual definitions attached to these descriptions are:

- Hyponatraemia is a plasma sodium level below 135 mmol/l and severe hyponatraemia a value below 120 mmol/l. In CAH this signifies dehydration and needs to be carefully treated with saline infusion.

- Hypernatraemia is a plasma sodium level above 145 mmol/l and severe above 150 mmol/l. This is unusual as the thirst mechanism drives water intake once the plasma sodium reaches 145 mmol/l.

- Hypokalaemia is defined as a plasma potassium level below 3.5 mmol/l. Hypokalaemia is associated with muscle weakness but the most important effect is that it leads to irregular heartbeats and cardiac arrest.

- Hyperkalaemia is defined as a plasma potassium level above 5 mmol/l. The main worry when potassium is high is cardiac arrest.

Understanding chloride and bicarbonate is more complex because this involves body systems which are involved with dealing with acids in the body and is beyond the scope of this book.

FURTHER READING

Ranke, M.B., Mullis, P.E., 2011. Diagnostics of Endocrine Function in Children and Adolescents, fourth ed. Karger, Basel.

SECTION TWO

When Things Go Wrong in Congenital Adrenal Hyperplasia

The focus of our regular review of young people with congenital adrenal hyperplasia is to prevent over or under treatment with glucocorticoid steroids.

Over treatment can lead to suppression of growth and under treatment leads to an increase in male adrenal androgens which will accelerate growth rate and maturity of the skeleton.

In addition to this, we now realise that the glucocorticoids which we use, might leave the person when exposed to too much of them, with other problems in terms of bone mineralisation, glucose levels and cholesterol. As a result, we have over the years spread our review of people with CAH to cover many of these different aspects.

In reality, we always hope there will be no problems with the congenital adrenal hyperplasia a child has, but this section not only outlines some of the things which can happen, but also gives an idea of what we might be able to do to make things right. As is so often the case in medicine, the important thing is not to let things become a problem in the first instance, which is why we have placed a great deal of emphasis in this book and in our clinical practice, on detailed assessments of glucocorticoid dosing using 24 hour profiles and follow up.

CHAPTER 9

Monitoring Long Term Outcomes

GLOSSARY

Acne A skin condition characterised by red pimples on the skin, especially on the face, due to inflamed or infected sebaceous glands.

Adrenal rests The presence of adrenal tissue in the testes. This tissue responds to ACTH stimulation leading to an increase in size. The rests are hard and irregular in shape and can be mistaken for testicular cancers. These can occur wherever there are adrenal cells, but mainly in testes and rarely ovaries. These are often referred to as Testicular Adrenal Rest Tissue or TART.

Cardiovascular health Blood pressure and cardiac function are two important components. Blood pressure is the easiest to measure and has the most important effect on long term health.

Cataracts Condition in which the lens of the eye becomes progressively opaque, resulting in blurred vision.

Cortisol The major glucocorticoid in humans. Made in the adrenal glands. Cortisol regulates over two thirds of human genes. Cortisol regulates blood glucose, muscle function, the body's response to infection, fat distribution and brain thought processes.

Diabetes Raised blood glucose due to lack of insulin (type 1) or impaired insulin action (type 2).

Dizziness Symptoms are often associated with mineralocorticoid deficiency and occur in conjunction with low blood pressure. Noted especially on standing up quickly from a sitting position.

Fertility The ability to form sperm in males and to create an egg in females.

Gastritis Inflammation of the lining of the stomach which can lead onto an ulcer.

Growth acceleration Increase in height usually expressed over a period of 1 year. Usually associated with an increased exposure to adrenal androgens or sex steroids. Often indicative of under replacement with hydrocortisone.

Growth arrest Complete cessation of growth in height. Often occurs with prednisolone or dexamethasone use.

Growth retardation Decrease in growth rate usually expressed over a period of 1 year and sometimes actual arrest of growth. Usually associated with over replacement of hydrocortisone.

Glycosuria Loss of glucose into the urine which occurs when blood glucose levels go above 10 mmol/l.

Congenital Adrenal Hyperplasia. http://dx.doi.org/10.1016/B978-0-12-811483-4.00009-X

Hirsutism Excessive body hair in men and women where body hair is normally minimal or absent, for example, appearance of facial hair in a female.

Hypercalciuria Increased excretion of calcium in the urine.

Hypertension A blood pressure reading greater than 95th centile for age and height.

Infertility Defined as the failure to achieve a clinical pregnancy after 12 months or more of regular unprotected sexual intercourse. In CAH this may arise in males, because of reduced sperm production due to the presence of adrenal rests, or in females, due to polycystic ovarian syndrome.

Ischemic bone necrosis Situation where blood supply to bone is interrupted leading to death of some bone cells.

Long term side effects Side effects from over and under replacement of cortisol which develop over many years and may not become apparent until later in life, such as infertility, adrenal rests, polycystic ovaries, short term memory loss, osteoporosis, obesity, diabetes, metabolic syndrome, coronary heart disease and hypertension.

Metabolic syndrome The collection of obesity, hyperlipidaemia, hypertension, raised insulin, type 2 diabetes which is associated with increased risk of heart disease and stroke.

Obesity Abnormal or excessive fat accumulation which may impair health. Usually estimated by body mass index (person's weight in kilograms divided by the square of their height in meters). For adults, obesity is a BMI greater than or equal to 30.

Osteoporosis A marked reduction of mineral in bone which weakens the bone structure thereby increasing the risk of fracture.

Over treatment Cortisol peaks too high from the dose being too high and doses taken too frequently, resulting in over stacking.

Polycystic ovaries This is a particular appearance where the ovaries are enlarged and filled with dense stroma in the middle, with lots of small cysts around the periphery of the ovary.

Short term memory loss Classic effect of glucocorticoids. Recall of recent events or recently learnt facts is impaired.

Short term side effects Side effects which occur within the first few years of inappropriate cortisol (hydrocortisone) replacement, such as growth acceleration, growth retardation, weight gain, short term memory loss, dizziness, headaches, hirsutism and acne.

Slipped epiphyses Condition where the cartilage on the hipbone becomes loosened and displaced. Produces a limp and requires urgent surgical assessment.

Toxic psychosis Altered mental state with confusion, hallucinations, e.g. strange voices and thought disorder.

Under treatment Inadequate levels of cortisol, doses taken too far apart. Poor distribution of cortisol over the 24 hour period.

Weight gain In paediatrics this is represented by an increase, during childhood, of more than 2.5–3 kg/year. Result of over treatment with hydrocortisone.

	END POINT	RATIONALE	MEASURE
SHORT TERM	1. Growth acceleration	1. Assess control	1. Acceleration greater than 2 cm/year needs attention
	2. Weight changes	2. Assess dosing	2. Weight gain in excess of 2 kg/year needs attention
	3. Correct dose for size	3. Optimise therapy	3. 1 and 2 above and blood tests
	4. Blood pressure	4. Treatment effects	4. Blood pressure and plot on centile charts
	5. Puberty	5. Timing can be altered in CAH	5. Special examination
MEDIUM TERM	1. Bone maturation	1. Rate of skeletal maturation	1. Yearly bone age
	2. Pubertal status	2. Early puberty or rapid progression	2. Tanner staging
	3. Hydrocortisone dose	3. Optimise therapy	3. Cortisol and 17OHP profiles over 24 hour period
	4. Fludrocortisone dose	4. Avoid high blood pressure	4. Plasma renin activity
	5. Testes and ovary health	5. CAH might influence how they work	5. Pelvic ultrasound for girls. Careful exam for boys
	6. Metabolic status	6. Insulin insensitivity and lipids	6. Fasting glucose, insulin and lipids
LONG TERM	1. Growth	1. Outcome	1. Final height within target height of parents
	2. Bone mineralisation	2. CAH/treatment effect on bone	2. DEXA scan
	3. Fertility	3. Effect of CAH	3. Check for regular menstrual cycle (girls) and adrenal rests in testes in boys
	4. Cardiovascular risk	4. CAH/treatment effect	4. Fasting glucose and insulin, blood pressure, fasting lipids

Figure 9.1 *Annual review plan. CAH, Congenital adrenal hyperplasia; 17OHP, 17-hydroxyprogesterone.*

ANNUAL REVIEW

When thinking about how we should monitor young people with congenital adrenal hyperplasia, we need to think firstly about where we want to be in the long term. This is a little bit like using a 'satnav' to get where you want to go. We simply work out the destination and then work backwards from that to construct a series of maps or events which have to be passed along the way to get to the destination. The nice thing about CAH maps or satnavs is that there is no annoying voice.

In Fig. 9.1 we write out the annual review plan and following the satnav analogy, we start thinking about the long term which we have broken down into the following four areas: growth, bone mineralisation, fertility and cardiovascular risk. We know all these are important because both the condition of CAH itself, particularly if it is not looked after well, as well as the treatments used, will impact upon all these four measures.

We have also said why we want to measure them and what actual measure we will use. We will be looking at this in a bit more detail as we go through this whole section about when things go wrong in CAH.

To get to these points we need to have a series of short and medium term measures. For example, with growth you can only get to final adult height by a series of increments in height. This means we need to measure height quite frequently which is why growth acceleration and indeed weight changes, come across in the short term measures.

When we think about bone mineralisation we are interested in both short and medium term measures which add together to produce an effect on the skeleton. These include in the short term, the correct dose of the steroids we use and also in the medium term puberty is achieved at the right time and is completed correctly.

Fertility might seem to be something that only happens to adults, but we know getting doses correct and avoiding being overweight, along with entering puberty at the normal time and progressing through it normally, are important factors which also determine how well the testes and ovaries will work.

Finally, knowing we have got the dose of steroid right will help us avoid problems with blood pressure, glucose and insulin and the combination of these can, if they are not looked after properly, cause long term problems with the heart and blood vessels.

As a result of this, the situation looks rather complicated, but if we break it down into the various sections then we can see that addressing these both in the short and medium term, will help us achieve where we want to get to in the longer term, which is healthy young adults.

SHORT TERM

Growth

Here we check that the rate of growth is optimal.

- No growth or slow growth can point to over treatment.
- Growth exceeding 2 cm in a year can indicate under treatment.

In both cases, doses need adjusting. What we do is try to keep growth on track by using 24 hour profiling to optimise the dose and these profiles have been successful in keeping growth on track. Using growth as a method to assess replacement of cortisol is a handy check; however, like many of these markers for assessments, the problem has already occurred.

We cover growth in Chapters 6 and 10.

Weight changes

Weight gain in excess of 2 kg/year needs investigation as does poor weight gain.

- Weight gain can be a sign of over treatment where the peaks of cortisol from dosing are too high, or if the cortisol distribution is not correct. You can get weight gain from the high peaks even with periods of no cortisol being in the blood.
- Weight loss can occur if the doses are too low.

We cover weight in Chapters 6 and 10.

Signs of early puberty

Any sign of axillary hair or body odour, should always be reported to your endocrinologist as these are signs of precocious (early) puberty. This is a sign of under treatment. We cover this in Chapters 7 and 11.

Bone age

This is an X-ray of the hand and is usually done annually after the age of 3 years. Again this assessment only shows the problem after the event, as in advanced bone age. This means for some period of time there has been under treatment. We cover bone age in Chapters 6 and 10.

Blood pressure

A 24 hour profile allows us to measure blood pressure at different points of the day and night. We look at these measurements with particular attention to fludrocortisone doses along with the plasma renin activity. High blood pressure can mean over treatment with mineralocorticoid replacement which would also give a low plasma renin level. Low blood pressure can be a sign of under replacement of either hydrocortisone or fludrocortisone. We cover blood pressure in Chapter 12.

MEDIUM TERM

Medium term means we look at keeping the normal progression of all the previously mentioned short term assessments on track and that all is progressing normally.

Puberty

To ensure that the progression of puberty is correct we scan the ovaries in girls. Boys have a sonogram of testes to check for adrenal rests. In boys, we also measure the size of the testes to assess the stage of their puberty. A 24 hour profile also allows us to measure the activity of the hormones that drive puberty, LH and FSH, which in the beginning are only active at night. We cover this in Chapters 7 and 11.

Metabolic state

To ensure that the glucocorticoids are not altering glucose and cholesterol, we check these every year. In addition to glucose, we measure insulin to make sure the pancreas is not under any stress which might lead to it not working properly and the person developing diabetes. This is covered in Chapter 12.

LONG TERM

Long term objectives are getting the dose as fine tuned as possible and we can only do this by looking at cortisol over 24 hours. The distribution of cortisol is also very important in achieving optimal growth and weight. If cortisol replacement is good, 17OHP levels will reflect this and androgen levels will also optimise.

Bone density

Once growth is almost complete we add a DEXA scan annually, or every 2 years, to ensure bone density is normal. This is to prevent osteoporosis from occurring due to long term use of steroids in adulthood. We cover this in detail in Chapter 13.

Fertility

During puberty and postpuberty we can measure LH, FSH, testosterone and estrogen levels in both males and females over the 24 hour period. This gives us a good indication of any adjustments which need to be made to ensure fertility is optimal.

We check for adrenal rests and polycystic ovaries. We cover this in Chapter 14.

Cardiovascular risks

24 hour profiles also allow us to test fasting glucose and insulin levels, fasting lipids as well as blood pressure checks both lying and standing, at certain intervals during the 24 hours. Therefore, we are able to optimise therapy and prevent many problems which can occur in later life.

Lying and standing blood pressure is useful as there is normally a drop of about 10 mm Hg when you stand up. Any more than this makes it possible there is under replacement with fludrocortisone. This can be complimented by the measurement of plasma renin activity lying and standing which should increase when standing.

We also like to measure blood pressure overnight as normally there is a 10% drop in blood pressure and we know that when this drop is absent, it is a good marker for the future development of hypertension. We cover this in Chapter 12.

FURTHER READING

Hindmarsh, P.C., 2009. Management of the child with congenital adrenal hyperplasia. Best Pract. Res. Clin. Endocrinol. Metab. 23, 193–208.

CHAPTER 10

Growth

GLOSSARY

Aromatase inhibitors A class of drug which block the conversion of testosterone to estradiol and androstenedione to estrone. Estrogens are the main factors in maturing the skeleton and advancing bone age.

Cortisol profile Measurement of cortisol in the blood at one hourly intervals to buildup a profile of what levels are achieved from treatment with hydrocortisone.

Gonadotrophin releasing hormone analogue Hormone which is produced by the hypothalamus and directs the pituitary gland to produce luteinising and follicle-stimulating hormones. Analogues (an analogue has a similar biochemical structure to the native molecule and is often altered slightly to enhance or decrease biological action), stay attached to the pituitary gland for long periods of time and cause the pituitary gland to stop producing luteinising and follicle-stimulating hormone.

Height velocity The rate of gain in height over a time period, usually 1 year.

GENERAL

There are two areas which can go wrong in terms of height and weight and these are caused by over or under treatment with hydrocortisone. Although we mention weight issues in the chapter we also cover this in more detail in Chapter 12.

OVER TREATMENT

Over treatment with glucocorticoids leads to the suppression of growth.

This means that the amount of height that is gained on a year by year basis is less than normal and if this continues for a very long period of time then adult height would be reduced.

This is where steroids have got their bad name from in terms of growth, but we have to remember that it is steroid use with very high doses of very powerful steroids, such as dexamethasone that often do this.

What we aim to do is to replace with steroid therapy, as close to what happens naturally in the body as is possible, hence avoiding or reducing the possibility that growth might be suppressed.

Congenital Adrenal Hyperplasia. http://dx.doi.org/10.1016/B978-0-12-811483-4.00010-6

The weight and height charts in Fig. 10.1 show what happens to the height and weight pattern when someone is receiving too much glucocorticoid. As you can see, the normal growth pattern illustrated by the blue solid line follows the 50th percentile, however, the red dashed line shows slow growth and over time the height drops below the next percentile. There is a critical dose of glucocorticoid which will suppress height gain. If the total hydrocortisone dose is greater than 30 mg/m^2 body surface area/day, then height gain will be suppressed. Over treatment is not good for height because if too much glucocorticoid is used, not only will the height gain be slow, but the actual growth plate itself can be damaged and this cannot be reversed Fig 10.8. For weight, the dose of glucocorticoid which leads to weight gain is approximately 20 mg/m^2 body surface area/day.

In the weight chart, the purple dashed line shows how the weight has increased well above where the normal progression should be (indicated by the solid blue line).

This combination of a reduction in height, coupled with an increase in weight, strongly suggests over treatment with glucocorticoids.

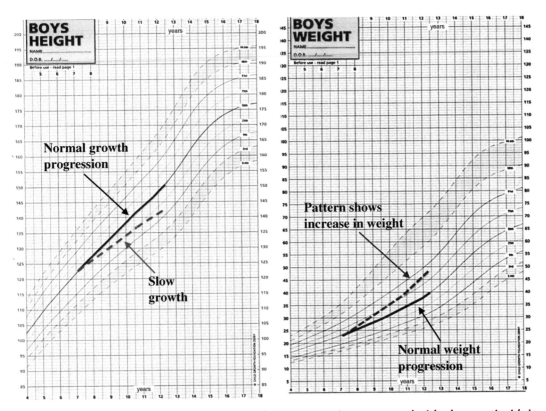

Figure 10.1 *The effect on height and weight when someone is over treated with glucocorticoids in CAH, shown by the dashed lines. (All charts copyright Child Growth Foundation reproduced with kind permission).*

What can be done?

1. Check with a 24 hour profile to see what is happening in terms of the distribution of cortisol as a result of hydrocortisone administration. Are the peaks too high? Is the level of cortisol in the blood too high generally over the 24 hours?

2. Work to reduce the total exposure to glucocorticoid whilst maintaining a good balance in terms of the other hormones which the adrenal glands produce, e.g. 17-hydroxyprogesterone and the adrenal androgens.

3. Until the hydrocortisone dose is adjusted, usual attempts to control weight such as diet and exercise, will not work.

UNDER TREATMENT

The weight and height charts in Fig. 10.2 show how under treatment affects height and weight. Growth is accelerated and often the child will appear far taller than their peers. Weight gain is slow and can result in the child being underweight.

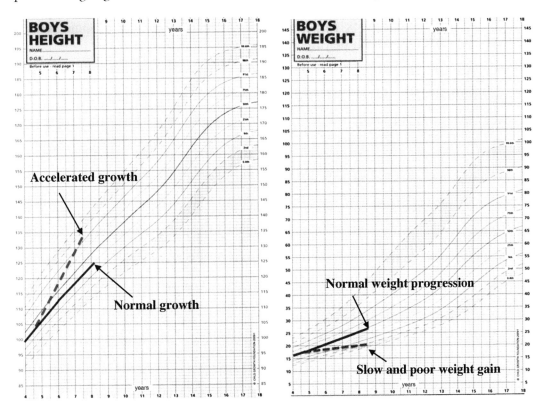

Figure 10.2 *The effect on height and weight when someone is under treated with glucocorticoids in CAH, shown by the dashed lines. (All charts copyright Child Growth Foundation reproduced with kind permission).*

Under treatment is more of a problem because the adrenal androgens will alter the maturity of the skeleton. This is where our bone age assessment comes in very useful, because it indicates the maturity of the skeleton and how much growth has actually taken place and therefore how much growth is available to the person (Fig. 10.3). Exposure to adrenal androgens leads to an acceleration in bone maturity which means there is less time in which to grow and we would then expect adult height to be reduced (Fig. 10.4).

HOW BONE AGE IS USEFUL IN MONITORING GROWTH

Bone age is really useful in helping us understand and manage growth in people with CAH. Bone maturation is influenced by the CAH condition itself as well as the treatment used.

1. Over treatment can lead to bone age delay and if doses which are too high are used, damage to growth plates can occur, again leading to less of an adult height achieved (Fig. 10.3, boy with delay in bone maturity).

2. Under treatment leads to acceleration in skeletal maturity which means growth is completed more quickly. As there is less time to grow, adult height will be less (Fig. 10.4, boy with mature skeleton).

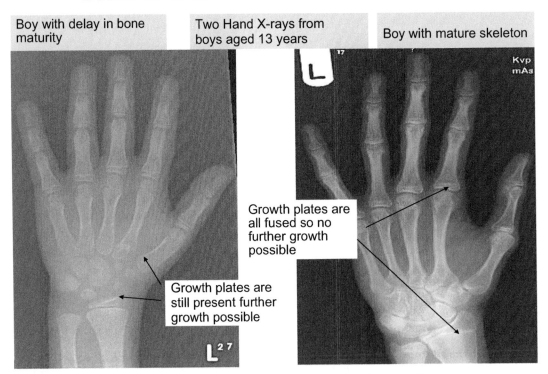

Boy with delay in bone maturity

Two Hand X-rays from boys aged 13 years

Boy with mature skeleton

Growth plates are all fused so no further growth possible

Growth plates are still present further growth possible

Figure 10.3 *Delayed bone age.*

Figure 10.4 *Advanced bone age.*

NON-CLASSICAL CAH (NCCAH) AND ADVANCED BONE AGE

This is what happens in non-classical CAH (NCCAH) (either SVCAH or LOCAH) as the presentation is later in life and not at birth. In NCCAH, bone age can be very advanced at diagnosis due to exposure to excess androgen production from the adrenals for a long period of time. In Fig. 10.5 we can see that bone age is in advance of the chronological age. In this situation, the advance in bone age means there is less time available to complete growth. If we look at the actual calculation, what has happened during this period of time is although the individual was destined to be 170 cm, the advance in bone age has meant that the height estimate has been reduced to 160 cm.

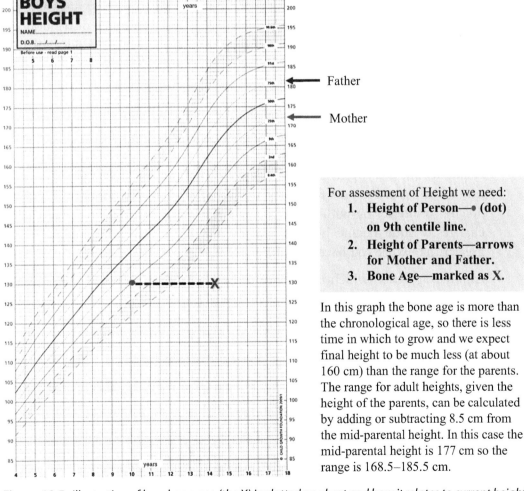

For assessment of Height we need:
1. **Height of Person—• (dot) on 9th centile line.**
2. **Height of Parents—arrows for Mother and Father.**
3. **Bone Age—marked as X.**

In this graph the bone age is more than the chronological age, so there is less time in which to grow and we expect final height to be much less (at about 160 cm) than the range for the parents. The range for adult heights, given the height of the parents, can be calculated by adding or subtracting 8.5 cm from the mid-parental height. In this case the mid-parental height is 177 cm so the range is 168.5–185.5 cm.

Figure 10.5 *Illustration of how bone age (the X) is plotted on chart and how it relates to current height by the dashed line connected to the red dot, which is current height. (All charts copyright Child Growth Foundation reproduced with kind permission).*

Remember, in NCCAH the adrenal glands can still produce cortisol but they only do this because the drive to cortisol production by ACTH from the pituitary gland is quite high. This means the adrenal glands are working very hard to produce cortisol which is often enough to keep the body happy, but because there is a partial block, the increased drive increases production of all steroids above the block which includes the androgens. Have a look at Chapter 4 to remind yourself of the pathways. Although the adrenal androgens are not as strong as testosterone they do affect bone maturity, making it advance more quickly, hence the older bone age. Although this is called NCCAH, once treatment with hydrocortisone is started, endogenous (natural production) cortisol production is switched off and the person needs the same approach to cortisol replacement as someone with SWCAH.

What can be done

1. Again a 24 hour profile will help us to work out the exact distribution of hydrocortisone during the 24 hour period and to determine periods when the individual might be under treated.

2. Readjust the hydrocortisone dosing to get better coverage.

3. The situation is not as easy as it may appear, because the bone age has advanced. Endocrinologists sometimes try to improve the situation by holding up entry into puberty as we discuss in Chapter 11 'using gonadotropin releasing hormone analogue' but this approach is not as effective as it might seem. The reason for this is the contribution of puberty to stature is relatively fixed at about 20–30 cm, so interfering with this at the end of growth is unlikely to make major changes to adult height, because the amount that needs to be manipulated is greater than what you have available.

4. Another approach which may prove to be a bit more successful is to stop the conversion of the adrenal androgens to female hormones. This takes place by an enzyme called aromatase (CYP19), which is present in many parts of the body but particularly in fat cells.

Bone maturation is dependent on the formation of estrogen both in males and females. This sounds surprising at first but there are many examples where estrogens cannot be made properly in males who go on to develop osteoporosis, but also continue to grow well into adulthood because their skeleton does not fuse.

An aromatase inhibitor is an agent which is used to stop the conversion of testosterone to estradiol (Fig. 10.6) and can be used to stop conversion of adrenal androgens to the various forms of estrogen (Fig. 10.7). We go into more detail on this in Chapter 12.

Studies on this are still in progress, but there are data to suggest that this approach might be advantageous in situations where bone age has become too advanced and the adult height is going to be compromised, as we have shown in Fig. 10.5.

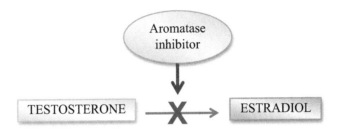

Figure 10.6 *The enzyme aromatase converts testosterone to estradiol and is blocked by aromatase inhibitors.*

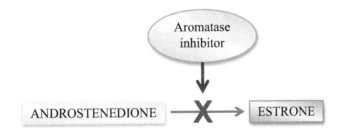

Figure 10.7 *The enzyme aromatase converts androstenedione to estrone and is blocked by aromatase inhibitors.*

5. Extra growth hormone has been tried to see if that will boost growth and ultimately adult height. Studies where growth hormone has been given to short but otherwise normal children, do not show any long term benefit for this approach. Growth hormone if used in CAH, must be used very carefully as it decreases the conversion of cortisone to cortisol which reduces the pool of cortisol that is in the blood, so dose changes to hydrocortisone will be needed.

There are some reports of success in situations where bone age is advanced in CAH, but unless the growth hormone is combined with some means of preventing advance in skeletal maturation, such as an aromatase inhibitor or holding up puberty, this approach is unlikely to be successful.

Over treatment with glucocorticoids can lead to the opposite effect on growth to under treatment (Fig 10.8).

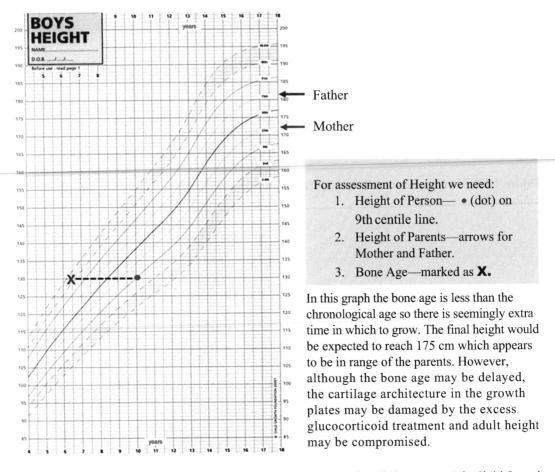

Father

Mother

For assessment of Height we need:
1. Height of Person— • (dot) on 9th centile line.
2. Height of Parents—arrows for Mother and Father.
3. Bone Age—marked as **X.**

In this graph the bone age is less than the chronological age so there is seemingly extra time in which to grow. The final height would be expected to reach 175 cm which appears to be in range of the parents. However, although the bone age may be delayed, the cartilage architecture in the growth plates may be damaged by the excess glucocorticoid treatment and adult height may be compromised.

Figure 10.8 *Illustrates the effect of delayed bone age on growth. (All charts copyright Child Growth Foundation reproduced with kind permission).*

This situation can occur when there is over treatment with suppression of adrenal androgens. The bone age is less than the chronological age so there is extra time to grow and the person ends up taller than expected from simply looking at their position on the growth chart. Care must be taken in this situation. Although the bone age may be delayed, the cartilage architecture in the growth plates may be damaged by the excess glucocorticoid treatment and adult height may be compromised. We talked about what to do about over treatment in an earlier part of this chapter.

FURTHER READING

Hindmarsh, P.C., 2009. Management of the child with congenital adrenal hyperplasia. Best Pract. Res. Clin. Endocrinol. Metab. 23, 193–208.

CHAPTER 11

When Things Go Wrong With Puberty

GLOSSARY

Adrenal androgen Male like hormones with a structure similar to testosterone. The two main androgens are dehydroepiandrosterone and androstenedione.

Aromatase inhibitors A class of drug which block the conversion of testosterone to estradiol and androstenedione to estrone. Estrogens are the main factors in maturing the skeleton and advancing bone age.

Gonadotrophin releasing hormone analogue Hormone which is produced by the hypothalamus and directs the pituitary gland to produce luteinising and follicle-stimulating hormones. Analogues (an analogue has a similar biochemical structure to the native molecule and is often altered slightly to enhance or decrease biological action), stay attached to the pituitary gland for long periods of time and cause the pituitary gland to stop producing luteinising and follicle-stimulating hormone.

Gynaecomastia Breast tissue development in males.

Non–classical CAH (NCCAH) Also known as late-onset CAH (LOCAH) Mildest form of CAH and often not detected until adolescence or sometimes as late as adulthood.

Simple virilising CAH (SVCAH) Presents in childhood with rapid growth, body hair development and body odour. Cortisol production is maintained by high ACTH drive.

GENERAL

When we consider how things might go wrong in puberty when having congenital adrenal hyperplasia (CAH), there is very little to be concerned about when considering the natural timing of puberty in boys and girls. In individuals who have optimal replacement, the timing of puberty is the same as the general population for both boys and girls. Problems arise when we think about children presenting with premature signs of puberty as in simple virilising CAH, as true puberty can often follow once treatment starts.

We have already talked a little about the two systems in the body involved in terms of making male like hormones. It might be a good idea to reread Chapter 7, our initial chapter on puberty if you need to remind yourself on this. If you remember, we said that it was the hypothalamic–pituitary–gonadal axis which controls the testes and ovaries and instructs them to make the appropriate hormones, either testosterone or estradiol.

Congenital Adrenal Hyperplasia. http://dx.doi.org/10.1016/B978-0-12-811483-4.00011-8

In addition, we know the adrenal glands can make androgens and in females without CAH, it is these androgens which cause pubic and axillary hair development. In males without CAH, these hormones are less important because testosterone is so potent and is produced by the testes.

In CAH if prepubertal females have been under treated with glucocorticoids and as a result have high adrenal androgens, they will develop pubic and axillary hair. Similar changes will take place in prepubertal males, although the penis may also enlarge slightly in the latter. In both situations, growth will accelerate and bone age will advance as we have described in Chapter 10. This situation needs to be brought under urgent control by carefully adjusting the glucocorticoid dose.

The message from this chapter is careful attention to glucocorticoid dosing both in timing and amount is extremely important. This can be easily checked by undertaking a 24 hour profile to determine the distribution of hydrocortisone throughout the 24 hour period and thereby titrate and fine tune the dosing schedule for the individual.

Regular assessment of height and weight will also guide the clinician as to whether there are problems with respect to the dosing schedule and indicate that more detailed studies using profiles are needed, see Chapter 10.

A similar situation arises in the presentation of simple virilising CAH (SVCAH) and non-classical CAH (NCCAH) also known as late-onset CAH (LOCAH), where the body has worked hard to keep the cortisol concentration reasonably normal but at the expense of increased adrenal androgen production.

These individuals usually present as tall children with an advance in bone maturation, development of body odour, the appearance of axillary and pubic hair and often acne. They need treatment with glucocorticoids.

There is no doubt that exposing a person to adrenal androgens leads to further problems, because these prime the hypothalamo-pituitary-gonadal axis so when the adrenal androgens are brought under control by readjusting the glucocorticoid dose, any effect of these adrenal androgens to suppress the hypothalamo-pituitary-gonadal axis will be lost. This axis will switch on and start to produce the normal changes associated with true puberty. This will compound the problem from the growth and bone age perspective.

The initial problem was tall stature with advanced bone maturation as well as pubic and axillary hair changes. If we now superimpose true puberty on top of this, we will get further growth acceleration, but at the expense of a marked acceleration in bone age leading to very short stature in the long term.

Furthermore, there will be progression in the secondary sexual changes with breast development in girls and enlargement of the testes and penis in boys. In girls, menarche (periods) will commence approximately 2 years after the first signs of puberty, namely breast bud development.

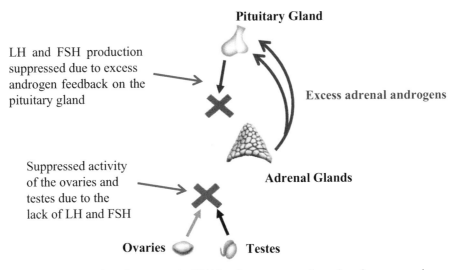

Figure 11.1 *Poor cortisol replacement in CAH leads to excess adrenal androgens and suppression of LH and FSH production by the pituitary but stimulation of the puberty clock in the hypothalamus.*

Fig. 11.1 illustrates that in CAH if cortisol is poorly replaced with too little glucocorticoid, ACTH levels rise which cause the adrenal glands to increase in size in an effort to make more cortisol. The enlarged adrenal glands will then produce excess adrenal androgens such as androstenedione and testosterone. These androgens then feedback on the pituitary gland suppressing the production of LH and FSH and switch off, or suppress gonad activity.

They will also stimulate (prime) the area of the hypothalamus containing the puberty system. This area will still not switch on completely until adrenal androgen production is normalised with optimal cortisol replacement. Once the adrenal androgens are normalised, the system is "ready" to go.

What to do?

1. We need to consider delaying the whole of the puberty process. This can be done by using gonadotropin releasing hormone analogue therapy.

   Gonadotropin releasing hormone analogue is a protein which is very similar in structure to the gonadotropin releasing hormone produced by the hypothalamus. Gonadotropin releasing hormone is a protein and proteins are made up of small building blocks called amino acids. Gonadotropin releasing hormone is made up of 10 amino acids and by altering one of these amino acids, the duration of action is prolonged.

   This means it sits on the gonadotropin releasing hormone receptor in the pituitary longer than the natural hormone. This stops the receptor from working properly as it only works well when it detects gonadotropin releasing hormone in discrete bursts. This constant occupation switches off the production of the two pituitary hormones LH and FSH.

   Switching these off, reduces the drive to the testes or ovaries and reduces the amount of sex steroid, either testosterone or estradiol, which is produced as can be seen in Figs 11.2 and 11.3. The effect of this is to slow down or stop any pubertal progress and overall reduce the rate of maturation of the skeleton.

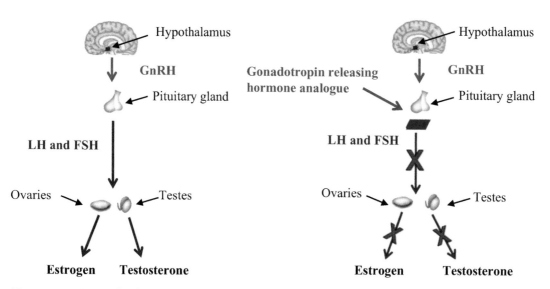

Figure 11.2 *Normal puberty production.*   Figure 11.3 *Puberty switched off.*

This therapy is extremely effective in holding up puberty and when the time comes for the normal onset of puberty, the therapy can be stopped, puberty will recommence and normal progression through puberty will ensue.

2. *Aromatase inhibitors* can be used to block estrogen thus making sure there is no estrogen formation (Fig. 11.4).

HOW AROMATASE INHIBITORS WORK

We have mentioned these aromatase inhibitors before so it is worth going over them again in a bit more detail. There are three estrogens which can be made and these are Estrone (E1), Estradiol (E2) and Estriol (E3).

- Estrone (E1) is formed from androstenedione by the action of the enzyme aromatase or CYP19.

- Estradiol (E2) is the most abundant estrogen and is formed from testosterone by the action of aromatase. You can see this step in Fig. 11.4.

- Estriol (E3) is only made in pregnancy from the special adrenal androgens the fetal adrenal glands make.

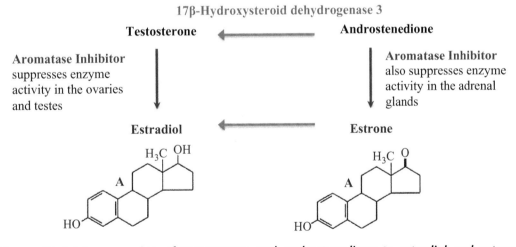

Figure 11.4 *Interconversion of testosterone and androstenedione to estradiol and estrone. Androstenedione is converted to testosterone and estrone to estradiol by the same enzyme 17β-hydroxysteroid dehydrogenase. Androstenedione and testosterone are converted to estrone and estradiol respectively by the addition of H_3C at point A by the aromatase enzyme.*

Estradiol has the highest levels in the blood and the amount of estrone produced is quite small. The aromatase inhibitors block the formation of all the estrogens and they are very specific drugs, which do not affect any other part of the body. So when you take them, the production or conversion of either testosterone to estradiol or androstenedione to estrone, is blocked. This is good because we know that estrogens are important to mature the skeleton. If we block estrogen formation, bone age will stop advancing rapidly, giving us a chance to try and improve the height of the child. So they are really helpful, in situations where bone age has advanced.

In males, we can use these medicines at any age as long as we carefully monitor the other effect estrogens have namely, making the bones denser and stronger. This means if we use these drugs, we need to carefully monitor bone mineral density with regular DEXA scans, which we discuss in Chapter 13. In females, we cannot use these drugs during the normal puberty years as they will block estradiol formation, which is essential for normal female development.

Aromatase inhibitors have very few side effects. Some people get stiff joints. The most important effect to monitor is bone mineral density because they might cause osteoporosis if used over very long periods of time, such as 10–15 years and only if they switch off estradiol production completely.

> *Please Note: If your child with CAH develops pubic or axillary hair or any of the other signs of puberty, such as the development of breast buds, body odour or acne before the normal onset age of puberty, which we go into detail in Chapter 7, then it is important to see your child's endocrinologist as soon as possible.*

DELAYED PUBERTY

Delayed puberty happens quite commonly in the general population, particularly in boys. The reason for this is unclear but it is something to do with how the body clock, which is involved in setting the timing of puberty, works. We know that this clock is very susceptible to changes, particularly if the child has a long standing illness because the clock gets reset to start late. This can happen in CAH although it is not very common nowadays.

The reason it was common in the past was because quite high doses of steroids were used which completely suppressed the system. When the system is suppressed we know that puberty can be delayed. As said, we don't really know why this happens in the general population and have perhaps even less of an idea why it happens in CAH, apart from the fact that it is often a reflection of over treatment at some stage.

Puberty that is only delayed by about 12–18 months doesn't usually need intervention to alter the timing. In some instances, particularly in boys, timing of puberty can be quite late by 2–3 years and because the puberty growth spurt is later in boys than girls, they can lag a long way behind their peers in terms of height. In these situations and it can be the case in girls as well, it is often helpful to speed up the start of the puberty process by giving very small doses of either female sex hormones in girls, or testosterone in boys.

Considerable care needs to be taken in this approach because if the dose of sex steroids used is too high, then rapid acceleration in the bone age might take place which would lead the individual to be shorter than they might otherwise have been, had no intervention taken place.

As such, this is a very specialised area in which very careful use of these drugs is required and if your child does have a delayed start to puberty, then a discussion with your endocrinologist is essential and careful regular follow up is needed in order to ensure that if any intervention is undertaken, there is no adverse effect on the maturation of the bones.

GYNAECOMASTIA

Gynaecomastia (breast development in males) is a common condition which causes boys' and mens' breasts to swell and become larger than normal. It is most common in teenage boys and older men. It is quite common during adolescence with up to 70% of males estimated to exhibit signs of gynaecomastia during their adolescence. Gynaecomastia also occurs in 25–60% of males over 50 years of age. The amount of breast tissue that can form ranges from a small amount around the nipples to more prominent breasts. One or both sides can be affected.

WHAT CAUSES GYNAECOMASTIA?

Gynaecomastia can have several causes.

Hormone imbalance

Gynaecomastia is caused by an imbalance between the sex hormones testosterone and estradiol. We mentioned before that males can make small amounts of the female hormones either from testosterone which forms estradiol or androstenedione which forms estrone. Estradiol is the more powerful form. It may seem odd that males make some female hormones but it is vitally important they do. People who cannot convert testosterone to estradiol develop severe osteoporosis.

The important thing which determines whether males develop breasts or not, is the ratio of testosterone to estradiol. Testosterone is converted to estradiol by the enzyme aromatase (Fig. 11.4). This is a relatively inefficient process with only about 10% conversion and as testosterone is normally high in males, testosterone levels will always exceed estradiol and it is this balance in favour of testosterone which stops the estradiol from causing breast tissue to grow.

During puberty boys' hormone levels vary. If the level of testosterone drops, then the balance shifts in the testosterone/estradiol ratio towards estradiol which causes the breast tissue to grow. Gynaecomastia at puberty usually clears up as boys get older and they get more and more testosterone production.

It is very important to realise that the growth in breast tissue is not due to extra body fat from being overweight, so losing weight or doing more exercise will not improve the condition. As men get older, they produce less testosterone, so this natural change can lead to excess breast tissue growth.

Other causes

Gynaecomastia can also be caused by the side effects of medication, such as anti–ulcer drugs like omeprazole, drinking too much alcohol or products, such as tea tree oil. The omeprazole effect is very rare. Alcohol seems to inhibit testosterone formation in the testes and tea tree oil has an estrogen like effect and appears to be an anti–androgen as well.

HOW DOES THIS RELATE TO CONGENITAL ADRENAL HYPERPLASIA?

As we know in CAH when receiving treatment the levels of adrenal androgens will be low. However, if cortisol replacement is poor and adrenal androgens rise, then problems with breast development in males can occur. This is because the adrenal glands will make a lot of androstenedione and a small amount of testosterone. Although androstenedione is a male like hormone it lacks the potency of testosterone. This means the male/female hormone balance will again tip in favour of estrogen.

Both of these androgens can be converted to estrone and estradiol, respectively. Estrone is a weak estrogen but the amounts can be high when androstenedione is high. Androstenedione is much weaker than testosterone so when we then think about the androgen to estrogen ratio, it will be tipped in favour of estrogen so breast development can take place (Fig. 11.5). Getting the androgen levels within normal range and the cortisol replacement optimal should tip the balance back but this is not always the case.

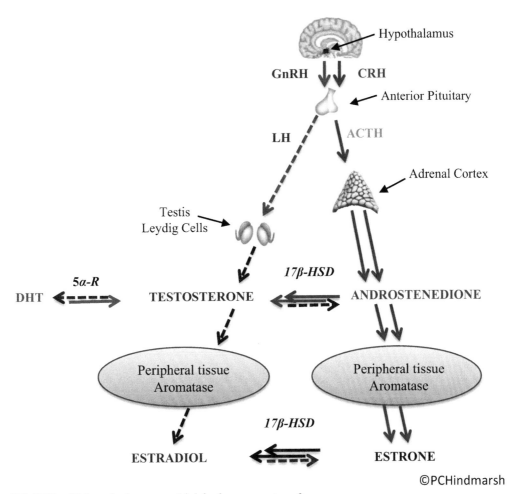

Figure 11.5 *The change in balance of androgen production in congenital adrenal hyperplasia if androstenedione is high leading to high estrone and a swing to higher amounts of estrogen than androgen.* Solid, double arrows in the adrenal pathway indicate over production and dashed arrows in the testes pathway indicate reduced production due to suppression of LH and FSH by the high adrenal androgens.

The reason for being cautious is that a large number of adult men with CAH do not have as good testosterone production from the testes, as might be expected. When cortisol replacement is poor, testosterone and androstenedione are often high as they are derived from the adrenal glands. When cortisol replacement is optimised, low testosterone values can be detected in the face of normal androstenedione values, implying that the testicular production of testosterone is not as good as it could be. Whilst it is true, technically the testosterone is within the lower half of the normal range and is often based on a single blood test which can be misleading. It is unclear why this happens because if the system is tested, there is usually good production of the pituitary testes regulating hormones, LH and FSH. However, if these hormones are measured over 24 hours, they are often less pulsatile than would be expected and often lower than a one-off measurement. Single blood testosterone measures may be misleading when not placed in this context.

One explanation could be that exposure of the pituitary to high levels of adrenal androgens in the womb and early in life, alters the functioning of the pituitary, setting it to produce fewer hormones later in life. There is very little research in this area, although it does seem to be a bigger problem judging by patient comments, than otherwise appears from medical literature.

TREATMENT FOR GYNAECOMASTIA

There are two approaches to treating gynaecomastia. Firstly, we can use medication that either blocks the formation of estradiol from testosterone, or those that block the action of estradiol. Arimidex, an aromatase inhibitor, is a blocker of testosterone to estradiol and is very effective at restoring the balance between testosterone and estradiol in favour of testosterone. Estradiol can also be blocked by using the estrogen receptor blocker, Tamoxifen, but overall the Arimidex approach is more specific and has the added advantage of raising testosterone levels as well.

Secondly, if these medical approaches do not work, then it is possible to reduce the breast tissue by surgery. The operation is straightforward in that breast tissue is sucked out using liposuction and there is almost no scar.

FURTHER READING

Dattani, M.T., Hindmarsh, P.C., 2009. Normal and abnormal puberty. In: Brook, C.G.D., Clayton, P., Brown, R. (Eds.), Brook's Clinical Paediatric Endocrinology. fifth ed. Blackwell Publishing, Oxford.

CHAPTER 12

When Things Go Wrong—Weight, Diabetes and Hypertension

GLOSSARY

Electrolytes A general term used to indicate the blood measurement of sodium, potassium, chloride and bicarbonate.

Fludrocortisone Cortisol modified with fluorine atom, which prolongs action on the mineralocorticoid receptor which retains salt and water.

High blood lipids Also known as hyperlipidaemia where cholesterol and triglycerides in the blood are raised. These lipids are known to lead to heart disease if raised for long periods of time.

High blood pressure A blood pressure reading greater than the 90th centile for age. Hypertension is defined as blood pressure reading greater than 95th centile for age.

Hydrocortisone Synthetic form of cortisol.

Metabolic Syndrome The collection of obesity, hyperlipidaemia, hypertension, raised insulin, type 2 diabetes, which is associated with increased risk of heart disease and stroke.

Plasma renin activity Measure of how renin from the kidney is converted to angiotensin. It is a measure of the blood volume and salt and water balance.

Type 2 diabetes mellitus Form of diabetes where insulin does not work as well as it should and is associated with high risk of diabetes complications, such as kidney failure, blindness and heart disease.

GENERAL

When glucocorticoids were first used in high doses for conditions other than CAH, it was quite clear they had the ability to increase body fat, blood pressure and blood glucose. In fact, the change in the latter was so great that often diabetes was associated with high dose glucocorticoid use. The combination of diabetes, weight gain and high blood pressure along with changes in blood cholesterol, are known in diabetes circles as the Metabolic Syndrome. This particular problem arises because insulin does not act so well and is exactly the same set of problems which arise with glucocorticoid use.

Congenital Adrenal Hyperplasia. http://dx.doi.org/10.1016/B978-0-12-811483-4.00012-X

Some people have referred to this as the CAH Metabolic Syndrome but the cluster of features is not due to CAH itself, but rather the treatment of the condition with glucocorticoids and fludrocortisone. One important point to note is the more potent the glucocorticoid is, the more likely there are to be problems with this constellation of features.

These observations reinforce the need to follow our annual review approach using the listings in Fig. 9.1. Each year we check a blood sample for fasting glucose, insulin and cholesterol to detect at an earlier stage, problems occurring in these three areas. In addition, we measure blood pressure on a four hourly basis so that we get an overall pattern, day and night, as to what is happening in this area. The reason we do this is that blood pressure, like cortisol, has a circadian rhythm. Blood pressure is lower overnight by about 10% and the loss of this drop in blood pressure, is the first sign of developing high blood pressure. Weight gain, or rather weight itself along with the calculation of body mass index, is undertaken at each clinic visit.

Using this approach and using lower doses with better distribution during the 24 hour period of glucocorticoid and mineralocorticoids, there is much less of a problem with weight gain, insulin and cholesterol in the United Kingdom. In fact, at our clinic we have not had any problems in these areas, largely because the doses we have used with glucocorticoids have decreased over time from the original schedule of 25 mg/m^2 body surface area/day down to the current value of about 10–12 mg/m^2 body surface area/day. This is important, as it means we have moved away from the two critical doses; 30 mg/m^2 body surface area/day, which was associated with poor height gain and 18–20 mg/m^2 body surface area/day, which was associated with marked weight gain. That is not to say that weight gain cannot take place on current dosing schedules because it can, particularly if the distribution of cortisol through the 24 hour period is not correct.

This is another reason for using 24 hour profiles as they allow us to get the dose and distribution of cortisol correct.

The effect on blood pressure has also been quite dramatic because about 10 years ago, high blood pressure and hypertension was noted in about 30% of the clinic population. With careful readjustment (using 24 hour profiles) and limiting the dose of mineralocorticoids based on plasma renin activity and blood pressure measurements, we have now reduced the number of people with hypertension to about 12%.

The messages from this section are clear:

1. Glucocorticoid and mineralocorticoid doses need to be carefully titrated against their biochemical markers. For glucocorticoids, this means determining overall exposure and the best way to do that is through 24 hour profiles. For mineralocorticoids, careful attention to plasma renin activity and blood pressure is required to keep the overall exposure to fludrocortisone to a minimum.
2. By using careful dose adjustment the issue of excessive weight can be avoided. This also requires clinicians not to use the more potent agents, such as prednisolone and dexamethasone, where possible.

WHAT TO DO IF PROBLEMS ARISE

Weight gain

Early weight gain is a sign of over treatment and we can resolve the issue by readdressing the amount of glucocorticoid given and the distribution of the glucocorticoid, using carefully constructed 24 hour profiles. Unless the dose of glucocorticoid is changed, trying to reduce weight by diet and exercise will not work.

GLUCOSE AND INSULIN METABOLISM

High blood glucose

Glucocorticoids affect the way the body handles glucose. This is how they got their name in that they are hormones from the adrenal cortex which affect glucose. The way in which they do this is to reduce the effect that insulin has on the cells in the liver, muscle and fat. Glucocorticoids make these cells less responsive to insulin. The body overcomes this to keep the blood glucose levels steady and normal, by increasing the amount of insulin produced by the pancreas. The pancreas has an enormous capacity to increase insulin, but if it is asked to do it over an extremely long period of time, such as 20–30 years, then the cells which make insulin in the pancreas, can fail and this can lead to diabetes. Fig. 12.1 shows the relationship between glucose and insulin in the fasting situation. The body likes to keep glucose within a very tight range between 3.5 and 5.6 mmol/l. To do this however, even in the fasting state, the pancreas makes variable amounts of insulin. The pancreas reads the blood glucose level every 13 minutes and then readjusts the amount of insulin produced to meet the needs of the body with respect to the amount of glucose available for energy.

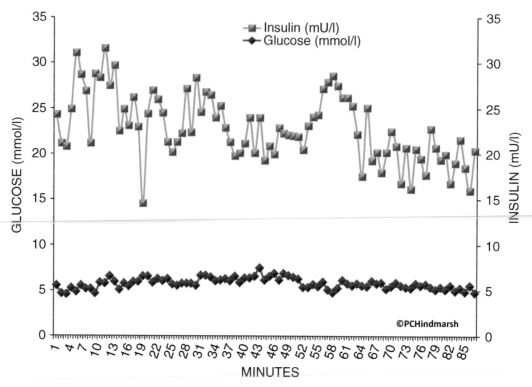

Figure 12.1 *The relationship between blood glucose in red and insulin in green over a 90 minute fasting period. Glucose is kept within a very tight range by insulin levels that pulse up and down.*

Insulin is very good at getting and keeping blood glucose levels in the normal range. When insulin levels are high and working less effectively then problems start to occur.

- Firstly, glucose cannot move into the cells as efficiently. There is a hierarchy for this. The liver becomes less responsive to high levels of insulin but the fat tissue does not, so the glucose is diverted into fat cells where it is converted and stored as fat.
- Secondly, the pancreas can produce more insulin for quite some time. However, the higher glucose values in the blood do damage the insulin-producing cells in the longer term and these cells also wear out so that less insulin is produced and the person develops diabetes.
- Thirdly, having persistently high insulin levels in the blood when the insulin cannot act properly, also leads to problems within the heart and circulation. Within the heart, it can lead to problems with circulation of blood through the small blood vessels, which may lead to heart attacks in the long term. In the circulation it can lead to high blood pressure or hypertension.

It is for these longer term reasons we really try to keep the fasting blood glucose levels normal (3.5–5.6 mmol/l) and also ensure the fasting insulin levels do not go higher than 25 mU/l.

We do this in our annual review where we check fasting blood glucose and insulin. We measure the levels of both glucose and its controlling hormone insulin and relate the two results. There are strict guidelines for diagnosing problems with glucose and they are shown in Fig. 12.2. We usually measure fasting glucose, but you can also see how people react to a glucose drink.

This is known as an oral glucose tolerance test and in this test we look at the glucose level, 2 hours after the drink. We use the glucose values to define whether the person has diabetes or not. There is also an intermediate category of impaired function, which leads onto diabetes unless treated. Generally, we find a fasting measure is sufficient.

	FASTING GLUCOSE (mmol/l)	2 HOURS AFTER GLUCOSE DRINK (mmol/l)
NORMAL	<5.6	<7.8
IMPAIRED	5.6–6.9	7.8–11.0
DIABETES	>7.0	>11.1

Figure 12.2 *American Diabetes Association Classification Scheme for glucose measurements.*

Once we have assessed the glucose level the next thing we look at is insulin. As glucocorticoids alter the way insulin acts you can have a normal blood glucose level, but high insulin value. As we said, too much insulin is not good and if the system is stressed for long enough to produce high levels of insulin, then the cells in the pancreas which produce insulin, will wear out, stop producing insulin and diabetes will develop.

What to do about high glucose

The first thing to do is to look at the amount of glucocorticoid which is being given. Again, we rely on our profile data to see if the amounts given are leading to too high cortisol peaks over the 24 hour period. If they are too high, then we need to take the following steps:

1. The first step is to try and normalise the cortisol levels by adjusting the hydrocortisone dose.

2. It might be necessary to think about changes to diet and this is particularly important if we find glucose levels indicate impairment of the way the body handles glucose, or diabetes itself. Often, with a strict diet and exercise approach, normalisation of glucose can be achieved and avoidance of progression to diabetes is possible.

3. The step after this is to use agents which are used classically in the management of type 2 diabetes. The mainstay of treatment is metformin. Metformin is a drug which makes the body more sensitive to the effects of insulin. Its main effect is on the liver and gut, but it also works on muscle and fat to a certain extent. Metformin action tends to oppose the effects of glucocorticoids, so it is a really good medication to use in situations where insulin has gone too high as a result of too much exposure to glucocorticoids. The medicine is taken once or twice a day and the effects on blood glucose and body weight which it also reduces, can be seen over a 6–12 month period.

Low blood glucose

Low blood glucose is also a problem in people receiving glucocorticoid treatment. The reason for this is glucocorticoids raise blood glucose, but if the glucocorticoid levels in the blood are low, e.g. during illness when the tablets might be vomited up, or if the distribution of glucocorticoid during the 24 hour period is incorrect so that there are periods when there is no glucocorticoid detectable in the blood, then blood glucose levels can fall.

The symptoms you get when blood glucose levels fall depend on how low the value is. We cover this in more detail in Chapter 19. Essentially, as blood glucose levels fall below 3.5 mmol/l the person feels shaky, dizzy, sweaty and unable to concentrate. If values fall below 2.6 mmol/l then loss of consciousness can occur.

What to do about low blood glucose

The most important thing in CAH is to try and prevent the occurrence of low blood glucose. This is why it is extremely important to ensure there is a good delivery of cortisol, not only by doubling the dose given, but by also giving an extra double dose at 4 a.m. (04:00) when we know that cortisol levels from the previous night's hydrocortisone dose are likely to be quite low, see Chapter 19. More at 4 a.m. and double dose during illness or trauma are two ways in which we can prevent hypoglycaemia.

If the child becomes hypoglycaemic which means they have a blood glucose test result reading of less than 4 mmol/l, then it is advisable to give 15 g of glucose. This glucose has to be what is called readily available, in other words neat glucose. You can find this in orange drinks and fizzy drinks, such as Coca-Cola (not diet or sugar free). For example, 100 ml of Coca-Cola contains exactly 15 g of glucose. Fig. 12.3 shows other things available which contain 15 g of glucose.

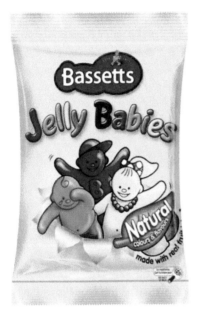

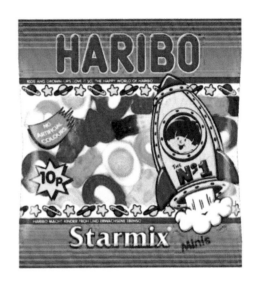

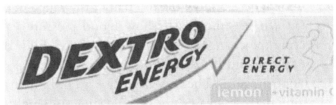

Figure 12.3 *Other items that contain 15 g of carbohydrate for use when blood glucose is low.*

We recommend they have this and then follow on regularly with sugary drinks throughout the period of illness. Giving 15 g of glucose will bring the glucose up very quickly and you should retest to make sure this has happened 15 minutes after giving the 15 g of glucose. If this has not raised the blood glucose, then repeat with a further 15 g of glucose and retest 15 minutes later.

If the child cannot tolerate any oral glucose you can always use the 'Glucogel' in the emergency pack, which you just squirt around the gums or into the cheek.

Glucose is absorbed very quickly this way and will rectify low blood glucose very quickly.

An emergency injection of hydrocortisone will also increase the blood glucose, but this is a slower process and the best thing is to get on top of the blood glucose problem quickly by giving some easily available glucose. If this is not tolerated or cannot be given, then give extra hydrocortisone either by doubling the tablets or by emergency injection. You should then give the Glucogel as this order of events ensures normalisation of the blood glucose will take place quickly and be sustained.

So if the child is having an adrenal crisis:

1. Give intramuscular hydrocortisone.
2. Then apply Glucogel to the gums and cheek.

BLOOD PRESSURE

The main problem we encounter is either high or low blood pressure. Before looking at this it might be worth seeing how blood pressure changes with age.

Figs 12.4 and 12.5 show the top half of the range of blood pressure for boys and girls. As you can see, the charts show blood pressure values increase steadily with age, reflecting the change in the body size of the child. Blood pressure is strongly related to body size and in particular body mass index. So the heavier you are the higher the blood pressure. The reason for this is not known. Certainly, the changes in blood pressure as age increases, relates to change in height. The rest we are really not sure about.

Nonetheless, these centile charts are extremely helpful because we consider anything over the 95th percentile as hypertension and this has important health consequences if not picked up and treated. This is why at our annual review, we always measure blood pressure four hourly to determine whether it is too high or too low. Measuring overnight also allows us to pick up blood pressure problems sooner, as the first sign of problems emerging is the loss of the normal 10% drop in blood pressure which takes place overnight.

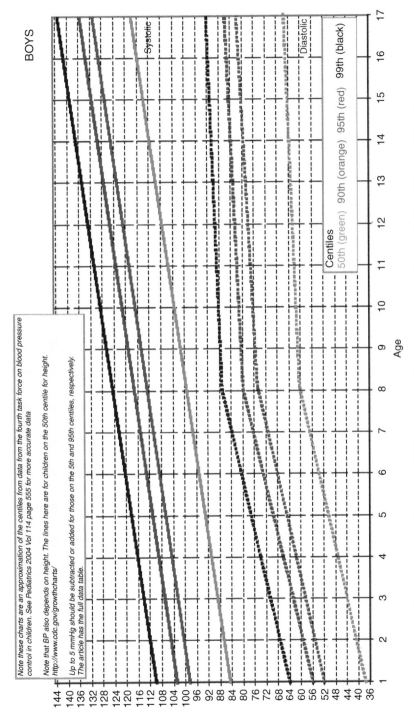

BOYS

Note these charts are an approximation of the centiles from data from the fourth task force on blood pressure control in children. See Pediatrics 2004 Vol 114 page 555 for more accurate data

Note that BP also depends on height. The lines here are for children on the 50th centile for height. http://www.cdc.gov/growthcharts/

Up to 5 mmHg should be subtracted or added for those on the 5th and 95th centiles, respectively. The article has the full data table.

Systolic

Diastolic

Centiles
50th (green)   90th (orange)   95th (red)   99th (black)

Age

Figure 12.4 Blood pressure chart for boys. (With permission from International Paediatric Blood Pressure Task Force).

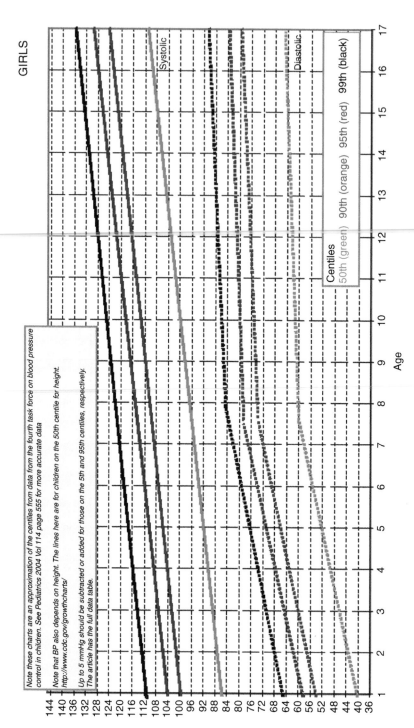

Figure 12.5   Blood pressure centile chart for girls. *(With permission from International Paediatric Blood Pressure Task Force).*

High blood pressure

High blood pressure is defined as blood pressure values between 90 and 95 centile. Hypertension is defined as the blood pressure values over the 95th centile. You will see that when blood pressure is recorded, there are two values, a value which is high followed by a value which is lower. These are known as systolic and diastolic blood pressures.

They are important because they tell us a lot about how the heart and circulation are responding. You can have high or low blood pressure in either the systolic or diastolic components, but the one that is really important is high systolic blood pressure.

What to do about high blood pressure

High blood pressure nearly always responds to reconsideration of the dose of glucocorticoid and in particular the dose of mineralocorticoid. Simply reducing these doses based on careful biochemical work is often all that is needed. Where high blood pressure or hypertension persists, it may be necessary to use the various drugs which block angiotensin formation or action.

Low blood pressure

Low blood pressure in the general population is actually quite common. In people with CAH however, we are always concerned that low blood pressure might indicate either under replacement with glucocorticoid or mineralocorticoid. Glucocorticoids and mineralocorticoids interact in the generation of blood pressure.

What to do about low blood pressure

We have already talked about the effect of mineralocorticoids, which help retain salt and water in the body and is one way blood pressure increases. If the dose of fludrocortisone is too low then the person will have low blood pressure and the symptoms of this are dizziness on standing from the sitting position. People often crave salt and will switch to salty foods. If this happens, then the first step is to check the plasma renin and sodium levels in the blood.

Oddly, glucocorticoids are also important in maintaining blood pressure as well. Glucocorticoids act directly on blood vessels and are also important for the effects of adrenalin on the blood vessels. Adrenalin acts generally to increase blood pressure. So if you are under dosed with glucocorticoids, you might also end up in a very similar situation as with low blood pressure. Incidentally, this is also why people with low cortisol often have a low heart rate as adrenalin is less effective. Glucocorticoids, particularly hydrocortisone, also have some mineralocorticoid action which affects water retention and this increases blood volume and pressure. Fig. 12.6 shows the interaction of changes in blood pressure on the renin–angiotensin system. In high blood pressure situations, we block the angiotensin converting enzyme so the body stops making angiotensin II which stops the kidney from absorbing water and salt, which brings down blood pressure.

High blood pressure from exposure to excess glucocorticoid or mineralocorticoid is a sign that the heart and blood vessels are being worked too hard and if untreated this can lead to atherosclerosis and congestive heart failure

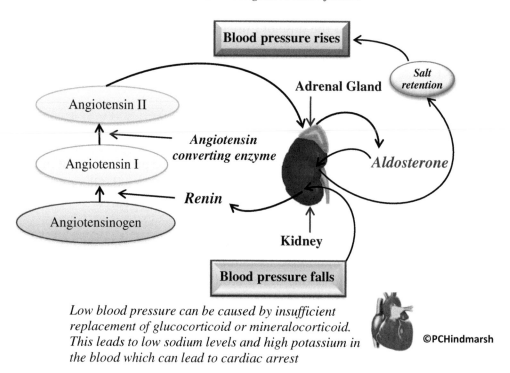

Low blood pressure can be caused by insufficient replacement of glucocorticoid or mineralocorticoid. This leads to low sodium levels and high potassium in the blood which can lead to cardiac arrest

©PCHindmarsh

Figure 12.6 *The renin-angiotensin system and how it reacts to high and low blood pressure.*

The situation is easily remedied because it simply requires careful attention to the biochemistry and readjusting the mineralocorticoid and glucocorticoid doses. Salt supplements are required in newborn babies to replace the salt which has been lost up to the point that they present. This is because in the newborn, the kidneys are normally less responsive to aldosterone than later in life. Normally the newborn needs 2 mmol sodium/kg body weight/day and breast milk or infant milk formulas only just deliver this amount. So if salt has been lost from the body, then extra supplements are required to normalise the sodium in the blood and to keep blood pressure normal. Sometimes, extra salt is needed to stabilise blood pressure in older children, particularly if they travel to hot climates with temperatures over 30°C. We discuss this further in our chapter on fludrocortisone (Chapter 32).

FURTHER READING

Charmandari, E., Weise, M., Bornstein, S.R., Eisenhofer, G., Keil, M.F., Chrousos, G.P., Merke, D.P., 2002. Children with classic congenital adrenal hyperplasia have elevated serum leptin concentrations and insulin resistance: potential clinical implications. J. Clin. Endocrinol. Metab. 87, 2114–2120.

Hindmarsh, P.C., 2014. The child with difficult to control congenital adrenal hyperplasia: is there a place for continuous subcutaneous hydrocortisone therapy. Clin. Endocrinol. (Oxf.) 81, 15–18.

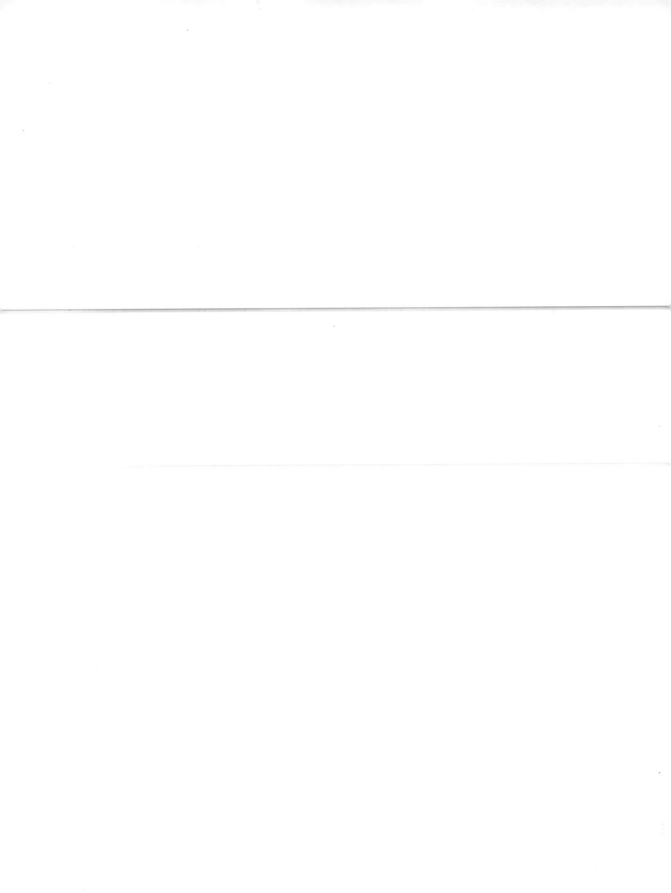

CHAPTER 13

When Things Go Wrong—Bone Density and Osteoporosis

GLOSSARY

Bone mineral density A measure of how much mineral is present in the bone.
DEXA A scan that measures the bone mineral density.
Fludrocortisone Cortisol modified with fluorine atom which prolongs action on the mineralocorticoid receptor which retains salt and water.
Glucocorticoids Group of steroid hormones (glucose + cortex + steroid) which regulate glucose metabolism and suppress inflammation.
Osteopenia This is milder form of reduction in bone mineral density compared to osteoporosis, which is defined on DEXA.
Osteoporosis A marked reduction of mineral in bone which weakens the bone structure thereby increasing the risk of fracture.

GENERAL

Osteoporosis is a term which is used to describe a reduction in the amount of mineral present in bone. The main mineral is calcium and in osteoporosis there is a loss of calcium deposited in the fine structure of bone. The reason osteoporosis is of concern, is that it is associated with weak bones and increased risk of fracture. One of the factors known to be associated with an increased risk of osteoporosis, is the use of glucocorticoids. It has to be said at the outset, the association of osteoporosis with glucocorticoid use, is with the high doses used in other illnesses, particularly for their anti-inflammatory action. These are doses which are much higher than those used in CAH. This makes it very difficult to be absolutely sure whether there is any effect on bone density, with glucocorticoid replacement therapy, in CAH. Certainly, in children the data is very hard to interpret whereas in adults, there is certainly some evidence to suggest that lower bone mineral density is a problem. Bone density refers to a measure of how much mineral is in bone. It can be assessed by X-ray technology on how much of an X-ray can pass through the bone.

Congenital Adrenal Hyperplasia. http://dx.doi.org/10.1016/B978-0-12-811483-4.00013-1

WHAT HAPPENS?

Glucocorticoids alter the number of cells within bone. The special bone cells that help form bone, are reduced in number during glucocorticoid treatment and although glucocorticoids also reduce the number of cells that resorb bone, these are less affected than the number of cells that promote bone formation. Overall, the net effect is to reduce bone buildup. Glucocorticoid induced osteoporosis predominately affects regions of the skeleton which have a certain type of bone named cancellous bone. The areas most abundant in cancellous bone are the spine and neck of the hip bone. Loss of bone mineral density with very high doses of glucocorticoids occurs in two phases. There is approximately a 10% loss within the first year and then a slower 3% loss thereafter. That said, most fractures occur within the first 3 months of starting treatment. If you do not incur a fracture during this first period, then you are likely to have little in the way of recurrent fractures.

However, it is important to realise that all this information comes from adult patients who have used very high doses of glucocorticoids and we simply do not know what the likely situation is going to be in people with CAH. Long term data in adults with this condition suggest there might be some problems.

CAH is likely to be different because the doses used are only replacement. We do not use very high doses for long periods of time, which is when most problems associated with glucocorticoid induced osteoporosis occur. In fact, there is no information to suggest that fracture risk in people with CAH, is likely to be any different to the general population.

In addition, as puberty is rarely altered in CAH, a good accumulation of bone mineral is likely to take place because of the normal production of the sex steroids from the testes or ovary. There is some suggestion that the slightly higher production of the male like hormones from the adrenal glands might also help strengthen the bones in CAH.

Finally, we must not forget the mineralocorticoid influence. Fludrocortisone has dexamethasone like effects and needs to be considered when looking at total daily glucocorticoid dose. In addition, running a low blood sodium leads to problems. Much of the sodium in the body is bound to bone, cartilage and connective tissue. Long standing low blood sodium levels have been shown to be a more potent cause of osteopenia, than Vitamin D deficiency. The activity of the cells which resorb bone is increased when sodium levels are low for periods of time and this is associated with the development of osteoporosis and fractures.

HOW WE CHECK BONE DENSITY?

We can monitor bone mineral density by using dual photon absorption (DEXA) scanning. The DEXA scan passes a small beam of X-ray through specific areas of the bone. The speed at which the beam goes through the bone is dependent on the density of the bone and this can be detected by a series of cameras that pick up the passage of the beam. A series of complex calculations are then done to work out from this, what the likely density of that part of the skeleton is. Fig. 13.1 gives an idea of the type of picture which can be obtained.

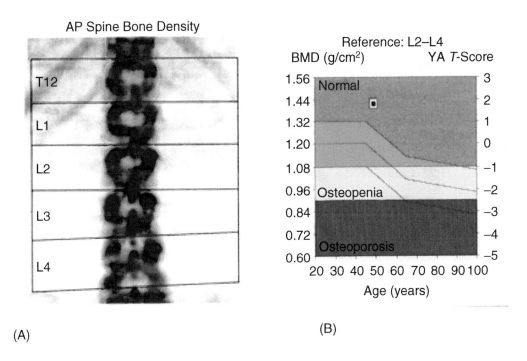

(A)

(B)

Region	Area (cm²)	BMC (g)	BMD (g/cm²)	T-score	Z-score
L1	11.6	14.8	1.278	1.2	1.5
L2	13.5	18.1	1.447	2.1	2.4
L3	13.5	20.9	1.543	2.9	3.2
L4	16.5	21.4	1.292	0.8	1.1
Total	54.1	75.2	1.417	2.1	2.1

(C)

Figure 13.1 *Actual dual photon absorption (DEXA) picture in top left (A) of spine with the actual value plotted on reference chart on right (B). A table (C) of the data for comparison with reference values is shown below the two pictures. BMC, Bone mineral content; BMD, Bone mineral density.*

A variety of ways of recording data are either as *T*-scores which show the individual's DEXA results compared to the ideal peak bone density of a healthy adult, or as a *Z*-score which compares the individual's DEXA results to the average reference range which is based on the same age, weight, height and gender of the general population as the individual. This means we can compare these results with those of the general population, as we do the height and weight results. A positive *Z*-score means good bone density. A value between 0 and −2 is satisfactory but between −1 and −2 is often referred to as osteopenia or low density. It is only when values get below −2, the risks of fracture increase and this area is termed osteoporosis.

Both the hips and the spine can be scanned and Fig. 13.2 shows the hip studies in an individual along with the *T*-scores and matched *Z*-scores.

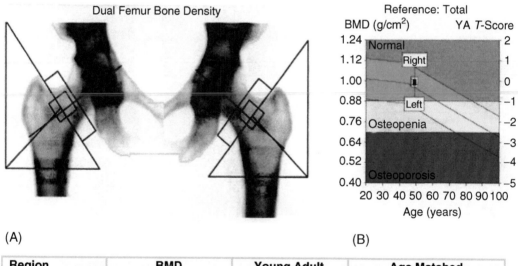

(A)   (B)

Region	BMD (g/cm²)	Young Adult (%)	T-Score	Age Matched (%)	Z-Score
Total Left	0.982	98	−0.2	102	0.2
Total Right	1.001	100	0.0	104	0.3
Total Mean	0.991	99	−0.1	103	0.3
Total Diff.	0.019	2	0.2	2	0.2

(C)

Figure 13.2 *Actual DEXA picture in top left (A) of hip with the actual value is plotted on reference chart on right (B). A table (C) of the data for comparison with reference values is shown below the two pictures.*

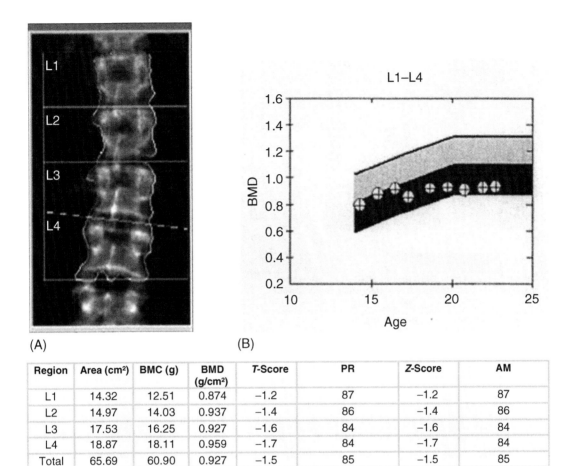

(A)   (B)

Region	Area (cm²)	BMC (g)	BMD (g/cm²)	T-Score	PR	Z-Score	AM
L1	14.32	12.51	0.874	−1.2	87	−1.2	87
L2	14.97	14.03	0.937	−1.4	86	−1.4	86
L3	17.53	16.25	0.927	−1.6	84	−1.6	84
L4	18.87	18.11	0.959	−1.7	84	−1.7	84
Total	65.69	60.90	0.927	−1.5	85	−1.5	85

(C)

Figure 13.3 *Actual DEXA scan of the spine (A) of someone who has congenital adrenal hyperplasia (CAH) and had a considerable amount of steroids. The actual value is plotted on the reference chart on right (B) and a table (C) of the data for comparison with reference values is shown below the two pictures. AM, Age matched; BMC, Bone mineral content; PR, peak reference.*

Figs. 13.3 and 13.4 show the effects on bone mineral density of the hip and spine in someone who has CAH and was prescribed large doses of dexamethasone for a period of time. The patient has had regular annual DEXA scans and the previous results can be seen plotted in the graphs and corresponding tables. Notice how the steroids have caused the scan data to flat line at lower values than was originally expected (Fig. 13.3B and 13.4B).

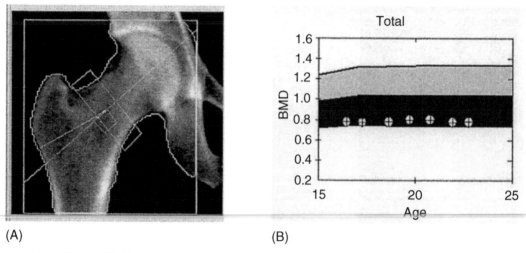

(A)   (B)

Region	Area (cm²)	BMC (g)	BMD (g/cm²)	T-Score	PR	Z-Score	AM
Neck	5.73	4.25	0.742	−1.4	80	−1.4	80
Troch	11.27	6.85	0.608	−1.3	78	−1.3	78
Inter	18.28	16.37	0.896	−1.7	75	−1.7	75
Total	35.27	27.47	0.779	−1.7	75	−1.7	75
Ward's	1.18	0.71	0.604	−1.9	73	−1.8	74

(C)

Figure 13.4 *Actual DEXA scan of the hip (A) of someone who has CAH and had a considerable amount of steroids. The actual value is plotted on the reference chart on right (B) and a table (C) of the data for comparison with reference values is shown below the two pictures. AM, Age matched; BMC, Bone mineral content; PR, peak reference.*

WHAT CAN BE DONE TO PREVENT OSTEOPOROSIS?

Measurements of Vitamin D and calcium can be quite useful and if either value is low, supplements are helpful. Other measures of bone turnover are not very useful.

Preventative treatment

All people should receive adequate calcium supplementation and this amounts to approximately 1200 mg/day in divided doses and adequate Vitamin D supplementation of between 800 and 2000 units/day. These are suggested to simply provide the optimum environment for laying down bone. Other than that, there is no preventative treatment recommended for those with CAH where the bone mineral density is normal. There are insufficient data to suggest any other interventions are necessary, even if bone mineral density is in the lower region (Z-score −1 to −2).

Treatment for established osteoporosis

The only effective treatment which helps with glucocorticoid induced osteoporosis is bisphosphonate therapy. This helps strengthen the bones. There are oral treatments available but often therapy is given as a course of intravenous infusions. Long term studies are needed to work out the best way to manage bone density for young people with CAH, who need long term glucocorticoid treatment.

Monitoring

To try and prevent problems before they occur, we suggest routine DEXA scans are started towards the end of the puberty growth spurt. The reason to wait until this point, is because growth itself upsets the actual density measures obtained, so adjustments have to be made for this. To avoid this additional problem, end of growth is a good time to start.

DEXA scans should then be carried out at 2 year intervals if the results are normal and there is good density, but a yearly scan may be needed to establish trends if density is found to be lower than it should be. There are other ways being developed to monitor bone density such as ultrasound and magnetic resonance imaging scanning. These may be useful in the future but at present we recommend DEXA. The radiation dose is very low and the important information gained about bone health far outweighs this minor exposure.

FURTHER READING

Hoorn, E.J., Liamis, G., Zietse, R., Zillikens, M.C., 2011. Hyponatremia and bone: an emerging relationship. Nat. Rev. Endocrinol. 8, 33–39.

Weinstein, R.S., 2011. Clinical practice. Glucocorticoid induced bone disease. N. Engl. J. Med. 365, 62–70.

CHAPTER 14

Fertility

GLOSSARY

Adrenal rests The presence of adrenal tissue in the testes. This tissue responds to ACTH stimulation leading to an increase in size. The rests are hard and irregular in shape and can be mistaken for testicular cancers. These can occur wherever there are adrenal cells but mainly in testes and rarely ovaries. These are often referred to as Testicular Adrenal Rest Tissue or TART.

Anovulatory A menstrual cycle in which an egg is not generated.

Follicle stimulating hormone (FSH) Hormone produced by the pituitary gland which is involved in sperm formation from the testes in males. In females, along with luteinising hormone, it is involved in egg selection and production of estradiol.

Luteinising hormone (LH) Hormone produced by the pituitary gland which generates testosterone from the testes in males. In females, along with follicle-stimulating hormone, it is involved in egg selection and production of estradiol.

Polycystic ovaries This is a particular appearance where the ovaries are enlarged and filled with dense stroma in the middle, with lots of small cysts around the periphery of the ovary.

Polycystic ovary syndrome Ovarian appearances on ultrasound in association with increased androgen production, irregular or absent menstrual cycles and often obesity.

GENERAL

As we discussed in Chapter 4 on how people with CAH present, we noted that females have normal ovaries and womb and males form normal testes.

Fertility therefore, should not be a problem in people with CAH because the structures necessary are present in both sexes. Indeed, females with CAH, if cortisol replacement is optimal and all other levels are within normal range, have their first period about 13 years of age which is only slightly later than the average of 12.4 years. The problems which arise relate to the degree of androgen production from the adrenal glands. The way in which high androgen levels resulting from suboptimal cortisol replacement upsets the hypothalamo-pituitary-gonadal axis which controls reproductive function, is complex and differs between males and females.

Congenital Adrenal Hyperplasia. http://dx.doi.org/10.1016/B978-0-12-811483-4.00014-3

FERTILITY IN FEMALES

In females, suboptimal cortisol replacement leads to an increase in adrenal androgen production. This increase in androgen, if there is a considerable amount, will suppress the hypothalamic-pituitary-gonadal axis. You might want to have another look at the chapter on puberty (Chapter 7) to think about how this system works.

Excess androgen from the adrenal glands suppress the pulsation of gonadotropin releasing hormone in the hypothalamus leading to reduced production of the two hormones, LH and FSH, from the pituitary gland. If adrenal androgen production is very high the axis will suppress completely, leading to a lack of ability to generate a surge of LH during the menstrual cycle and a failure to ovulate.

Fig. 14.1 shows the two systems: the hypothalamo-pituitary-ovary system and the adrenal glands. When cortisol replacement is optimal in CAH, adrenal androgen production, particularly androstenedione, is low. No feedback takes place to the hypothalamus and the hypothalamo-pituitary-ovary system works to generate estradiol. When adrenal androgens rise (Fig. 14.2) they feedback on the hypothalamus. This causes the hypothalamo-pituitary-ovary system to switch off leading to no estradiol production.

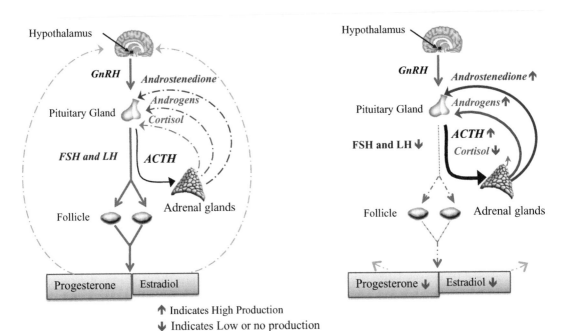

↑ Indicates High Production
↓ Indicates Low or no production

Figure 14.1 *The hypothalamo-pituitary-ovary system and the adrenal glands working when adrenal androgen is low.*

Figure 14.2 *When the androgen production is high the hypothalamo-pituitary-ovary system is switched off.*

In this situation, the way to rectify the problem would be to optimise cortisol replacement so adrenal androgen production is reduced to normal values. The cortisol replacement would need to be carefully adjusted by using a 24 hour profile to assess not only the cortisol, but also 17OHP and androstenedione levels.

Unfortunately, manoeuvres such as this do not often lead to full restoration of fertility. The reason for this is not clear, but what seems to happen is the way the ovary functions after exposure to adrenal androgens, changes.

POLYCYSTIC OVARY

When we look at the ovary using ultrasound studies (Fig. 14.3) what we often find is an appearance known as a polycystic ovary. In this situation, the ovary is slightly larger than normal and the follicles which are usually present in the ovary, are dotted like a necklace around the edges of the ovary. Contained within the ovary is a dense soft tissue called stroma.

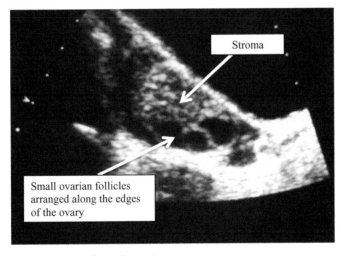

Figure 14.3 *Ultrasound picture of a polycystic ovary.*

This characteristic picture is also associated with a slight change in the balance of the hormones, so that generally speaking, slightly more LH is produced compared to FSH. This appears to be a continuous feature throughout the menstrual cycle and the end result is that periods become irregular and when they do occur, they are often heavy. The reason for this is although the female hormone estradiol is produced which continues to stimulate the endometrium, the formation of progesterone which is associated with regular menstrual cycles is upset, leading to the irregularity in cycle length. During these cycles the normal ovulatory events do not seem to take place as regularly as in normal cycles and as a result fertility is compromised due to reduced egg production.

This situation is very difficult to rectify from the CAH standpoint.

Normalising androgen levels is useful in such situations, but it does not seem to overcome the inherent problem that has been generated within the ovary and it is often necessary in these situations, to work with a reproductive endocrinologist to manipulate the hypothalamic–pituitary–ovarian axis to promote ovulation.

FERTILITY IN MALES

In males a slightly different scenario arises. In situations of suboptimal cortisol replacement where adrenal androgens are very high, a certain amount of testosterone will be generated from the adrenal glands and is often sufficient coupled with the other adrenal androgens produced to compensate for the loss of testicular testosterone.

Looking at Figs 14.4 and 14.5 we can see what would happen if adrenal androgen concentrations became very high.

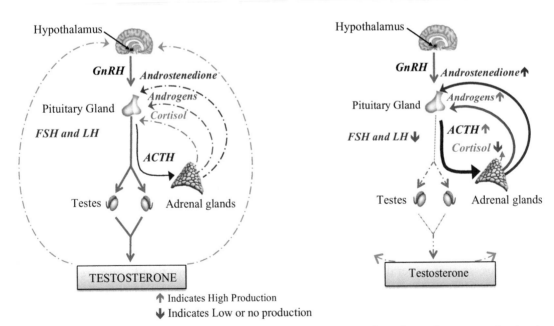

↑ Indicates High Production
↓ Indicates Low or no production

Figure 14.4 *The hypothalamo-pituitary-testes system and the adrenal glands working when adrenal androgen is low.*

Figure 14.5 *When the androgen production is high the hypothalamo-pituitary-testes system is switched off.*

As in females, the hypothalamo-pituitary-gonadal axis would switch off due to the feedback of adrenal androgens dampening down gonadotropin releasing hormone pulses. This leads to a reduction in testicular testosterone production and spermatogenesis. The fall in testicular testosterone may not be noticed, because it may be compensated by the increased production of adrenal androgens (Fig. 14.6).

The switching off of the hypothalamo-pituitary-gonadal axis will also reduce the production of FSH and because this hormone is particularly involved in sperm formation infertility will result, due to a marked reduction in the sperm count and size of the testes.

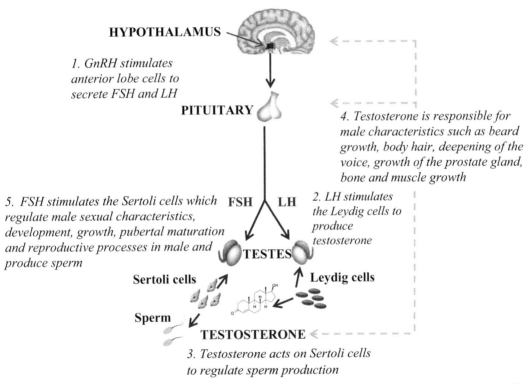

HYPOTHALAMUS

1. GnRH stimulates anterior lobe cells to secrete FSH and LH

PITUITARY

4. Testosterone is responsible for male characteristics such as beard growth, body hair, deepening of the voice, growth of the prostate gland, bone and muscle growth

5. FSH stimulates the Sertoli cells which regulate male sexual characteristics, development, growth, pubertal maturation and reproductive processes in male and produce sperm

FSH   LH

2. LH stimulates the Leydig cells to produce testosterone

TESTES

Sertoli cells   **Leydig cells**

Sperm

TESTOSTERONE

3. Testosterone acts on Sertoli cells to regulate sperm production

Figure 14.6 *Control of sperm production in the testes by the pituitary hormones LH and FSH and by the production of testosterone within the testes.*

The testes are filled with tiny coiled tubes called seminiferous tubules. The tubes are lined by Sertoli cells as well as sperm stem cells called spermatogonia. Sertoli cells are stimulated into action by FSH and interact with the spermatogonia to get sperm production underway. Situated close by are the Leydig cells which make testosterone. Testosterone is produced by LH. Some of the testosterone goes out into the blood and some remains to stimulate the maturation of sperm. Therefore, anything that alters FSH production will alter sperm production as intratesticular testosterone is controlled by LH production. Anything which dampens down the hypothalamic–pituitary–testicular axis and reduces testicular testosterone formation, will also impact indirectly on sperm formation due to the loss of the generation of intratesticular testosterone.

The interaction of the testes and adrenal axis is therefore extremely important. It tells us that getting cortisol replacement optimal is critical in the care of males with CAH, as it is for females with CAH. Simply using testosterone or androstenedione as the marker for cortisol replacement in CAH is inadequate, as this will not tell us exactly how cortisol is replaced nor guarantee adequate intratesticular generation of testosterone. Let's have a look at this in a bit more detail.

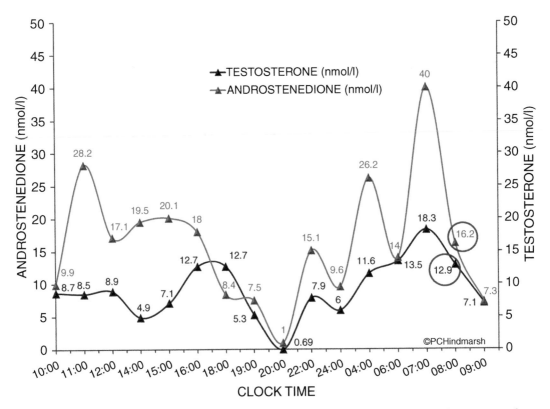

Figure 14.7 *Measures over 24 hours of testosterone and androstenedione with spot sample at 08:00 highlighted in red circles.*

If we study the androstenedione levels in this postpubertal male (Fig. 14.7) which were taken over a 24 hour period and consider that a one-off sample had been taken at 08:00 h, the result of 16.2 nmol/l would indicate under replacement. However, if a one-off sample had been taken on the same day but an hour later at 09:00 h, the result 7.3 nmol/l would suggest that cortisol replacement was optimal. Similarly, if the sample had been taken several hours before at 07:00 h where the level of androstenedione was 40 nmol/l, we would say that this patient was under treated (Fig. 14.8).

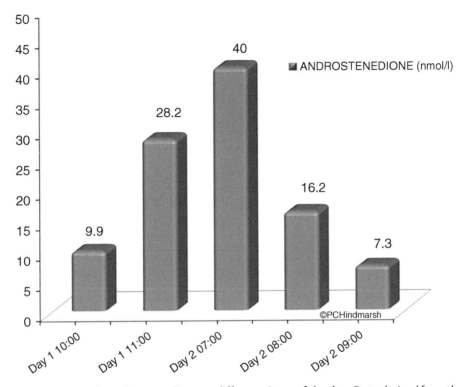

Figure 14.8 *Variation in androstenedione at different times of the day. Data derived from the profile in Fig. 14.7.*

If we look at the testosterone levels which were taken during the same profile (Fig. 14.7) and consider that a one-off sample of testosterone was taken at 08:00, the result of 12.9 nmol/l would point towards low testosterone, that the patient is over treated and cortisol replacement should be decreased. However, decreasing the cortisol would not raise testosterone from the testes, any increase would come from androgen production and testosterone would be made by the adrenal glands. Had the sample been taken at 07:00, the testosterone level of 18.3 nmol/l (Fig. 14.9) would be considered to be within normal range and no adjustments to cortisol replacement needed.

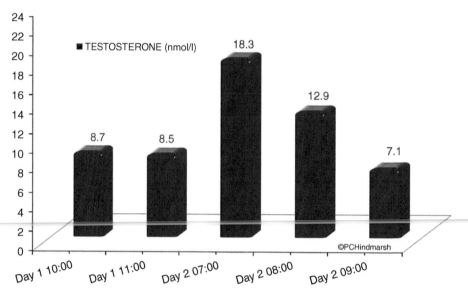

Figure 14.9 *Variation in testosterone at different times of the day.* Data derived from the profile in Fig. 14.7.

When we add the cortisol levels of this patient to the profile data (Fig. 14.10), we can see there are good levels of cortisol and in fact what this patient needs is an altering in the timing of their doses, not an increase or decrease.

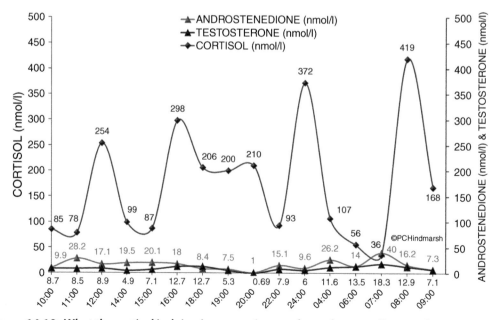

Figure 14.10 *What the cortisol is doing in comparison to the androstenedione and testosterone.*

When we go back and look carefully at the cortisol measurements at the times of these morning samples (Fig. 14.11), we can see the cortisol and testosterone do not relate; this is because testosterone production at this age (postpubertal) should be from the testes and not from the adrenal glands. We can see that at 07:00 androstenedione is very high at 40 nmol/l and testosterone is also at its peak at 18.3 nmol/l; however, cortisol is low at 36 nmol/l and testosterone is adrenal driven rather than coming from the testes.

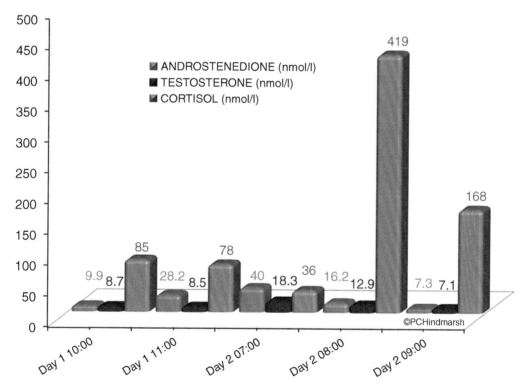

Figure 14.11 *Cortisol, testosterone and androstenedione. Data derived from the profile Fig. 14.10.*

The variation of both androstenedione and testosterone over the 24 hour period does not correlate closely enough to cortisol levels to give an indication of overall cortisol replacement (Fig. 14.10). This serves to highlight the importance of getting cortisol right and also interpreting all measures in the light of what cortisol is doing during the 24 hour period. We discuss this further in Chapter 24.

ADRENAL RESTS (TESTICULAR ADRENAL REST TISSUE-TART)

A more serious problem can happen in males with CAH when cortisol replacement is suboptimal, resulting in high androgen levels; this is the activation of adrenal rests which occur in the testes. Adrenal rests are adrenal cells which are present in the testes. These appear in the testes because of the way the gonads and adrenal glands develop at the very early stage of development. You might want to have a look at Chapter 2 showing where the adrenal glands and gonads form close to each other in the primitive streak (Fig. 2.2). As some of the adrenal cells can get into the testes, there is a possibility they will respond to ACTH in the same way adrenal cells in the adrenal glands do. Normally, this does not matter as long as ACTH concentrations are low.

In males, where cortisol replacement is suboptimal resulting in high circulating ACTH concentrations, the high ACTH will stimulate the adrenal rest tissue in the testes and over time will lead to the enlargement of these cells. This enlargement is known as adrenal rests and is given the abbreviation TART (Testicular Adrenal Rest Tissue) (Fig. 14.12).

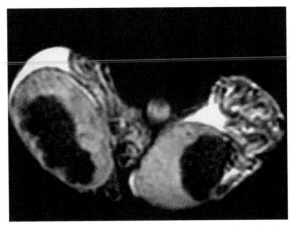

Figure 14.12 *Picture of testes showing the dark black irregular shaped adrenal rest tissue.*

The tissue which forms is quite hard and craggy and can often be mistaken for a testicular tumour. TARTs are sometimes referred to as testicular adrenal tumours. These are not malignant but the size they can grow to, can produce serious problems with respect to the remainder of the testicular tissue which can essentially be squashed and malfunction. The presence of TART, is associated with a poor outlook for long term fertility. It is important to realise that TART can arise in anyone who has high ACTH levels and is not only found in CAH.

Not all adrenal rests are palpable and it is important that males have sonograms. TART can appear in young boys.

What can be done for males is to optimise cortisol replacement. If adrenal androgens have been suppressing the hypothalamo–pituitary–gonadal axis, the good news is that spermatogenesis will resume, once the hypothalamo–pituitary–gonadal axis has been released from the suppressing effect of the adrenal androgens.

The situation with respect to TART however, is not so good and the likelihood of fertility ensuing in an individual with TART, no matter how optimal the cortisol replacement is after the development of the TART, is very poor indeed. Large doses of potent glucocorticoids such as dexamethasone may shrink the TART. The role for surgery is unclear. If a young man has TART, careful review with an urologist is needed.

PREGNANCY IN A PERSON WITH CONGENITAL ADRENAL HYPERPLASIA

In this section we are going to consider some general points about pregnancy in a woman with CAH. We have already discussed in Chapter 3 about the genetic risks of a baby having CAH. In addition, we have mentioned the idea of antenatal treatment to reduce the chance of having an affected virilised female child. This practice is falling out of favour due to a higher incidence of brain defects in the children treated.

It is possible for a woman with any form of CAH to fall pregnant. The most important point is that the pregnancy is best planned because of the genetic issues raised in Chapter 3 and also to ensure that adrenal androgen levels are optimal. The reason for this is to increase the chances of egg production and fertilisation by sperm, ensure normal ovarian hormone production until the formation of the placenta (after birth) takes place and to reduce the exposure of the baby to maternal androgen.

The baby might not have CAH but if the mother's adrenal androgens are high, these can transfer to the baby across the placenta and affect a normal female baby.

The changes in the mother, particularly the high estradiol concentrations, mean the proteins which carry cortisol around in the blood will be increased. If these carrier proteins, such as cortisol binding globulin are increased, then unless the hydrocortisone dose the mother takes is altered, there will be less free cortisol present and adrenal androgens will increase.

During pregnancy, the mother should be switched to hydrocortisone if not already on it. Hydrocortisone does not cross the placenta whereas dexamethasone does. Dexamethasone may harm the baby in terms of short term memory development, later risks of hypertension and diabetes as well as recently reported brain development problems.

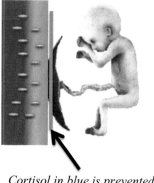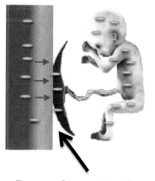

Cortisol in blue is prevented from crossing the placenta by the enzyme 11-beta hydroxysteroid dehydrogenase type 2 which inactivates cortisol

*Dexamethasone in yellow can cross into the baby as it is **NOT** inactivated by the enzyme 11-beta hydroxysteroid dehydrogenase type 2*

Figure 14.13 *The enzyme 11-beta hydroxysteroid dehydrogenase type 2 prevents cortisol getting across the placenta into the baby.*

The situation in pregnancy is that the level of cortisol in the mother is about 10 times greater than in the baby. We would expect cortisol to move across the placenta into the baby to equal things out. However, the baby in the womb needs to have a low cortisol level to allow structures to develop. This means the placenta blocks cortisol moving across. It uses the enzyme 11-beta hydroxysteroid dehydrogenase type 2 to inactivate cortisol to cortisone in the placenta (Fig. 14.13).

If the enzyme was missing, cortisol from the mother would cross the placenta into the baby and lead to poor growth and development. Dexamethasone is not inactivated by the enzyme and so can get into the baby. This is why it was used to switch off a CAH affected baby's adrenal glands but there are problems with this as mentioned previously and this is why it is no longer recommended.

Pregnancy needs to be managed jointly by an endocrinologist and an obstetrician. During delivery, stress doses of hydrocortisone will be needed especially if a caesarean section is required.

FURTHER READING

Otten, B.J., Stikkelbroeck, M.M., Claahsen-van der Grinten, H.L., Hermus, A.R., 2005. Puberty and fertility in congenital adrenal hyperplasia. Endocr. Dev. 8, 54–66.

CHAPTER 15

Sleep and Mood Alterations

GLOSSARY

Depression A clinical condition characterised by disturbances in mood, appetite and sleep.

Light/dark cycle Cyclicity in the function of a number of brain components which appear to follow light and dark, rather than an exact linkage to a 24 hour clock.

SLEEP

Sleep is conventionally broken down into various stages depending upon brain activity. This is shown in Fig. 15.1.

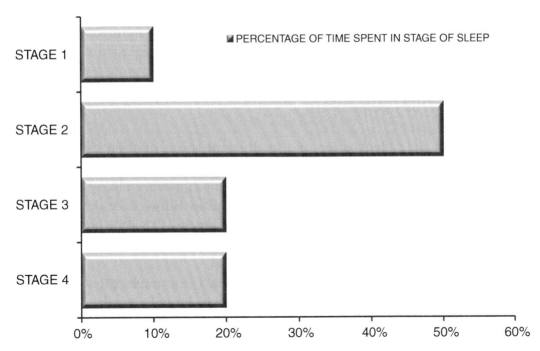

Figure 15.1 *Illustration of the time course of the stages of sleep.*

Congenital Adrenal Hyperplasia. http://dx.doi.org/10.1016/B978-0-12-811483-4.00015-5

Stage 1

Stage 1 is the beginning of the sleep cycle; it is a relatively light stage of sleep and can be considered a transition period between wakefulness and sleep. This period of sleep lasts only a brief time (around 5–10 minutes). If you wake someone up during this stage, they might report that they weren't really asleep.

Stage 2

Stage 2 sleep lasts for approximately 20 minutes. Body temperature starts to decrease and heart rate begins to slow.

Stage 3

During this stage, people become less responsive and noises as well as activity in the environment may fail to generate a response. It also acts as a transitional period between light sleep and a very deep sleep.

Stage 4

Most dreaming occurs during the fourth stage of sleep which is known as rapid eye movement (REM) sleep. REM sleep is characterised by eye movement, increased breathing rate and increased brain activity. REM sleep is also referred to as paradoxical sleep because while the brain and other body systems become more active, muscles become more relaxed. Dreaming occurs because of increased brain activity, but voluntary muscles become paralysed.

The amount of time spent asleep and in different stages of sleep varies. Infants spend more time sleeping and spend a greater percentage of sleep in REM sleep compared with older children and adults. For example, newborn babies sleep about 16 hours/day and spend about 50% of that time in REM sleep. Older people (50–85 years old) sleep only 5.75–6 hours/day and spend 13.8–15% of that time in REM sleep.

Sleep is also associated with the release of hormones. For example, growth hormone tends to be released the most during Stage 4 sleep which might be where the idea of good sleep and growing came from.

ACTH and cortisol tend to appear during Stage 3/REM sleep. However, the relationship between sleep stage and ACTH/cortisol release is not clear cut and

ACTH/cortisol are more attuned to the light/dark cycle than sleep itself. The clock genes in the hypothalamus that regulate ACTH release, work almost independently of sleep itself receiving their cues from day/night lengths. The association of sleep with the release of many hormones, for example ACTH/cortisol and growth hormone is close but sleep itself does not necessarily trigger the release of these hormones.

We also do not understand if the hormones themselves influence the stages of sleep or rather the time spent in various stages of sleep. The situation is made even more complex because our natural day/night rhythm is not actually 24 hours but something slightly less (about 23 hours roughly), which means that we need to readjust every now and again to fit the 24 hour cycle. If we do not readjust, then the sleep/wake cycle gradually gets out of synchrony and then we experience difficulties getting off to sleep or going to sleep at different times of the day. This is quite a problem in the elderly where this disrupted pattern is common.

We also need to understand what people mean when they say they cannot sleep properly. Sleep studies have revealed two broad categories. People who cannot get off to sleep and people who get off to sleep, but wake later in the night and cannot get back to sleep.

The first group responds well to melatonin therapy. Melatonin is a hormone that appears to be released in the evening/early night and is involved in getting you off to sleep. It is probably the hormone that works to reset or resynchronise the sleep/wake cycle.

The second group is more complicated to treat as melatonin does not seem to work very well in this group. The best treatment for this group seems to be the benzodiazepine group of drugs (the class of sleeping tablets such as Valium). These are not without their own problems and side effects, but are effective in this particular group of individuals.

It has often been stated that people receiving glucocorticoid treatment have problems getting off to sleep. In adult practice this idea is so engrained that patients are advised to take their last dose of medication at 18:00 (6 p.m.). This raises the question as to whether the way in which glucocorticoids are replaced affects how people sleep. It is of interest that when we are going off to sleep our cortisol levels are at their lowest. Whether this is important to get off to sleep is not at all clear.

This raises two possibilities:

1. Either you do not need glucocorticoids to go to sleep and you should not have any in the blood stream which is the adult dosing argument.

   or

2. You do need some cortisol around and this amounts to evening cortisol levels of about 80–100 nmol/l.

This is important to resolve because if you dose at 18:00 (6 p.m.) with hydrocortisone, you will be without cortisol in the blood for a very long period of time and there will be no cortisol present from midnight, which is the time cortisol levels naturally start to rise. Many of the treatment regimens in children and young people use glucocorticoids given late in the evening and usually this dose can be quite high, particularly if reverse circadian dosing is employed. As you can see in the 24 hour profiles that we have throughout this book, the normal circadian rhythm has low amounts of cortisol from about 21:00 through to about midnight (Fig. 15.2). However, there is always some cortisol present in the blood stream.

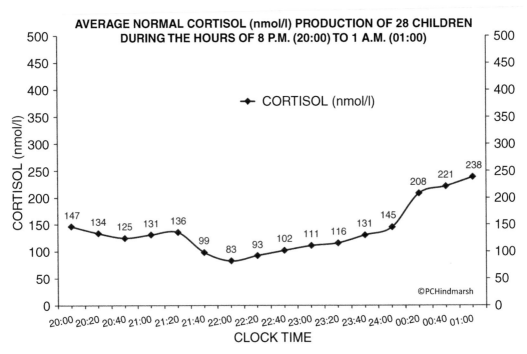

Figure 15.2 *Cortisol in the blood between 20:00 (8 p.m.) and 01:00 (1 a.m.) in a normal child.*

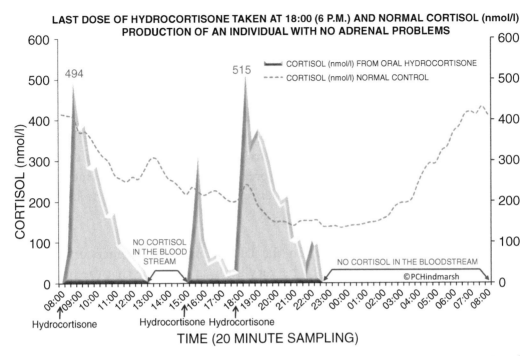

Figure 15.3 *Cortisol in the blood after a dose of hydrocortisone given at 18:00 or 6 p.m.* Note the periods of time with no cortisol when superimposed upon the normal cortisol production (dashed light blue line) from an individual without adrenal problems.

Fig. 15.3 shows the effect of dosing with hydrocortisone at 18:00 (6 p.m.). The peak is achieved quickly and by the late evening there is very little cortisol present.

What we can see in the graph are three things:

1. Firstly, the patient does not have any cortisol in the blood from 21:00 onwards until the next dose in the morning, a period of some 10–11 hours. This is in contrast to what should be happening, if we are trying to mimic the normal circadian rhythm.

   In CAH, this would mean that the strong ACTH drive at this period of time would make the adrenal glands produce a lot of adrenal androgens so both ACTH and androgen levels will be high at this stage. This may also explain for example, why patients with Addison's disease complain of increased pigmentation (see Chapter 16), this occurs because they will have a very high ACTH drive at this stage. Latest studies show that some male patients with Addison's disease have been found to have adrenal rest tissue in the testes (TART) which occur due to high levels of ACTH.

2. Secondly, in this way of treatment all the dose is distributed between 08:00 and 21:00. Even then the schedule has not quite mimicked the circadian rhythm as there is a period of time when there is no cortisol when there should be some present.

3. Thirdly, by putting the entire daily dose over this time frame the peaks are very high (related to the second point). This means that for some of the day there is *over* exposure and for some of the day *under* exposure. Over exposure during the day when we are eating, is likely to lead to the situation where more insulin is needed to be produced by the pancreas, this will drive fat generation, weight gain and diabetes, whereas the under replacement periods lead to high ACTH and androgen levels.

In contrast, when we are dosing in the late evening with glucocorticoids the circulating concentration can often be very high, at the time that the person may be going off to sleep (Fig. 15.4). You may remember, we call cortisol the 'get up and go' hormone and it is quite possible that having these high concentrations late in the evening when we want to get off to sleep, upsets that process.

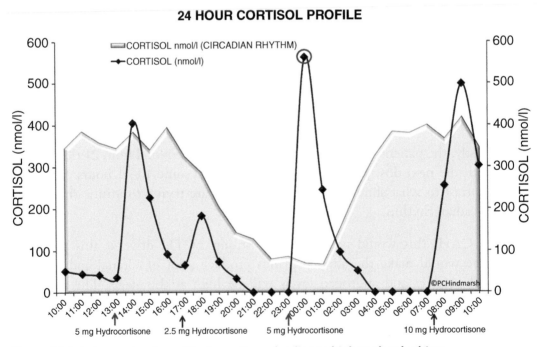

Figure 15.4 *Late evening dose of hydrocortisone leading to high peak at bedtime.*

This may well be the case when the more potent glucocorticoids such as prednisolone or dexamethasone are used. But what is the evidence that sleep really is disrupted?

There are a number of carefully constructed sleep studies that have investigated this question. The overall message is very clear. It does not matter if you take your hydrocortisone medication as in Fig. 15.4.

The time to start, sleep quality and duration of sleep is not affected and that is irrespective of the reason that you are taking the hydrocortisone tablets. This is a really important piece of information.

It means that we can replace as close to the circadian rhythm as we possibly can without worrying about sleep issues. This point is also supported by questionnaire results from people taking hydrocortisone for different conditions such as CAH, Addison's disease and hypopituitarism. Fig. 15.5 shows the answers to how you sleep.

The important message from Fig. 15.5 is that it does not matter what time the last dose is taken, there is no difference in ability to get off to sleep. The group that has the least problems in falling asleep is the CAH group, who always take their medication as late as possible. Many of these are children who have a fair amount of cortisol in the blood stream before going off to sleep and wake at midnight to take a further dose of hydrocortisone, before going straight back to sleep.

WHAT WE CAN DO ABOUT THIS?

There is no need to take the last dose at 18:00 (6 p.m.) and the last dose should be taken as late as is possible, ideally around midnight, as this would better mimic the circadian rhythm. It is probably better to avoid using the more potent glucocorticoids, prednisolone and dexamethasone. Sometimes giving melatonin, which helps sleep onset, can be useful if taken around an hour before going to bed. Avoiding stimulants such as caffeine before bed can be helpful. If these simple remedies do not work then a consultation with a doctor specialising in sleep disorders can be very helpful.

CAH - PARTICIPANTS WHO HAVE NO PROBLEM FALLING ASLEEP & TIME THE LAST DOSE OF THE DAY IS TAKEN

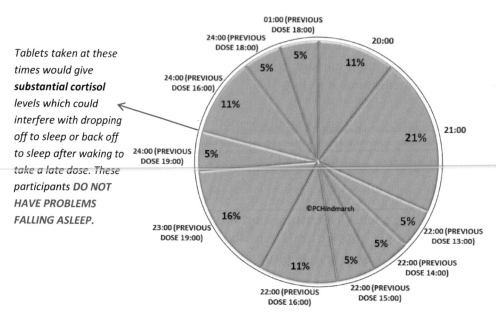

*Tablets taken at these times would give **substantial cortisol** levels which could interfere with dropping off to sleep or back off to sleep after waking to take a late dose. These participants DO NOT HAVE PROBLEMS FALLING ASLEEP.*

CAH - PARTICIPANTS WHO HAVE PROBLEMS FALLING ASLEEP & TIME THE LAST DOSE OF THE DAY IS TAKEN

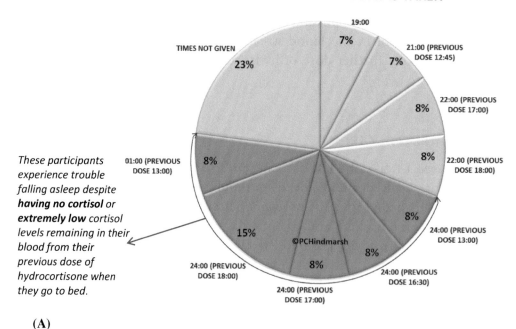

*These participants experience trouble falling asleep despite **having no cortisol** or **extremely low** cortisol levels remaining in their blood from their previous dose of hydrocortisone when they go to bed.*

(A)

Figure 15.5 *(A) Effect of timing of last dose taken at night and difficulty in falling asleep in patients with congenital adrenal hyperplasia.*

ADDISON'S - PARTICIPANTS WHO HAVE NO PROBLEM FALLING ASLEEP & TIME THE LAST DOSE OF THE DAY IS TAKEN

*Tablets taken at these times would give **substantial cortisol** levels which could interfere with dropping off to sleep but these participants DO NOT HAVE PROBLEMS FALLING ASLEEP*

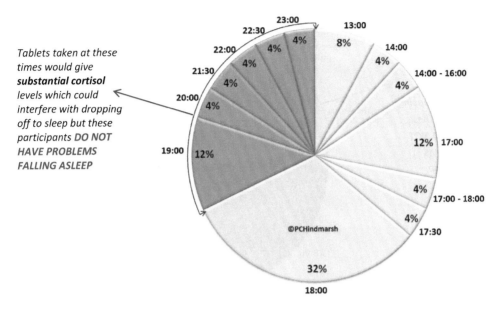

ADDISON'S - PARTICIPANTS WHO HAVE PROBLEMS FALLING ASLEEP & TIME THE LAST DOSE OF THE DAY IS TAKEN

Participants who have trouble falling asleep however, doses taken at these times would leave very low cortisol levels or no measurable cortisol in the blood when going to bed. The participants would be cortisol deficient until the next morning when their hydrocortisone dose is taken.

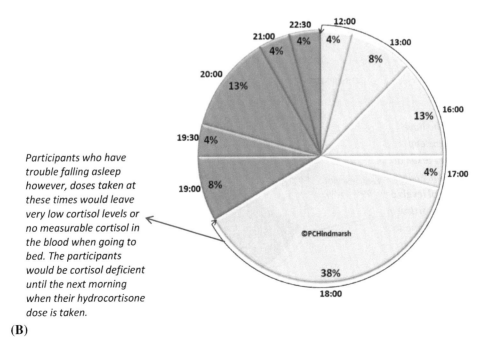

(B)

Figure 15.5 *(B) Effect of timing of last dose taken at night and difficulty in falling asleep in patients with Addison's disease.*

HYPOPITUITARISM - PARTICIPANTS WHO HAVE NO PROBLEM FALLING ASLEEP & TIME THE LAST DOSE OF THE DAY IS TAKEN

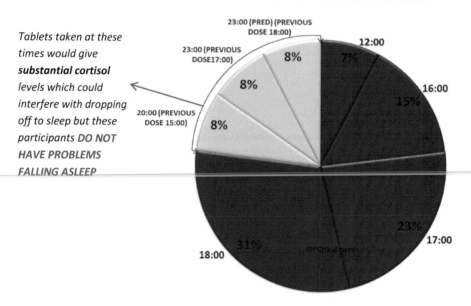

*Tablets taken at these times would give **substantial cortisol** levels which could interfere with dropping off to sleep but these participants DO NOT HAVE PROBLEMS FALLING ASLEEP*

HYPOPITUITARISM - PARTICIPANTS WHO HAVE PROBLEMS FALLING ASLEEP & TIME THE LAST DOSE OF THE DAY IS TAKEN

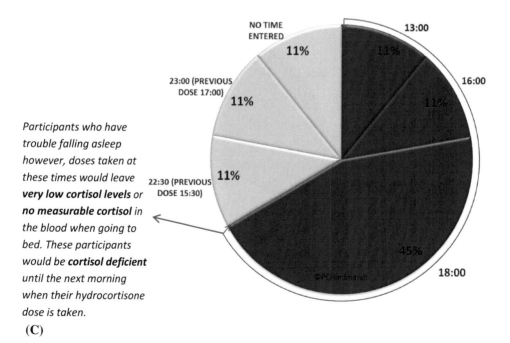

*Participants who have trouble falling asleep however, doses taken at these times would leave **very low cortisol levels** or **no measurable cortisol** in the blood when going to bed. These participants would be **cortisol deficient** until the next morning when their hydrocortisone dose is taken.*

(C)

Figure 15.5 *(C) Effect of timing of last dose taken at night and difficulty in falling asleep in patients with hypopituitarism.*

MOOD ALTERATIONS

Over many years it has been observed that in certain situations such as depression, cortisol levels are altered. Fig. 15.6 shows average cortisol levels in patients with depression and controls (people without depression). Overall, the circadian patterns are very similar but the depressed patients produce about 20% more cortisol during the 24 hour period than the control group.

In people experiencing chronic stress, the circadian rhythm is maintained, albeit cortisol concentrations remain at a higher level. Whether the altered amount of cortisol in these situations leads to the depression/chronic stress or is a secondary effect of whatever causes the problem in the first place, is not clear.

We know for example, if young animals are food restricted in the first few months of life, they increase their cortisol production and this change can be permanent. This would imply that it is the event that alters the cortisol rather than the other way around.

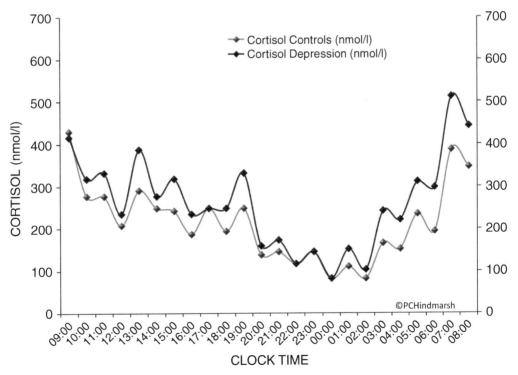

Figure 15.6 *24 Hour average cortisol profiles in patients with depression (purple line) and those without depression (blue line).*

Where it is more evident is in Cushing's disease. In this condition the pituitary gland, instead of producing ACTH in a circadian pattern, produces ACTH all the time so that there is a constant high level throughout the 24 hour period. This is often associated with depression which usually reverses once the condition has been treated. So it is possible, persistent high levels of glucocorticoids can lead to mood alterations such as depression.

Although mood changes can be associated with any of the glucocorticoids, both prednisolone and dexamethasone appear to have higher rates of mood changes associated with their use.

With prednisolone in particular there are reports of becoming depressed on this medication and we also know that both dexamethasone and prednisolone do seem to alter short term memory particularly when taken in high doses. Dexamethasone because of the rather long exposure from oral dosing seems to be very prone to these problems.

Both over and under treatment can cause problems with behaviour and mood. We know very little about this and more research is needed. Under treatment leads to problems in two ways, lack of cortisol is associated with a general slowing in activity and reduced energy levels. It is also associated with low blood glucose and this in itself can lead to mood changes, irritability, loss of concentration and lethargy.

CONCLUSIONS

To try and minimise sleep and mood disturbances, hydrocortisone is probably the preferred glucocorticoid. Careful adjustment of the dose and duration of exposure to high concentrations can be best achieved, using the 24 hour profile approach that we talk about frequently throughout the book. We have found sometimes by simply lowering the cortisol peaks achieved will often improve hyperactive behaviour.

FURTHER READING

Abali, Z.Y., Saka, N., Erol, O.B., et al., 2014. Adrenal rest tumors in patients with primary adrenal insufficiency. European Society for Paediatric Endocrinology Abstracts. 82, P-D-1-3-12.

García-Borreguero, D., Wehr, T.A., Larrosa, O., Granizo, J.J., Hardwick, D., Chrousos, G.P., Friedman, T., 2000. Glucocorticoid replacement is permissive for rapid eye movement sleep and sleep consolidation in patients with adrenal insufficiency. J. Clin. Endocrinol. Metab. 85, 4201–4206.

Machin, P., Young, A.H., 2004. The role of cortisol and depression: exploring new opportunities for treatment. Psychiatric Times. Available from: http://www.psychiatrictimes.com/articles/role-cortisol-and-depression-exploring-new-opportunities-treatments

German, A., Suraiya, S., Tenenbaum-Rakover, Y., Koren, I., Pillar, G., Hochberg, Z., 2008. Control of childhood congenital adrenal hyperplasia and sleep activity and quality with morning or evening glucocorticoid therapy. J. Clin. Endocrinol. Metab. 93 (12), 4707–4710.

CHAPTER 16

Abdominal, Skin and Other Problems

GLOSSARY

Enteric formulations A coating applied to a drug to prevent breakdown in the stomach and delivery of the drug at a point further down the gut.

Gastric ulcers and erosions Breakdown of the normal lining of the stomach. This allows the stomach acid to act on the exposed area leading to pain. If the erosion or ulcer occurs over an underlying blood vessel then gastric bleeding can occur which can be severe.

Immunosuppression Dampening down the immune response to inflammation which is useful to prevent inflammatory diseases such as arthritis.

Proximal myopathy Weakness of the muscles of the upper leg or arm. Classic effect of excess glucocorticoids. Patients usually cannot raise themselves up from squatting position.

Striae Purple/reddish stretch marks. Glucocorticoids cause thinning of the skin and striae appear when the collagen and elastin fibres in the skin, tear. Where the fibres break this allows the blood vessels below, to show through giving the red or purple colour initially. When the blood vessels eventually shrink the fat below the skin is visible which gives the stretch marks a silvery white colour.

STOMACH PROBLEMS

Virtually all glucocorticoids have problems associated with stomach upsets. This usually takes the form of inflammation of the lining of the stomach called gastritis. Occasionally, this can be more severe and lead to stomach ulcers (Fig. 16.1). The symptoms are often upper abdominal pain, particularly after ingestion of food and some people also complain of heartburn. These symptoms arise due to the effects of the glucocorticoids themselves on the stomach wall where they can produce small ulcers.

Ideally, it would be best to stop the medication to allow the ulcers to heal but clearly when we need to give medicines such as glucocorticoids for life, this is not going to be possible.

Congenital Adrenal Hyperplasia. http://dx.doi.org/10.1016/B978-0-12-811483-4.00016-7

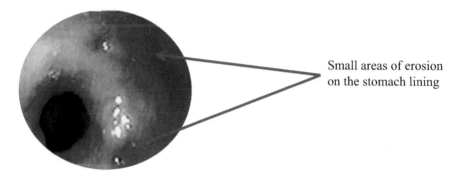

Small areas of erosion
on the stomach lining

Figure 16.1 *Endoscopic examinations show small areas of erosion on the lining of the stomach caused by gastritis.*

The only way to tackle this particular problem is to use some of the enteric coated glucocorticoids that are available. These protect the stomach wall from the effects of the glucocorticoids because they prevent breakdown of the tablet until it reaches the small bowel. Unfortunately only prednisolone comes in this format and has other problems as we have talked about because it is a potent glucocorticoid. It is important to note, the enteric coat also affects the absorption and delivery of the glucocorticoid.

What to do?

One practical solution is to always take glucocorticoids with food and never on an empty stomach.

Another approach is to use medicines called antacids, which reduce the production of acid in the stomach. There are a variety of these available. Many are extremely effective in reducing acid production and alleviating symptoms.

A further approach if stomach problems are severe, is to bypass the oral route altogether and deliver hydrocortisone using the pump system which we describe in Section Three.

CONSTIPATION

Constipation is a particular problem in children and this may relate in part, to the effect of the mineralocorticoid, fludrocortisone. Fludrocortisone acts on the kidney to retain salt. It also acts on the large bowel to promote a similar absorption of sodium or salt from the content of the large bowel. Because salt will move into the body across the bowel wall, it will also take water with it. This means the consistency of the stool formed will have less water in it and become increasingly thicker as it moves through the large bowel. The end result is the generation of small stools which are often quite hard and difficult to pass. In small children, the situation becomes increasingly difficult because once they realise that going to the toilet is painful, they tend to avoid doing so which makes the constipation worse.

What to do?

In addition to keeping to a high fibre diet and ensuring there is good fluid intake, one can also use laxatives or a stool softener to improve the consistency of the stool. In addition, it is also worth checking the plasma renin activity as a way of monitoring the fludrocortisone dose and reducing the fludrocortisone dose to a level which allows for a plasma renin activity towards the upper end of the normal range.

SKIN PROBLEMS

Skin problems can occur with CAH. These take several forms, the most important of which is acne (Fig. 16.2).

Acne develops when too much oil (sebum) is produced from the sebaceous glands within hair follicles. These glands are very sensitive to androgens. As part of the androgen effect, dead skin cells lining the hair follicles are shed which causes them to block the secretion of oil from the sebaceous glands. Acne spots are of course common in puberty but usually settle. They will generally also settle in CAH if cortisol replacement is optimised and androgen levels normalised. However, if they do not, advice from a dermatologist might be needed.

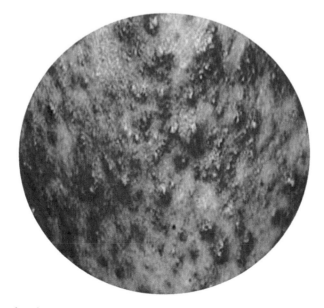

Figure 16.2 *Acne vulgaris.*

In young children, acne can often be a sign of under treatment and in non–classical CAH it can be one of the symptoms of the condition itself.

Acne can also be caused by high steroid doses and this is known as steroid induced acne (Fig. 16.3). It occurs when high doses of steroid are used, especially when using prednisolone or dexamethasone. Once the dose is lowered the acne may clear, if not again advice from a dermatologist might be needed.

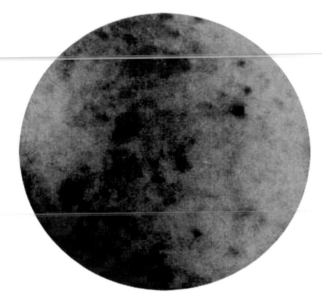

Figure 16.3 *Steroid induced acne.*

HYPERPIGMENTATION

Another way inadequate cortisol replacement can show itself in the skin is with increased tanning. This is because ACTH levels rise very high and when they are high, the skin tans, turning a yellowy brown colour. This can be seen particularly in skin creases (Fig. 16.4). The colour disappears when cortisol replacement is optimised and high ACTH levels normalised.

This happens because ACTH is derived from a polypeptide precursor called proopiomelanocortin (POMC). POMC is also the precursor for several other hormones, one of these being melanocyte stimulating hormone (MSH), so if you make more POMC to produce more ACTH, you will also make more MSH. MSH stimulates melanocytes and the main function of melanocytes is to produce melanin.

Melanin is what gives skin its colour (pigment), so when this level is high, the skin will darken.

Sometimes the tanned appearance will appear all over the body; however, it can often be more localized in areas subjected to pressure, like skin folds, knuckles as well as the gums. These are often referred to as ACTH patches.

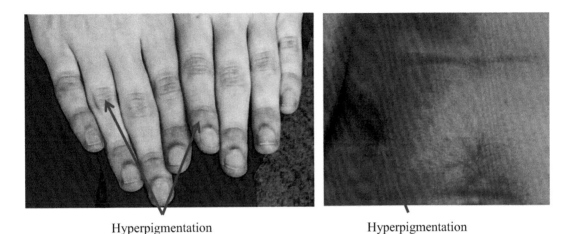

Hyperpigmentation   Hyperpigmentation

Figure 16.4 *Hyperpigmentation on the knuckle joints in a patient with CAH who had high ACTH levels.*

STRIAE (STRETCH MARKS)

Over treatment with steroids also leads to stretch marks. These are purple/red in colour (Fig. 16.5). The remedy is to adjust the glucocorticoid dose and although they do fade in time, they do not completely disappear. Stretch marks are more common when using dexamethasone and prednisolone because they are far more potent glucocorticoids than hydrocortisone.

Stretch marks can be likened to scarring and appear when the collagen and elastin fibres in the skin, tear. Where the fibres break this allows the blood vessels below to show through, which is why the stretch marks are red or purple when they first appear. The blood vessels eventually shrink and the pale coloured layer of fat below the skin is visible, which gives the stretch marks the silvery white colour. High levels of glucocorticoids can cause these tears in the collagen and elastin fibres when the skin is stretched.

Stretch marks also appear when there is a rapid increase in weight which stretches the tissues. These stretch marks are usually more white coloured.

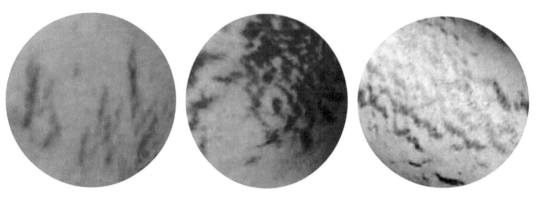

Figure 16.5 *Striae – stretch marks.*

THIN SKIN AND BRUISING

Thin skin and bruising has a similar cause to stretch marks (Fig. 16.6). The thin skin itself is a direct effect of glucocorticoids on the collagen and elastin fibres in the skin. These are often closely linked and one of the effects of glucocorticoids as previously mentioned, is to break up the tight bonding between these fibres. This leads to less strong skin and a reduction in the underlying protection that skin with these dense fibres, provide the blood vessels underneath. The blood vessels which can be damaged are small capillaries and venules. These are thin walled structures and are very susceptible to minor trauma. This explains why the slightest knock or bump often leads to problems and quite extensive bruising, arising to damage to these fragile vessels.

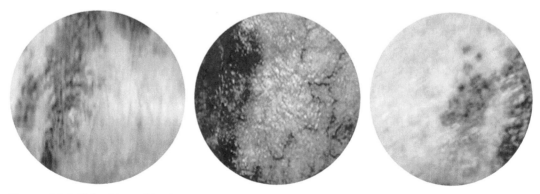

Figure 16.6 *Thin skin and bruising.*

MUSCLES

Muscle mass is also influenced by glucocorticoids. If glucocorticoid concentrations are high for a long period of time, then muscle wasting takes place. Muscle strength is lost and although this is generalized, it is more pronounced in the upper arms and upper legs. This is known as proximal myopathy and is characteristic of the use of high doses of glucocorticoids.

Interestingly, muscles can also be affected to a certain extent in CAH, when there is high adrenal androgen production as the muscle mass can actually increase in a similar way to the way anabolic steroids are used in sports doping. It has to be said that adrenal androgens have to be raised to a very high amount to get this effect and for a long period of time before the muscular changes can take place. However, it is important to realise that having high androgens can cause many long term health side effects in CAH, particularly with fertility.

Oddly, low or no cortisol leads to muscle weakness as well. The reason for this is not clear but may be something to do with cortisol action on the muscle fibres and how they slide together. This can also be accompanied by muscle aches and easy fatigue on exercise which may also be due to poor glucose delivery to provide energy.

High levels of cortisol resulting from taking high doses of glucocorticoids can damage muscle. This leads to a myopathy where the function and strength of the muscle tissue is reduced. This is reversible if detected early, but if long standing high levels are encountered over several years, full recovery may not occur.

The main effect is on the muscles of the upper part of the arm and leg. This is called a proximal myopathy. The most common feature is the person finds it difficult to stand upright from the squatting position. Using high dose of glucocorticoids for illness will not cause this kind of damage, it is only when constantly high doses are used over a long period of time, will the damage occur. As expected, the more potent glucocorticoids such as prednisolone and dexamethasone are more likely to cause these problems.

IMMUNE MODULATION

Glucocorticoids play a critical role in the functioning of the immune system. In the amounts we encounter on a day to day basis, glucocorticoids exert a permissive or enhancing effect on the influence of components of the immune system on fighting infections. In this situation glucocorticoids are extremely helpful. Even when we double the dose of glucocorticoids as in stress, these doses all serve to enhance the effect of the immune system in dealing with whatever has caused the upset, whether it is infection or trauma.

It is only when high doses of glucocorticoids are used for their anti–inflammatory action that problems with the immune system arise. In fact, part of the anti–inflammatory effect is mediated by upsetting the immune system. This is why we try to avoid excessive doses of glucocorticoids for long periods of time because immune problems will follow.

HAIR AND VOICE CHANGES

Deepening of the voice can take place when adrenal androgen concentrations are high for very long periods of time. Unfortunately, when this happens there is very little that can be done because the changes produced in the voice box are irreversible. Careful voice training, concentrating on breathing techniques and the projection of the voice, can help with this but it is better to avoid this situation in the first instance.

Likewise, high doses of glucocorticoids can lead to loss of hair and this can be seen particularly when using prednisolone. In addition, hair loss can follow from high levels of androgens and is often referred to as male pattern balding. Again, rather like the voice changes, once hair loss has taken place it is very difficult to gain any significant regrowth, even if there is optimal cortisol replacement with suppression of the adrenal androgen levels.

EYES AND BRAIN

High doses of glucocorticoids can lead to calcifications in the lens of the eye and cataract formation. These can be avoided by using optimal replacement doses of glucocorticoid and to avoid the most potent agents such as prednisolone and dexamethasone.

Brain effects can also ensue. Short term memory problems are associated with prednisolone and with doses often not much higher than 10 mg per day. This raises the interesting question of whether dosing should be increased in stressful situations such as school examinations. The general advice is probably not to, because although exams are 'stressful', they are usually associated with an increase in adrenalin, rather than a change in cortisol. As such, it is probably better not to double dose for examinations given the effect of high levels of glucocorticoids on short term memory and memory recall, it is probably not the best scenario for an exam!

Other effects on the brain include benign intracranial hypertension. Benign intracranial hypertension is caused by water retention in the spaces around the brain. It is extremely rare but has been associated with glucocorticoid use. If it should happen and it is more likely to happen if there is a sudden change to a high dose, then it is simply resolved by reducing the high dose back to the original starting dose. A careful buildup to whatever dose is required should then be undertaken.

BONE DEATH

In rare occasions, particularly when there is associated obesity, slippage of the coverings of the femur (epiphysis) can occur. The femur is the long bone, the thigh bone. The epiphysis can slip quite easily, especially in individuals who are overweight and that is why there is a lot of emphasis on monitoring weight and body mass index. Glucocorticoids have not been directly implicated in slipped upper femoral epiphysis and it is probably more a secondary effect of the increase in body weight, rather than an effect of the glucocorticoids on the cartilage.

High doses of glucocorticoids can be associated with the death of some bone cells in certain areas, particularly again the head of the thigh bone. This is known as avascular necrosis and again the linkage with glucocorticoids is not that strong. Nonetheless, it is always wise to carefully assess the dosing schedules of glucocorticoids and this is the reason we take great care in titrating the dose of glucocorticoid exactly so we neither overdo or underdo the dosing schedule.

THE HEART

Glucocorticoids affect heart function. Mineralocorticoids do as well, but it is more because they alter blood pressure which alters the work that the heart has to do, so the mineralocorticoid effect is indirect as it is mediated by changes in blood pressure. For example, if blood pressure decreases in CAH because of under replacement with fludrocortisone, then the heart will have to beat faster and pump harder to keep blood pressure and circulation up.

With glucocorticoids, the situation is a bit more complicated. Hydrocortisone also has a certain amount of water retaining effect and this will also tend to increase blood pressure. If excess hydrocortisone is present, then the main problem is similarly retention of water and if the heart is not in a very good state, this can lead to poor function and heart failure. This is extremely rare in children but can be a problem in older adults.

The more important issue is under replacement with glucocorticoids, because the heart function, particularly the heart rate and to a certain extent how hard it forces blood into the circulation, is very dependent on the amount of glucocorticoid. For example, in people who do not have any glucocorticoid, the heart rate can be extremely slow. This in itself leads to problems with faints and funny turns. In other people, the heart does not pump blood fast enough so that there is a backlog of blood in the lungs leading to shortness of breath and even further back, swelling of the legs can take place. All these changes need to be interpreted of course, with the important effect that glucocorticoids have on the heart where they act in conjunction with adrenalin. Glucocorticoids are important for the production of adrenalin from the adrenal glands and also for facilitating the action of adrenalin on the heart.

This is in part the reason why, when glucocorticoids are very low, the heart rate slows. The interaction of glucocorticoids and adrenalin is important for the maintenance of blood pressure and this again is another reason why under replacement with glucocorticoids, can lead to problems because of the lack of good tone in the blood vessels.

CONCLUSIONS

In all of these situations it is clear that careful attention to the dosing schedule is important. We will be considering the use of profiles as we get into Section Three as a way of monitoring hydrocortisone replacement. It is by the use of these profiles that we can carefully adjust the dosing schedule ensuring peaks of cortisol are not excessive and that there are no periods when cortisol replacement is suboptimal.

These periods can occur at different times of the day and that is why we go for a 24 hour profile approach to ensure we understand what is happening with the doses of glucocorticoid we use. Profiles sound as though they are quite a big event, but in fact we only take about an egg cup full of blood over a 24 hour period. For that we get an immense wealth of information regarding the dosing of glucocorticoids and can better fine tune therapy.

We will be looking at some of the advantages of 24 hour profiles and how they have improved the dosing schedules in clinical practice in Section Three.

FURTHER READING

Belvederi Murri, M., Pariante, C., Mondelli, V., Masotti, M., Atti, A.R., Mellacqua, Z., Antonioli, M., Ghio, L., Menchetti, M., Zanetidou, S., Innamorati, M., Amore, M., 2014. HPA axis and aging in depression: systematic review and meta-analysis. Psychoneuroendocrinology 41, 46–62.

Carey, R.M., 2010. Aldosterone and cardiovascular disease. Curr. Opin. Endocrinol. Diabetes Obes. 17, 194–198.

Collaer, M.L., Hindmarsh, P.C., Pasterski, V., Fane, B.A., Hines, M., 2015. Reduced short term memory in congenital adrenal hyperplasia (CAH) and its relationship to spatial and quantitative performance. Psychoneuroendocrinology 64, 164–173.

De Winter, R.F., Van Mehert, A.M., De Rijk, R.H., Zwinderman, K.H., Frankhuijzen-Sierevogel, A.C., Weigant, V.M., Goekoop, J.G., 2003. Anxious-retarded depression: relation with plasma vasopressin and cortisol. Neuropsychopharmacology 28, 140–147.

Minetto, M.A., Qaisar, R., Agoni, V., Motta, G., Longa, E., Miotti, D., Pellegrino, M.A., Bottinelli, R., 2015. Quantitative and qualitative adaptations of muscle fibers to glucocorticoids. Muscle Nerve 52, 631–639.

SECTION THREE

Treatment for Congenital Adrenal Hyperplasia

The third part of this book looks at how we treat congenital adrenal hyperplasia. We are going to focus on the use of glucocorticoids (mainly hydrocortisone) and mineralocorticoids (9 alpha-fludrocortisone) to replace the cortisol and aldosterone which is lacking. This section focuses on the reasons in the way these medications are administered.

It will also concentrate on how best to monitor replacement therapy because it is important that these medications are used in the right amounts and not given in higher doses because it will bring with it, all the problems associated with steroid use.

In addition, we are going to consider some of the practical aspects of these treatments, particularly with respect to the administration of medicines in schools and also what happens in special circumstances, such as sick days and during travel abroad.

We are not going to consider in this section the aspects of congenital adrenal hyperplasia care which require surgery. We will describe how to manage situations of stress of which surgery is one, but it is not the purpose of this book to explore the complexities of surgical procedures used to correct the appearance of the external genitalia. We believe that this aspect of care is better described and considered in several books written by our surgical colleagues.

CHAPTER 17

History of Steroid Development

GLOSSARY

Anti-inflammatory glucocorticoids Glucocorticoids such as hydrocortisone but more often prednisolone and dexamethasone used for their anti-inflammatory properties, not as replacement cortisol. This treatment is usually prescribed in short high doses and if taken for longer periods, cortisol production may be compromised. Patients who are not usually cortisol compromised need to be weaned off slowly to avoid this.

Cortisone acetate Inactive form of cortisol. Needs to be converted into cortisol in the liver.

Fine tuned Adjustment of hydrocortisone dosing either by timing or amount to mimic the normal cortisol circadian rhythm.

Glucocorticoids Group of steroid hormones (glucose + cortex + steroid) which regulate glucose metabolism and suppress inflammation.

GENERAL

As hormones became identified with various glands in the body, many scientists and doctors realised that extracts from these glands could contain hormones which might be useful in the treatment of endocrine disorders. Following the success of the isolation of insulin from the pancreas in the 1920's, attempts were made to extract hormones from other glands in the body.

Very crude adrenal extracts were tried in the 1930's but the yield of useful substances were quite small. We now know that the adrenal glands make cortisol in response to any ACTH that is present. As such, the adrenal glands do not store very much cortisol, so attempts to get cortisol from adrenal glands themselves were unlikely to yield much of the drug. In 1935, chemists could isolate the compound from bile acids in the urine of oxen. Elaborate chemical procedures, involving 38 steps, were required to make important human steroids. In 1938 a gram of natural cortisone was worth $100 (1938 dollars!).

It took until the late 1940's to get to a position where the structures of the hormones made by the adrenal glands were known. It was possible to synthesise (manufacture) the adrenal steroids. The first steroid to be devised was cortisone, the inactive form

Congenital Adrenal Hyperplasia. http://dx.doi.org/10.1016/B978-0-12-811483-4.00017-9

of cortisol. Cortisone was first identified by the American chemist Edward Calvin Kendall who was a researcher at the Mayo Clinic, for which he was awarded the 1950 Nobel Prize for Physiology and Medicine, along with Philip S. Hench and Tadeus Reichstein. This was produced as cortisone acetate. Cortisone is an inactive glucocorticoid and requires conversion in the liver by an enzyme called 11beta-hydroxysteroid dehydrogenase type 1 (11β–HSD1) into cortisol (Fig. 17.1).

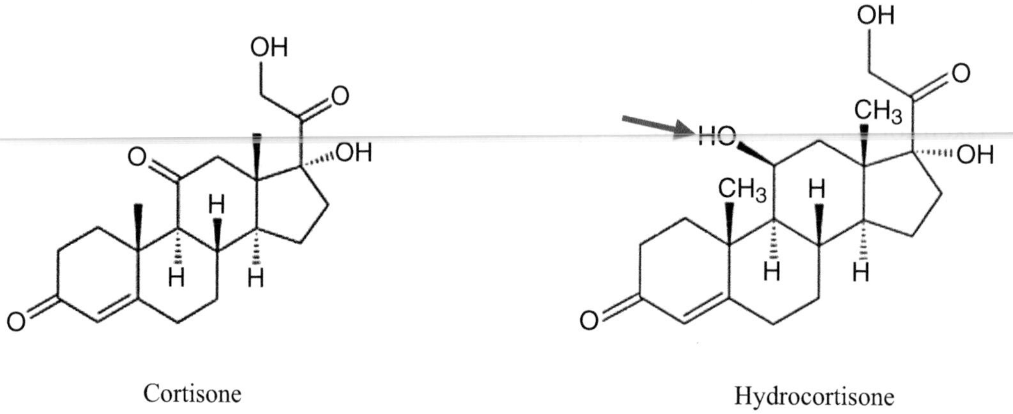

Cortisone   Hydrocortisone

Figure 17.1 *The chemical structures of cortisone and hydrocortisone or cortisol.*

Plant extracts were also used in the initial phases of creating the corticosteroids. This had started in the late 1930's when Russell Marker published a study in 1939 on sarsasapogenin, a plant extract which is used to make the drink sarsaparilla. The following year he published studies on diosgenin, which is a steroid crystalline compound called a saponin. Saponins are a class of chemical compounds which produce foam in water and are extracted from a Mexican yam species of the genus Dioscorea Diosgenin.

From diosgenin, he was able to synthesize the human hormone testosterone in eight steps and progesterone in just five steps. Marker made plans to use yams for mass production of human steroids, but proposals were rejected by the pharmaceutical companies, who saw no need for the venture. The important thing about these chemicals is they have structures similar to the glucocorticoid family. The structure of sarasapogenin was pivotal in the chemical modification that led to the production of progesterone. From that and knowing about diosgenin, it was then a question of making the modifications necessary to take these structures and convert them into structures which were like the naturally occurring steroids in the adrenal glands, ovaries and testes.

In 1942, Marker moved to Mexico. A company called Syntex was commissioned to make steroids from Mexican yams, using Marker's process. After a while, Marker left the company taking with him the key process steps and it was left to George Rosenkranz, who worked out the missing step. Rosenkranz took yams and was able to make progesterone, then testosterone and finally the female hormone estrone, leading him to say, "Adam goes into the test tube and Eve comes out".

All of this work in Mexico occurred while major pharmaceutical companies in the United States were trying to make hydrocortisone from the adrenal glands of 2,200,000 hogs. This was a high priority treatment for arthritis. Once again, Marker made another important discovery; he identified a yam saponin called botogenin. This compound has an oxygen atom located at the carbon-12 position. Upjohn Chemists used microorganisms to convert this compound into a useful form, because they could easily move the oxygen to the carbon-11 position.

This procedure opened the door for advanced corticosteroid production. About 66 pounds of fresh yams (two or three yam tubers) could yield one pound of diosgenin and eventually, through botogenin, about two ounces of cortisone.

Cortisone was first produced commercially by Merck & Co. On 30 September 1949, Percy Julian announced an improvement in the process of producing cortisone from bile acids which eliminated the need to use osmium tetroxide, a rare, expensive and dangerous chemical.

Despite all these limitations, there is no doubting how effective this treatment was. Rather like insulin therapy in patients with diabetes introduced some 30 years earlier, the effects of cortisone acetate were equally as dramatic. Lives were saved.

Congenital adrenal hyperplasia was no longer a condition associated with an almost 100% mortality. Lawson Wilkins in the United States pioneered this therapy and Fig. 17.2 shows the title of one of the scientific papers he wrote demonstrating the full effect of this new cortisone acetate in the management of young children with congenital adrenal hyperplasia.

In the United Kingdom in the early 1950's, John Cornforth and Kenneth Callow at the National Institute for Medical Research collaborated with Glaxo to produce cortisone from hecogenin extracted from sisal plants.

FURTHER STUDIES ON THE TREATMENT OF
CONGENITAL ADRENAL HYPERPLASIA
WITH CORTISONE

Pediatrics 1952; 10: 397

IV. Effect of Cortisone and Compound B in Infants
with Disturbed Electrolyte Metabolism

By John F. Crigler, Jr., M.D., Samuel H. Silverman, M.D.,
and Lawson Wilkins, M.D.
Baltimore

IN PRECEDING papers [1-7] the effect of cortisone on various phases of the syndrome of congenital adrenal hyperplasia has been reported. This paper will, therefore, be limited to a discussion of the treatment of infants with this disease who have an associated abnormality of the salt-regulating mechanism of the adrenal. Although this disorder has been recognized for a number of years, its diagnosis and treatment is often a difficult problem; and in general, the prognosis has been poor. With the advent of cortisone, which is capable of controlling the adrenal overactivity and thus preventing the excessive growth and virilization, the outlook is more encouraging. Accordingly, there is need for greater alertness in recognizing the abnormality and for a better understanding of the disturbed electrolyte metabolism, which is the primary cause of death. This paper is a report of data* accumulated over a 20 month period during studies on three infants with this disease.

Figure 17.2 *One of a series of reports by Lawson Wilkins on the treatment of congenital adrenal hyperplasia.* Reproduced with kind permission of the Editor of Pediatrics.

DOSING AND GROWTH

The doses of cortisone acetate used were high. This largely stemmed from the fact that estimates of how much cortisol was needed during the 24 hour period, were quite crude. They were based largely on attempts at measuring how much cortisol appeared in the urine, because at that stage it was not possible to measure hormones in blood samples. This was not to take place until the early 1970's and even then it was acknowledged that measuring steroids by special methods in blood, was difficult.

Initial doses of cortisone used were about 40 mg/m^2/24 hours.

The doses were actually calculated to give a normal growth rate. The reason growth rate was used as one of the markers of how effective the medication was and against which to titrate the dose, was after cortisone acetate was introduced by Lawson Wilkins. It became apparent over the next 5–10 years that glucocorticoids had marked effects on growth. Too much led to growth suppression.

As the 1960's evolved the aim of therapy was to titrate the dose against growth rate and assessment of skeletal maturity. The problem with this was the doses which allowed for a normal growth rate and a normal advance in skeletal maturation were quite high.

For example, when hydrocortisone became available it was noted a normal growth rate could be observed with the dose at 24 mg/m²/24 hours, which was similar to the dose which also allowed a normal progression in terms of skeletal maturity.

Neither of the doses derived, necessarily equalled the cortisol production rate from normal adrenal glands. An understanding of that had to wait until methods were available in the 1970's for the accurate and precise measurement of cortisol in blood samples.

Another way early doses were titrated, was to compare the effects of various doses on the excretion of metabolites of 17-hydroxyprogesterone in the urine. These methods were not as precise as the methods we have today and overall in the late 1950's and through the 1960's, the doses of cortisone acetate and subsequently hydrocortisone when it was introduced, were much higher than our current dosing schedules.

HYDROCORTISONE

Hydrocortisone came into use because of the problems with cortisone acetate as conversion in the liver from cortisone to cortisol was required (Fig. 17.3). The net effect of this was to reduce the potency of the steroid which meant more had to be given and probably with it, an increase in the side effect profile depending on the variability of the conversion of cortisone to cortisol.

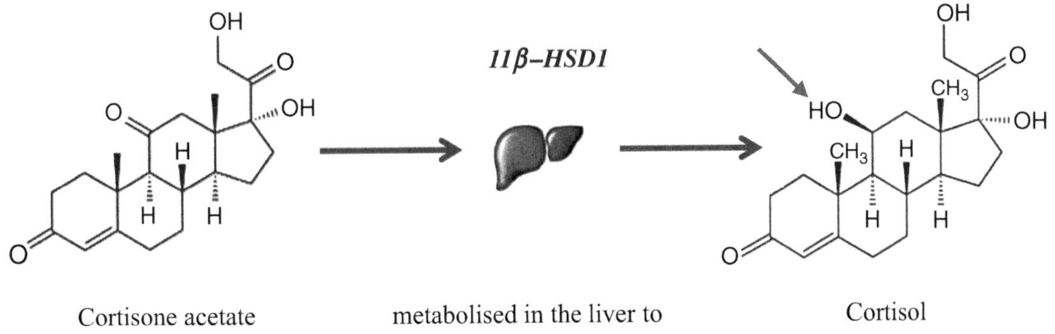

11β–HSD1

Cortisone acetate   metabolised in the liver to   Cortisol

Figure 17.3 *Cortisone acetate (inactive) has to be metabolised in the liver by the enzyme 11β-hydroxysteroid dehydrogenase type I to its active form of cortisol which limits its potency.*

The side effect profile of glucocorticoids in those early days was mainly growth suppression and weight gain. In the 1970's as better methods became available for the measurement of the adrenal steroids in blood, it was possible to start to determine how cortisol naturally appeared in the blood and what the normal daily production rate might be.

It is quite amusing looking back at a talk from the 1970's discussing the measurement of cortisol, where they make the point 'blood is easily collected but plasma levels reflect adrenal corticoid activity only at the moment. Because of the episodic nature of cortisol secretion, isolated values maybe misleading'. This is quite an interesting quote from a chemical pathology book making the point which we have reiterated ever since, that single measurements of steroid hormones are unhelpful, in the determination of cortisol status and the delivery of hydrocortisone.

With the ability to determine cortisol production rates, it became clear the dosing schedules used and still operative in the 1970's and early 1980's were too high. Although the total hydrocortisone dose had come down to about 15–18 mg/m^2/24 hours, it was still nowhere near the estimated natural cortisol production rate of 8 mg/m^2/24 hours.

Methods for monitoring CAH still relied on 24 hour urine measurements which made it very difficult to determine how to alter the timing of doses of hydrocortisone or indeed the amount.

By the beginning of 1980's several textbooks advocated hydrocortisone doses between 10 and 20 mg/m^2/24 hours which is still a considerably wide range. Again, the majority of these studies used growth rate as the marker for determining how effective treatment was.

In the light of the height and weight problems which had already become apparent, there was an increasing drive to reduce the total exposure to hydrocortisone. A variety of newer monitoring methods were introduced, such as blood spot 17OHP measurements which could be done at home and mailed to hospitals. However, these did not consider the amount of cortisol in the blood at the same time.

Despite these changes and suggestions cortisol replacement remained suboptimal and doses high. The reason for this is largely because of the infrequent sampling methods used and a lack of appreciation of aligning the measurements closely with the hydrocortisone dosing schedule. In addition, the majority of studies only measured 17OHP and not cortisol.

We know 17OHP levels can look quite good yet there can be both over and under treatment during a 24 hour period. This is especially evident when a twice daily dosing schedule was used (see Fig. 17.4).

In CAH it is important to measure both the cortisol and the 17OHP.

FREQUENCY OF ADMINISTRATION OF HYDROCORTISONE

Through the 1990's doses between 10 and 15 mg/m^2/24 hours became more common but the frequency of administration of hydrocortisone remained relatively fixed at twice daily. This largely stemmed from the limited observations of the circadian rhythm where a large dose in the morning was thought to be required, but physicians also realised that overnight suppression of ACTH was required, therefore a large dose was also given in the evening.

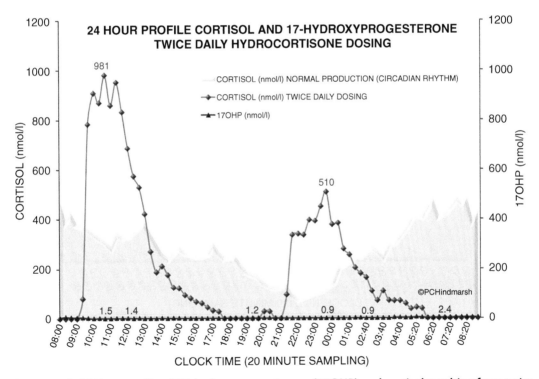

Figure 17.4 *24 Hour profile of 17-hydroxyprogesterone (17OHP) and cortisol resulting from twice daily administration of hydrocortisone showing high peaks with periods of under treatment.*

When we study cortisol derived from the two daily doses of hydrocortisone (blue line) plotted against the circadian rhythm (light blue area) as illustrated in Fig. 17.4, it is evident that the two large doses produced very high peaks of cortisol, causing over exposure to cortisol. On a daily basis, this over exposure leads to short and long term side effects. Many of these side effects are well documented in recent studies conducted in adults with CAH.

The 17OHP depicted in Fig. 17.4 (purple line) is so suppressed by the very high peaks of cortisol, that even when there is no cortisol in the blood stream for several hours, it does not rise very high. It was standard practice to increase the dose, not the frequency of dosing if the 17OHP level increased, which only produced higher cortisol peaks and in some cases this resulted in 17OHP production being totally 'switched off!' (Fig. 17.5).

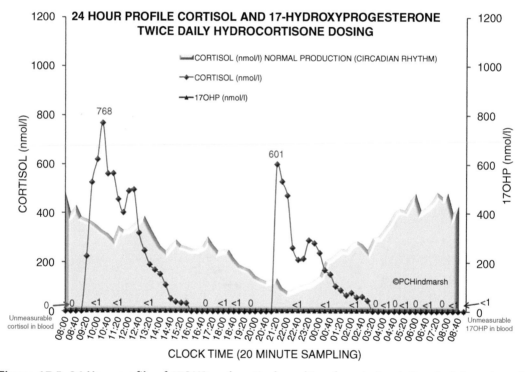

Figure 17.5 *24 Hour profile of 17OHP and cortisol resulting from twice daily administration of hydrocortisone. Note the high cortisol peaks, followed by long periods of time without any cortisol present when the circadian rhythm shows there should be cortisol present. Note there was no measurable 17OHP.*

Like many situations in endocrinology, it was only when the normal circadian rhythm of cortisol became better understood, that different dosing schedules could be attempted. One point that had already been observed with insulin therapy was that better blood glucose control could be achieved by giving smaller doses more frequently.

Initial studies in CAH using 3 times a day regimens which were reported towards the end of the 1990's, suggested this could also apply to CAH and gradually the 3 times a day regimen was introduced (Fig. 17.6). At the turn of the millennium it became apparent that consideration had to be given, not only to the amount of drug administered, but also to how it was handled within the body. Studies started to demonstrate that the clearance of hydrocortisone differed between individuals and that better individualisation of the dosing schedule was going to be required.

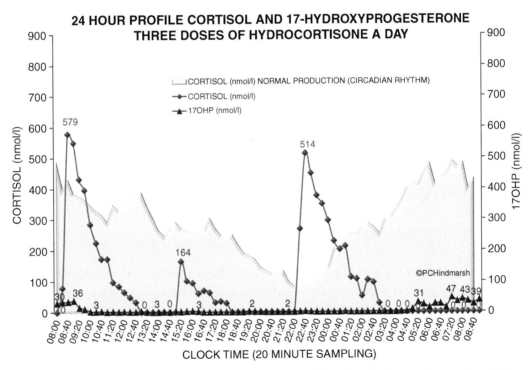

Figure 17.6 *24 Hour profile of cortisol and 17OHP resulting from hydrocortisone given 3 times per day.*

As 17OHP levels are the only measurement taken (and still are by most centres, either by blood spots or one-off blood tests), the measurements in Fig. 17.6 would have shown good control. However, when the cortisol replacement levels are considered, there are periods of under treatment where this patient is totally cortisol deficient, as well as periods of over treatment, where high peaks are obtained when cortisol production is naturally lower.

24 HOUR PROFILES AND DOSAGE CHANGE

Beginning in the early 2000's, it became apparent that 24 hour profiles might provide a better way of assessing drug delivery. The frequent sampling in these studies allowed for a better definition of the peak of cortisol achieved after the intake of hydrocortisone, along with the assessment of how long the high concentrations were obtained and also a useful insight into how fast the individual's cortisol level came down to the baseline value. The ability to also measure other hormones at the same time from the same sample of blood, such as 17OHP, allowed for a better understanding of the dynamics of the cortisol and 17OHP interaction.

This allowed individuals to have a better tailoring of cortisol dosing, so the peak concentrations achieved were not excessive and also there was adequate cover with cortisol during the periods of time when required.

These profiles allowed for a better approximation of the hydrocortisone dose to the attainment of the gold standard which is to mimic the circadian rhythm (the body's normal production) of cortisol. The introduction of these detailed studies allowed for a further reduction in the dose of hydrocortisone used, as well as giving a better distribution of cortisol. By the end of the first decade of the 21st century it was not unusual for doses to have reduced to 10–12 mg/m²/24 hours with some individuals receiving far less than this, whilst achieving better cortisol replacement. This tailoring of the dosing schedule was also associated with lesser effects on body mass index and weight gain.

Over a period of 10 years using this method, we have normalised weight despite the fact that in the general population, weight of course has been increasing steadily. This reduction in hydrocortisone dose and better distribution of cortisol from the more frequent dosing schedules, is also associated with better blood pressure measurements in children and young people.

SEARCH FOR BETTER METHODS OF DELIVERING CORTISOL

The '3 times a day per dosing' schedule is under question. The reason for this is there is accumulating information to suggest that the distribution of cortisol in the 24 hour period, as measured on profiles, will be better achieved by 4 times daily dosing regimen than a 3 times one. Empirically, this has also been observed in the dosing schedules for children where it has been clear, a 4 times per day regimen is required for those under the age of 3 years.

More recently, people have tried to think about delayed or slow release preparation of hydrocortisone. Although these preparations may mimic the circadian rhythm, patients will still suffer from the problem resulting in differences between individual rates of absorption and clearance (Chapter 20). It is important to note that individualisation of therapies will still be required using 24 hour profile data. It is imperative to include careful consideration of both cortisol and 17OHP levels in the individual and dosing should not be calculated using only 17OHP measurements.

It will be important to consider the peak of cortisol, the distribution of cortisol from the preparation and how long cortisol lasts, as the half-life is so variable in individuals (we discuss half-life in detail in Chapter 20).

What the history of dosing has shown, is that you cannot use 17OHP measurements, even if taken before each dose, to determine how much cortisol is in the blood. Getting cortisol levels optimal in replacement is very important as it has multiple effects in the body as shown in Chapter 1 Fig. 1.8.

An extremely promising approach is to again utilise technology derived from diabetes to deliver hydrocortisone. Insulin pump therapy has become the mainstay for achieving good control in diabetes and the same technology can and is being used to deliver hydrocortisone. The advantage of this method is that the pump can continuously infuse varying doses at different times of the day. Clearance and individual handling of cortisol can be worked into the rates and can better mimic the circadian rhythm of cortisol. We consider this further in Chapters 21 and 28 in which the practicalities of this approach are discussed in more detail.

PREDNISOLONE AND DEXAMETHASONE

Prednisolone and dexamethasone which share the same ring structure as cortisol, were not derived initially in their own right. The prototype molecule was in fact 9 alpha-fludrocortisone, the drug we use to replace aldosterone. The chemists were searching for a stronger more potent form of hydrocortisone and introduced the fluorine atom into cortisol. This certainly made the cortisol more potent and it did indeed have the power that dexamethasone has.

It also had an effect on blood pressure and salt and water retention, so although the chemists were trying to design a potent glucocorticoid, the side effects precluded its use for this. We now use it for its salt retaining properties. It was from this that further modifications took place to generate dexamethasone and further work was done to make prednisolone, both of which had longer durations of action and were more potent. These improvements however, were not necessarily associated with a better outcome, because the increase in the duration of action had to be offset against the increase of potency, which in children led to quite marked growth suppression. Essentially, these drugs had a limited place in paediatric practice.

In fact, the main reason for developing prednisolone and dexamethasone was for their potent anti-inflammatory action and not as adrenal replacement therapy.

Both prednisolone and dexamethasone have less water retaining effects compared to hydrocortisone, which was the limiting factor in the amount of hydrocortisone that could be used in arthritis. Prednisolone and dexamethasone have remained as the main anti-inflammatory medications since they were introduced and neither has supplanted hydrocortisone for adrenal replacement therapy. We discuss this further in Chapter 18.

FURTHER READING

Crigler, J.F., Silverman, S.H., Wilkins, L., 1952. Further studies on the treatment of congenital adrenal hyperplasia with cortisone. Pediatrics 10, 397.

CHAPTER 18

Glucocorticoid Treatment

GLOSSARY

Albumin Protein made in the liver. Binds lots of molecules other than cortisol.

Cortisol binding globulin A protein made by the liver which attaches itself to cortisol and carries it around the body. This is known as bound cortisol. 90–95% of cortisol is bound in this way with 5% in the free state. The free cortisol is the biologically active cortisol. In blood tests we measure bound and free cortisol and this is called total cortisol.

Duration of action The time over which a drug or hormone produces a biological effect (i.e. the inflammatory effects of hydrocortisone last for approximately 8–12 hours, which is longer than the drug is in the system).

Glucocorticoid receptor A docking station to which cortisol can attach and be transported into the nucleus of the cell.

Glucocorticoid response element Part of a gene which interacts with cortisol presented by the receptor. The response element can increase or decrease the protein that the gene codes for.

Glucocorticoids Group of steroid hormones (glucose + cortex + steroid) which regulate glucose metabolism and suppress inflammation.

Half-life The time taken for the level of a drug or hormone in the blood, to fall by half the value.

Nucleus Part of the cell which stores all the cells genes.

GENERAL

As we mentioned earlier in the book, glucocorticoids refer to particular steroids produced by the adrenal glands which increase blood glucose concentrations. For practical purposes, when we are considering replacement therapy, there are three mainstays of glucocorticoid replacement. These are hydrocortisone, prednisolone and dexamethasone. These three steroids are very closely related to each other from a structural perspective. Fig. 18.1 shows the structure of the common glucocorticoids: hydrocortisone, prednisolone and dexamethasone. The red arrows point to changes made to the hydrocortisone atom in order to form prednisolone (double bond) and dexamethasone (double bond and fluorine atom). These changes make these two

Congenital Adrenal Hyperplasia. http://dx.doi.org/10.1016/B978-0-12-811483-4.00018-0

steroids stronger acting than hydrocortisone. The red 'F' is a fluorine atom which is added and this prolongs the action of dexamethasone.

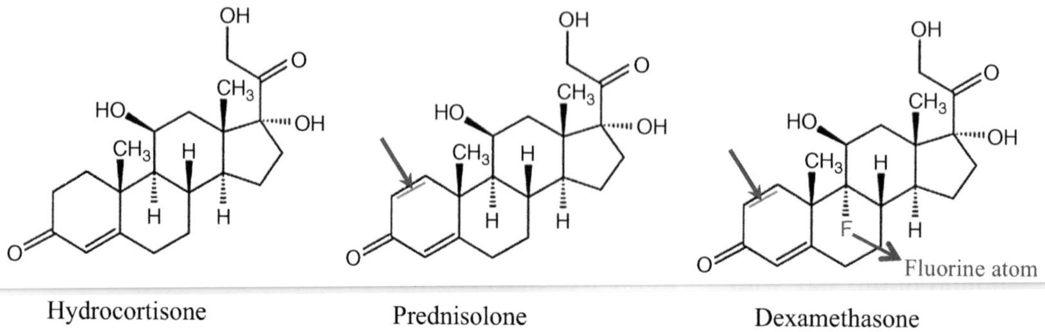

Hydrocortisone   Prednisolone   Dexamethasone

Figure 18.1 *The structures of hydrocortisone, prednisolone and dexamethasone.* *Prednisolone differs from hydrocortisone by the presence of a double carbon bond (red arrow) and dexamethasone differs from prednisolone by the introduction of a fluorine atom.*

Generally speaking, hydrocortisone is the preferred glucocorticoid for replacement therapy of cortisol in CAH. Hydrocortisone replaced cortisone acetate which was used in the early years of CAH treatment. The problem with cortisone acetate was that it is needed to be metabolised in the liver to cortisol, which limited its potency. Prednisolone is slightly stronger than hydrocortisone and dexamethasone is considerably more potent than both of them.

We will see further in this section actual profiles of hydrocortisone. Prednisolone has a very similar profile to hydrocortisone but its duration of action is much longer. The potency of prednisolone is much greater in terms of growth suppression. This limits its use in pediatric practice and has proven very difficult to use in a way which does not inhibit growth.

Dexamethasone has received some popularity recently because it is thought that it can be given once (but needed more than likely twice) a day. The main problem with dexamethasone, is that in the current form, it has an extremely flat profile. This means whilst it could easily be titrated to match the troughs of the circadian rhythm, at other times of the day the individual is under treated. Equally, if one tried to match the peaks there would be times of the day when over treatment would result. Although there have been reports of successful use, these have been associated with increased weight gain in the individuals and at this stage dexamethasone is not used as the first line of treatment in CAH.

HOW DO GLUCOCORTICOIDS WORK?

Glucocorticoids, whether made by the adrenal glands or if taken as tablets, enter into the blood stream and most of the glucocorticoid becomes attached to proteins which are present in the blood. These proteins are known as carrier proteins or binding proteins. There are two main ones for the glucocorticoids, cortisol binding globulin (CBG) and albumin.

These binding proteins carry cortisol to the various tissues of the body. It is only the unbound cortisol (free cortisol) which is active. We have talked a lot about steroids produced by the adrenal glands. When these steroids are produced they are immediately passed into the blood stream. However, the body is quite good at removing them from the blood stream and breaking them down, particularly in the liver. To prevent too much loss immediately after production, the body has within the circulation, a pool of special proteins attracted to the steroid family. These proteins attach themselves (bind) to the steroids, which means there is now a pool of steroid in the blood attached to the protein, which is really useful as it prevents rapid breakdown in structures such as the liver. The blood can then carry the steroid attached to the protein, to the various places around the body where the steroid needs to act.

CORTISOL BINDING GLOBULIN

Cortisol is no exception to this rule and it attaches itself to a special protein called cortisol binding globulin (CBG). This means that in the blood at any particular point, there is cortisol which is not attached to any protein known as free cortisol and cortisol which is attached to CBG is known as a bound cortisol (Fig. 18.2).

Free Cortisol

Cortisol Binding Globulin (CBG)

©PCHindmarsh

Figure 18.2 *The interaction in the blood between cortisol and cortisol binding globulin (CBG).*

When we carry out a blood test, we measure both the free and the bound cortisol and this is called the total cortisol concentration (Fig. 18.3). In fact, we do not always call it this, we simply refer to it as the plasma cortisol concentration but to be technically correct, we should really call it the total plasma cortisol concentration.

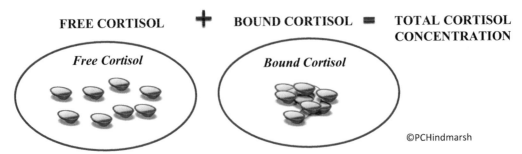

FREE CORTISOL ✛ BOUND CORTISOL ▬ TOTAL CORTISOL CONCENTRATION

Free Cortisol

Bound Cortisol

©PCHindmarsh

Figure 18.3 *Actual sticking of free cortisol onto CBG in the blood which yields bound cortisol.*

This means when we are interpreting cortisol levels we have to remember some is free and some is bound. Under normal circumstances this does not matter too much, but when CBG levels change, e.g. in people who take the oral contraceptive pill (Fig. 20.7), then the total cortisol concentration we measure will change as well. Using the oral contraceptive pill as an example, we know if we measure cortisol levels in the individual taking the pill, the plasma cortisol concentration, in other words total plasma cortisol concentration, will be high because more CBG is present which will bind more cortisol, raising the total cortisol concentration. What happens is the free cortisol concentration does not change much, at least initially. If you are taking hydrocortisone however, unless the dose is changed, more cortisol will be taken up and bound so there will be less free cortisol.

This becomes important because it is free cortisol which carries out all the action around the body. If more of your cortisol is bound, there is less free, so you might develop symptoms of being cortisol deficient even though when you measure and look at the total cortisol concentration, it looks normal because the extra is bound.

This all adds extra complexity but is extremely important to understand, because it influences many of the things we do with hydrocortisone replacement. We have seen one example with the oral contraceptive pill. Another example, is the whole question of whether you should double or triple or quadruple doses during illnesses. We all know that the standard teaching is to double the cortisol dose. The question is, what does doubling the dose, tripling or even quadrupling the dose achieve?

The answer is perhaps surprising at first. If you double and particularly triple the dose, e.g. go from 10 mg per day of hydrocortisone to 30 mg per day, you do not triple the amount of cortisol in the blood. So although you might triple the dose, in fact the cortisol concentrations in the blood barely double. This happens because of the presence of the binding proteins. When you give more cortisol, if you start to exceed blood levels of 450–500 nmol/l then the proteins (CBG) to which cortisol can attach, become saturated. In other words, there is a limit to how much cortisol can stick onto the protein. Once this threshold is reached there will be an increase in the amount of free cortisol, but because this is removed very easily by the liver and the kidney, the amount of total cortisol you actually achieve will not go up proportionately with the amount you are taking. This means if you double the dose of hydrocortisone when unwell, you probably will just about double the cortisol level. Although it might be tempting to triple the dose, this will not lead to a triple level of cortisol in the blood as the threshold will be exceeded and the extra cortisol that is being taken, will be lost in the urine. CBG plays a vital role in helping with the way cortisol works.

The real reason why we have these proteins, is not simply to act as a buffer and store, but because cortisol itself does not dissolve very easily in the blood. CBG binds up to 90% of all cortisol in the blood, which means there is only about 4–10% free in the blood to get into cells to act. The way in which cortisol attaches itself to CBG varies considerably between individuals, but even more importantly it is also influenced by body temperature. As body temperature increases, e.g. during a fever, the amount of cortisol which attaches itself to CBG decreases, so this becomes really important when we have a fever because the free cortisol that becomes available, particularly to the local tissues, nearly triples. This is a really interesting and important observation, because it is one of the ways in which the body protects itself and gets cortisol out to where it needs to be working in situations of stress and illness. So, although we do not necessarily double or triple the amount of cortisol in the blood when we double or triple the hydrocortisone dose, what will happen, particularly in local tissues, is that free cortisol will actually increase, so this is a very handy protective way the body has to ensure that during illness, the tissues of the body get exactly the right amount of extra cortisol they need.

What we are now going to consider is how cortisol instructs the cells of the body to do all the things that it is capable of. Nearly two thirds of human genes are regulated by cortisol. Cortisol influences our genes by instructing them to switch off or on and make proteins.

Free cortisol can cross easily into cells. Within the cell is a special docking station for cortisol, the cortisol receptor. On attaching to the receptor, the cortisol receptor complex moves into the nucleus of the cell. The nucleus contains all the genes that we have and once in there, the cortisol receptor complex attaches to specific parts of genes known as glucocorticoid response elements. It is through this attachment that cortisol then influences the gene to switch on and produce the proteins that it codes for, or to switch off (Fig. 18.4).

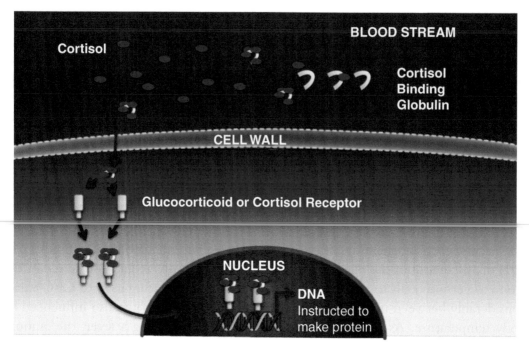

Figure 18.4 *Cortisol gains entry into the cell where it docks with a special glucocorticoid or cortisol receptor.* *This complex moves into the nucleus of the cell and attaches to a glucocorticoid response elements on DNA. This attachment tells the gene to make the mRNA that goes on to form the protein that cortisol regulates.*

HOW DO THE GLUCOCORTICOIDS COMPARE?

Glucocorticoids can be compared in a number of ways. From a drug action perspective we can think of them in terms of how long they last in the body. You may hear people talking about the potencies of the various glucocorticoids. This idea of how strong a glucocorticoid is, came about because of the need to standardise the use of these agents for their anti–inflammatory properties. It became apparent that dexamethasone had a greater anti–inflammatory effect than hydrocortisone and also possibly less of an effect on blood pressure. The glucocorticoids were then rated on this anti–inflammatory property. This rating system worked well in terms of comparing the dosages of drug needed to combat inflammation. However, it became clear that a different rating scale was needed when considering the effect of glucocorticoids on growth. Fig. 18.5 shows that compared to hydrocortisone, prednisolone and dexamethasone are 5 and 80 times more likely on a dose for dose basis, to suppress growth. Note also that the duration of action and peak of action differ. These relate to the half-life of the drug which is the time taken for 50% of the drug to disappear from the blood stream.

Glucocorticoid	Hydrocortisone	Prednisolone	Dexamethasone
Half-Life in Blood (hours)	1.5	2–3	3.5–4.5
Duration as Glucocorticoid (hours)	~6	~8	~12
Duration of Inflammatory Action (hours)	~8–12	~12–36	~36–54
Time to Peak Level (hours)	1–2	3–4	Rather flat profile
Growth Suppressing Effect	1	5	80
Dosing Effect on Growth (mg)	30	6	0.35–0.45

Figure 18.5 *Table comparing the duration and peak of action of the three glucocorticoids hydrocortisone, prednisolone and dexamethasone along with effects in dosing terms on growth.*

The data help us start to determine what the window for dosing with glucocorticoids in CAH should be. We know that we require approximately 12 mg of hydrocortisone/metre square body surface area/day (we write this as 12 mg/m^2/day) to suppress ACTH production and therefore switch off the adrenal glands. The actual growth suppressing dose of hydrocortisone is approximately 30 mg/m^2/day, so there is quite a wide gap (we call this the therapeutic window) between the dose we need to produce an effect and the dose that will produce a side effect, in this case growth suppression. For weight gain the weight gaining dose is 18–20 mg/m^2/day, even doubling the dose for illness, e.g. will still be within this therapeutic window.

The data also tell us that when we are working out glucocorticoid replacement doses, we must include all steroids which have a glucocorticoid effect. For example, fludrocortisone which is given to help retain salt because it is a mineralocorticoid, also has the same glucocorticoid potency as dexamethasone, so we need to include it in the calculations when we are thinking of how much glucocorticoid is needed to suppress the adrenal. Fifty micrograms of fludrocortisone has the same effect as 4 mg of hydrocortisone, so this is important to factor into the calculations, otherwise over treatment can easily happen.

As hydrocortisone is the mainstay of glucocorticoid treatment in CAH, the rest of this section deals with this medication in detail.

FURTHER READING

Hindmarsh, P.C., 2009. Management of the child with congenital adrenal hyperplasia. Best Pract. Res. Clin. Endocrinol. Metab. 23, 193–208.

Speiser, P.W., Azziz, R., Baskin, L.S., Ghizzoni, L., Hensle, T.W., Merke, D.P., Meyer-Bahlburg, H.F., Miller, W.L., Montori, V.M., Oberfield, S.E., Ritzen, M., White, P.C., 2010. Congenital adrenal hyperplasia due to steroid 21-hydroxylase deficiency: an Endocrine Society clinical practice guideline. J. Clin. Endocrinol. Metab. 95, 4133–4160.

CHAPTER 19

Glucose and Cortisol

GLOSSARY

Adrenalin A catecholamine that raises blood pressure and heart rate, as well as providing a rapid increase in blood glucose. This produces a rapid increase in blood glucose over a 30–60 minute period.

Cortisol The major glucocorticoid in humans. Made in the adrenal glands. Cortisol regulates over two thirds of human genes. Cortisol regulates blood glucose, muscle function, the body's response to infection, fat distribution and brain thought processes.

Glucagon Produced in the pancreas and instructs the liver to release stored glucose into the blood stream. This produces a rapid increase in blood glucose over a 30–60 minute period.

Growth hormone A protein made by the pituitary gland, which is secreted in bursts particularly overnight. It causes cartilage to divide and expand in size under the influence of its target protein insulin-like growth factor-1.

More@4 During periods of illness a double dose equal to the usual morning dose, to be taken at 4 a.m. (04:00), followed by normal double morning dose to be taken at the usual time. This additional dose is taken to prevent hypoglycaemia occurring in the early hours of the morning.

GENERAL

Blood glucose is maintained at a very constant level between 4 and 6.5 mmol/l. Occasionally, it may dip slightly lower than this to 3.5 mmol/l in young children who fast overnight. The tight regulation of glucose is brought about by an interaction between hormones which raise blood glucose, namely glucagon, adrenalin, cortisol and growth hormone and the only hormone that can reduce glucose, which is insulin. This is why diabetes occurs and is quite common, because there is only one hormone available to bring down blood glucose, compared to the four which are available to increase it. In this section, we are going to consider blood glucose and the way in which cortisol interacts with various systems to maintain blood glucose levels within a very tight range.

Congenital Adrenal Hyperplasia. http://dx.doi.org/10.1016/B978-0-12-811483-4.00019-2

GLUCOSE AND CORTISOL INTERACTION

As we have shown in earlier chapters, cortisol appears in the blood with a circadian rhythm. In other words, there are times of the day when cortisol concentrations are high and others when they are low. It is interesting when we look at this rhythm, that the times when cortisol concentrations are high or rising, are times when the body is subject to periods when food is usually absent. For example, during the night/early morning period cortisol levels start to rise very late at night and peak in the early hours of the morning. Given that during this period there is no food intake, this rise in cortisol is probably protective in that it increases the amount of glucose available to the body. This would mean we can go to sleep safe in the knowledge that our blood glucose will remain steady because cortisol will be working on different tissues, in particular fat, to liberate glucose and therefore energy.

Blood glucose is extremely important for all parts of the body, especially the brain. Unlike other parts of the body, the brain is totally dependent on blood glucose. The stores of glucose in the brain in the form of glycogen are very low and would only last 20 minutes. It is therefore imperative the brain has easy access to a ready supply of glucose and is why so many hormones are available to raise blood glucose and prevent it from going low, an event known as hypoglycaemia.

WHAT HAPPENS THEN IN CONGENITAL ADRENAL HYPERPLASIA?

People, particularly newborns with CAH before the diagnosis is made, are susceptible to hypoglycaemia. Cortisol plays an important role in raising blood glucose but the most important factors which raise blood glucose quickly are glucagon and adrenalin. Growth hormone and cortisol have a much slower effect (2–4 hours to have a maximum effect) on raising blood glucose.

In CAH where cortisol is missing and if hypoglycaemia occurs it, is not possible for the body to be able to get out of difficulty very easily.

As long as there is a steady input of glucose from food then all will be well. As we know however, before diagnosis particularly in the newborn period, a crisis might take place and part of the crisis is the person vomits. Any vomiting which takes place will mean that the steady stream of glucose the body needs, will be interrupted and because the stores of glycogen in the newborn and young infant are very low, hypoglycaemia will ensue very quickly. This is why, in an adrenal crisis particularly in the young, blood glucose is low.

However, there is another problem in this situation.

It might be thought that adrenalin and glucagon are still present and will be able to raise the blood glucose quickly. Under normal circumstances this would be the case. However, because of the way the adrenal glands are constructed, adrenalin, which is made by the adrenal glands, needs local cortisol production to ensure adequate amounts of adrenalin are made. The blood flow in the adrenal glands goes from the outside right through to the middle (Fig. 19.1).

Cortisol producing cells are located in the outside layer known as the cortex, whereas the adrenalin producing cells are in the medulla i.e. the middle of the adrenal glands. If cortisol production cannot take place in these outer cells, cortisol cannot be released into the small blood vessels that run between the cortex and the medulla, meaning that adrenalin production is compromised.

Adrenalin production is not completely abolished but is reduced and this creates problems for the individual, not only have they lost cortisol which they could not make anyway, but because of this loss of cortisol, production of adrenalin is also impaired. This double hit leaves the individual very susceptible to hypoglycaemia developing.

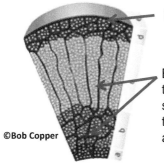

©Bob Copper

Blood flows in below the capsule

Blood flows though small vessels in the cortex collecting the adrenal steroids including cortisol and carries them to the centre or medulla of the adrenal glands

a. Medulla
b. Zona Reticularis
c. Zona Fasciculata
d. Zona Glomerulosa
e. Capsule

Figure 19.1 *Blood flow in the adrenal glands. Blood comes in via the adrenal artery which branches and supplies firstly the entire capsule or surface of the gland. Blood then moves into the cortex and collects the adrenal steroids including cortisol and carries them down to the centre or medulla of the adrenal glands. The blood then leaves the adrenal glands through the adrenal veins.*

GLUCOSE AND EXERCISE

Incidentally, we also see this problem influencing the body's response to exercise. Exercise causes a natural rise in glucose in the blood stream and post exercise there is often a slight rise observed. This glucose rise is not observed in individuals with CAH despite good cortisol replacement. If we measure cortisol after taking tablets, either as a normal dose or double dose prior to exercise, we do not see the rise in blood glucose during or after exercise. This effect is due to the lack of adrenalin or epinephrine production from the adrenal gland.

This can be seen in these pictures where doctors have studied cortisol, glucose and epinephrine (adrenalin) in individuals with CAH, undertaking 20 minutes of standard exercise (Fig. 19.2).

Participants had good cortisol levels due to having taken their tablets and cortisol does rise slightly in normal individuals following exercise. The glucose blip which occurs approximately 10–20 minutes after exercise is finished, is not due to lack of cortisol, because cortisol levels are very similar in those with CAH and those who do not have the condition.

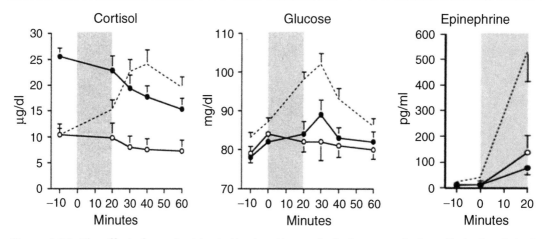

Figure 19.2 *The effect of exercise (shaded bar) on the cortisol, glucose and adrenalin (epinephrine) response. Patients with congenital adrenal hyperplasia are shown receiving low (open circles) and high (closed circles) dose of hydrocortisone. The response of people without congenital adrenal hyperplasia is shown by the dotted line. (Reproduced with permission from Green-Golan, L., Yates, C., Drinkard, B., VanRyzin, C., Eisenhofer, G., Weise, M. and Merke, D.P., 2007. Patients with classic congenital adrenal hyperplasia have decreased epinephrine reserve and defective glycemic control during prolonged moderate-intensity exercise. J. Clin. Endocrinol. Metab. 92 (8), 3019–3024).*

The big difference is in the epinephrine (adrenalin) panel where there is reduced production which explains the lack of glucose rise. This interaction between cortisol and adrenalin is extremely important for the full effects of adrenalin production.

The situation can become even worse if there are lots of hypoglycaemic episodes, because the adrenalin response becomes naturally blunted in its own right.

What all this means for an individual with CAH requiring cortisol treatment, is during periods of stress such as illness or trauma, they will be very susceptible to developing hypoglycaemia. This is most likely to occur in children because their glycogen stores where reserve glucose is held, are very low. Anything which upsets the normal delivery of glucose to the blood stream such as from food, is likely to lead to problems.

MORE AT 4 A.M.

Further, in CAH we know that the dosing schedule does not always equal that of the circadian rhythm. We have seen there is a period of time from about 4 a.m. (04:00) through to when the first dose is given at 6 a.m. (06:00), where cortisol levels are extremely low and often undetectable.

This leaves the individual with potential problems in terms of waking with hypoglycaemia, because just when cortisol concentrations should be increasing or high to keep blood glucose up, in individuals receiving cortisol by tablets, levels are actually falling or are undetectable.

This is the reason why we have suggested individuals should have 'More at 4 a.m.'.

In other words, during periods of illness we recommend they receive a double dose equal to the usual morning dose at 4 a.m. (04:00), followed by their normal double morning dose at 6 a.m. (06:00) or 7 a.m. (07:00). This is to tide them over and prevent developing hypoglycaemia in the early hours of the morning. Fig. 19.3 illustrates this.

When we look at the data in Fig. 19.3, we can see the last dose in the evening is taken at 8 p.m. (20:00) just before this young patient's bedtime and the next dose is given at 7 a.m. (07:00) on waking.

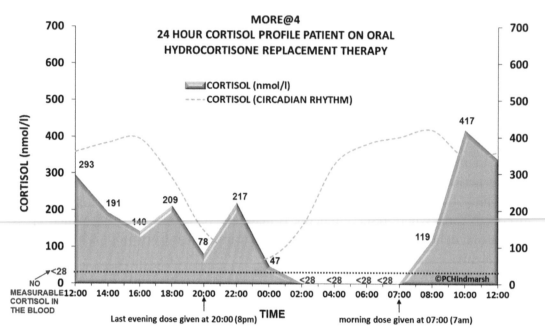

Figure 19.3 *Cortisol levels overnight resulting from the last dose given at 8 p.m. (20:00) showing the period in the early hours of the morning where there is no measureable cortisol in the blood.*

The profile shows this patient is without any measurable cortisol in the blood from 2 a.m. (02:00) for a period of 5 hours until the morning dose is taken at 7 a.m. (07:00). If we compare cortisol levels the adrenal glands would naturally produce during this period, (blue dashed line) it is easy to see the difference in how little is present, compared to how much the body should have in the blood stream.

We must also remember that increasing the last dose taken at 8 p.m. (20:00), or even doubling the dose will not make the 8 p.m. (20:00) dose last longer. What will happen is cortisol will peak higher and in illness, the body needs this extra cortisol. However, between 2 a.m. (02:00) and 7 a.m. (07:00) the patient will still be cortisol deficient and vulnerable to hypoglycaemia as well as adrenal crisis.

The data in Fig. 19.4 show even though this older patient takes their last dose of hydrocortisone at 11 p.m. (23:00), there is no cortisol in the blood from 4 a.m. (04:00). Again, doubling or tripling the 11 p.m. (23:00) dose will not make cortisol last longer and cortisol levels will fall dangerously low or become totally undetectable at the time where we can see the normal cortisol production is high. We also need to remember in illness the body needs extra cortisol during this period where there is none.

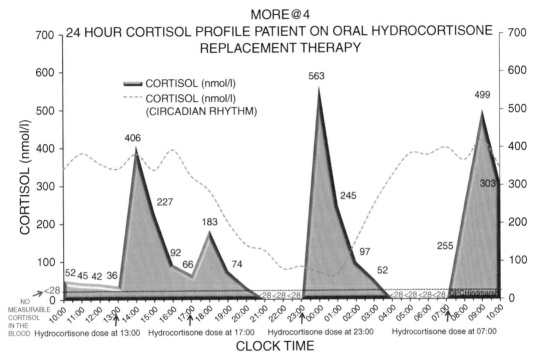

Figure 19.4 *Cortisol levels during the night when the dose is given later at 11 p.m. (23:00). As cortisol from hydrocortisone only lasts for approximately 6 hours, there is still a period of time in the early hours when cortisol cannot be measured in the blood.*

Therefore it is important, no matter what time of day the last dose is given, to give an extra double dose at 4 a.m. (04:00) to prevent low blood glucose levels.

These observations also mean people with CAH should not fast for periods longer than 6 hours. Consequently, if they have to fast for a surgical procedure then a glucose drip may be needed if the fast is for more than 6 hours.

We have also seen that if cortisol levels are maintained within the normal circadian rhythm, the blood glucose remains at a constant value. Fig. 19.5 shows this for a person on pump therapy where glucose is constant throughout the 24 hour period.

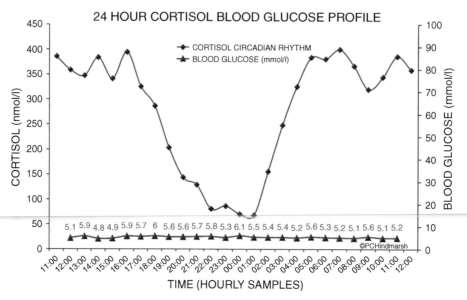

Figure 19.5 *Blood glucose is constant throughout the 24 hour period although the circadian rhythm of cortisol is maintained using pump therapy.* This illustrates the value of mimicking as close as is possible the circadian rhythm with replacement therapy.

WHAT HAPPENS IN THE BODY WHEN BLOOD GLUCOSE FALLS?

Blood glucose can fall either because there is too much insulin present or too little of the hormones adrenalin, glucagon, growth hormone or cortisol (Fig. 19.6). Low blood glucose is known as hypoglycaemia meaning low (hypo) glucose.

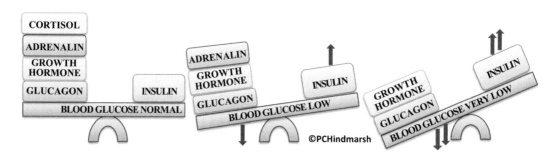

Figure 19.6 *On the left the normal balance between insulin, adrenalin, glucagon, growth hormone and cortisol when blood glucose is normal.* The middle panel shows an increase in insulin and reduction in adrenalin, glucagon, growth hormone or cortisol leading to low blood glucose. The right panel shows the more common situation in adrenal problems where insulin is switched off or is still present but adrenalin and cortisol are missing. The result is very low blood glucose.

Fig. 19.7 shows the changes which take place in the body when blood glucose starts to drop low. As blood glucose decreases from 5 to 4 mmol/l, insulin is switched off.

This is a 'sensible' event which occurs as it stops the only hormone which can reduce blood glucose from being produced.

If the switch off of insulin does not help the problem, then the next step in the process is to switch on the hormones which increase blood glucose, or what are known as the counterregulatory hormones. These are glucagon, adrenalin, growth hormone and cortisol.

Glucagon and adrenalin as previously stated, act quite quickly whereas growth hormone and cortisol have a much slower effect on blood glucose.

Sequence of Response to Falling Arterial Plasma Glucose

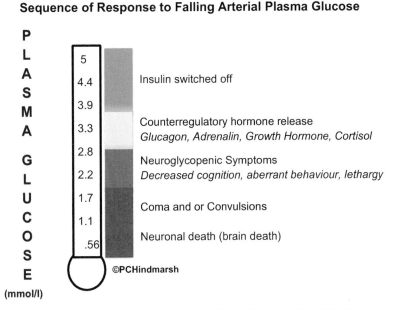

Figure 19.7 *Sequence of events which take place as blood glucose levels fall.* To convert to blood glucose units used in North America (mg/dl) multiply by 18.

As blood glucose drops a little further down to 3.3 mmol/l, a series of additional signs and symptoms become apparent in the person. These can be divided into two types. Firstly, those associated with the effects of low blood glucose on the brain such as inability to do tasks in the classroom, behavioural changes and ultimately seizure and coma if the blood glucose falls too low.

Secondly, other signs and symptoms are due to the activation of various alert systems in the brain, which are designed to draw attention to the fact there are problems taking place in the body. These are called neurogenic affects and rely on a variety of nerve systems to lead to an increase in heart rate, sweating, a feeling of hunger and increase in blood pressure. These effects are all trying their best to alert the person to what is taking place so they will be able to do something about the changes such as increase food intake.

Low blood glucose is a particular problem in children, as glucose is an essential source of energy for brain function, brain reserves of glycogen do not last long and reserves of alternative fuels to provide energy for the cells are limited. Even fasting overnight in children who do not have any problems at all, can deplete the stores.

We have mentioned some of the signs and symptoms which occur when blood glucose is low, but it is often very difficult for young children in particular to recognise these and they are often unable to communicate how they feel to adults. Due to this, it is sensible for parents to have small blood glucose testing systems so during periods when the child is unwell, they can measure blood glucose and if necessary, take appropriate action to raise the blood glucose value.

BLOOD GLUCOSE MEASUREMENT

There are a number of systems available for testing blood glucose. They all rely on taking a finger prick blood sample and measuring how much glucose is in the blood using a test strip. These are very handy little meters and are pocket sized (Fig. 19.8). They are very accurate and give a result very quickly, within 30 seconds. However, it is important to ensure that they are properly setup and the blood test strips are in date.

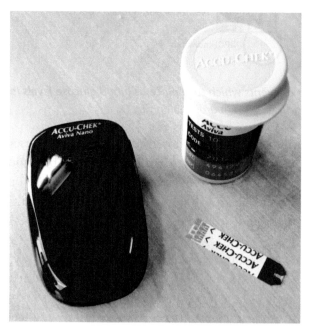

Figure 19.8 *Example of blood glucose meter and the test strip for blood glucose testing.*

WHAT TO DO IF BLOOD GLUCOSE IS LOW?

The most important thing in CAH is to try and prevent low blood glucose happening. This is why we have such strict rules regarding sick days because it is extremely important to ensure there is a good delivery of cortisol, not only by doubling the dose which is usually given, but also giving an extra double dose at 4 a.m. (04:00), when we know that cortisol levels from the previous night hydrocortisone dose are likely to be low. More at 4 a.m. (04:00) and double dose during illness or trauma are both ways in which we can prevent hypoglycaemia.

If however, the child becomes hypoglycaemic which means a blood glucose test reading less than 4 mmol/l, then it is advisable to give 15 g of glucose. This glucose has to be what is called 'readily available' in other words neat glucose. This can be found in orange drinks and in fizzy drinks such as Coca-Cola (not diet or sugar free). For example, 100 ml of Coca-Cola contains exactly 15 g of glucose. We recommend they have this and follow on with regular sugary drinks, throughout the period of illness.

Giving 15 g of glucose will increase the glucose very quickly and you should retest, to make sure that the increase has happened, 15 minutes after giving the 15 g of glucose. If this has not raised the blood glucose, then repeat with a further 15 g of glucose and retest 15 minutes later. If the child cannot tolerate any oral glucose you can use the 'Glucogel' in the emergency pack which you squirt around the gums or into the cheek. Glucose is absorbed very quickly this way and will rapidly rectify low blood glucose. Glucogel, formally known as 'Hypostop' raises sugar levels very quickly and provides a fast acting energy boost in the form of Dextrose Gel (40% dextrose). It comes in a tube which contains 10 g of fast acting glucose and we recommend one full tube to be applied around the gums.

An emergency injection of hydrocortisone will also increase the blood glucose but as we have said, it is a slower process, so the best solution to get on top of the blood glucose problem quickly is to give some easily available glucose. If this is not tolerated, or cannot be given, then give extra hydrocortisone either by doubling the tablets or by emergency injection. You should then give the Glucogel, as this order of events ensures normalisation of the blood glucose will take place quickly and be sustained.

So if the child is having an adrenal crisis:

1. Give intramuscular hydrocortisone.
2. Then apply Glucogel to the gums and cheek.

CONCLUSIONS

Hypoglycaemia is not a common problem in CAH, but is one to look out for when the child becomes unwell and normal supplies of glucose through food become compromised. In addition, during trauma and sickness, cortisol requirements do increase and double dosing of cortisol is required along with 'More at 4'. These preventive measures should be sufficient in the majority of situations to avoid hypoglycaemia.

Hypoglycaemia in CAH is a little more complex than just cortisol deficiency, because the production of adrenalin, which is one of the hormones the body uses to get out of problems very quickly when hypoglycemia occurs, is compromised in its production, so there is a double hit in the way that young people with CAH can respond to hypoglycaemia. Awareness of the problem is extremely important.

Modern blood glucose testing is easy to do at home and simple rules of giving small amounts of glucose to increase blood glucose, the untoward effects of hypoglycaemia, can be avoided.

FURTHER READING

Butler, P.C., Rizza, R.A., 1989. Regulation of carbohydrate metabolism and response to hypoglycemia. Endocrinol. Metab. Clin. North Am. 18, 1–25.

Green-Golan, L., Yates, C., Drinkard, B., VanRyzin, C., Eisenhofer, G., Weise, M., Merke, D.P., 2007. Patients with classic congenital adrenal hyperplasia have decreased epinephrine reserve and defective glycemic control during prolonged moderate-intensity exercise. J. Clin. Endocrinol. Metab. 92, 3019–3024.

CHAPTER 20

Hydrocortisone

GLOSSARY

Absorption rate Speed at which a drug is taken up from the gut. Derived from the time when taken as a tablet to the time a peak level is achieved in the blood.

Clearance How fast or slow the body removes a drug from the circulation.

Cortisol The major glucocorticoid in humans. Made in the adrenal glands. Cortisol regulates over two thirds of human genes. Cortisol regulates blood glucose, muscle function, the body's response to infection, fat distribution and brain thought processes.

Duration of action The time over which a drug or hormone produces a biological effect (i.e. the inflammatory effects of hydrocortisone last for approximately 8–12 hours, which is longer than the drug is in the system).

Half-life The time taken for the level of a drug or hormone in the blood, to fall by half the value.

WHAT IS HYDROCORTISONE?

Hydrocortisone is a synthetic preparation of the steroid hormone cortisol. Hydrocortisone is a glucocorticoid because by definition it increases the amount of glucose in the blood. We looked at the glucose cortisol relationship in Chapter 19. Hydrocortisone also has some salt retaining properties which distinguishes it from prednisolone and dexamethasone as they do not have the same salt retaining property.

Hydrocortisone comes in various forms and the one used in replacing cortisol are tablets that are taken orally. There are other preparations which are administered either by subcutaneous infusion using the pump method, intramuscular injections, or intravenously as well as suppositories. Each preparation works differently once administered and we discuss the other preparations in more detail in Chapter 27.

ORAL HYDROCORTISONE

How much of an oral dose gets into the body?

There are two parts to this question, first what is in a hydrocortisone tablet and second what happens once the tablet has been taken.

Congenital Adrenal Hyperplasia. http://dx.doi.org/10.1016/B978-0-12-811483-4.00020-9

1. Hydrocortisone comes in tablet form and the tablets contain lactose monohydrate, pregelatinised starch, calcium stearate as well as hydrocortisone usually in the acetate form. The additional agents are known as fillers and are used usually to bulk out the tablet. Different manufacturers use different fillers and the amount of hydrocortisone in a tablet from different manufacturers can vary. Although the packet may say 10 mg, there is an acceptance it may vary by plus or minus 8–10%. This means it is very important that once you start using a particular brand, you stay with that brand otherwise the levels you get may vary.

2. As taking hydrocortisone on an empty stomach can cause problems such as gastritis (inflammation of the stomach wall) and in the long term stomach ulcers, it is best taken after food, or with milk. The way hydrocortisone appears in the blood, depends on whether the tablet is taken on an empty stomach or not and absorption can be slowed slightly, if the tablet is taken with food. When we measure cortisol in the blood after taking a hydrocortisone dose, the picture we get looks something like that in Fig. 20.1. The dose taken here was a high dose and the cortisol peak amount is variable not only due to the individual's size and metabolism (Fig. 20.10), but also the time of day (Fig. 23.7) and whether there is any cortisol left in the system on which the dose would stack (Figs 21.7 and 21.8). So the important thing is what the pattern looks like rather than the absolute amount attained. We will look at fine tuning doses to get the peak right later.

Hydrocortisone is absorbed very quickly from the gut. In fact, the absorption is usually very efficient and generally, almost 95% is absorbed. The graph shows it takes approximately 1–2 hours for hydrocortisone to peak and approximately 6 hours before it is fully eliminated from the blood stream.

When you take hydrocortisone orally (Fig. 20.2) the tablet is absorbed very quickly from the gut; it then passes from the gut into the liver via the hepatic portal system. From here it passes from the liver through the venous circulation into the right side of the heart. It then flows through the pulmonary arteries through the lungs and back through the left side of the heart. It then passes through the aorta which is the main artery in the body, into circulation.

So this tells us a lot about how hydrocortisone is absorbed but not everyone is the same.

The time when the peak is achieved can vary between 20 and 180 minutes, so this individual variation in absorption needs to be factored into the dosing schedule and we do this using our profile work.

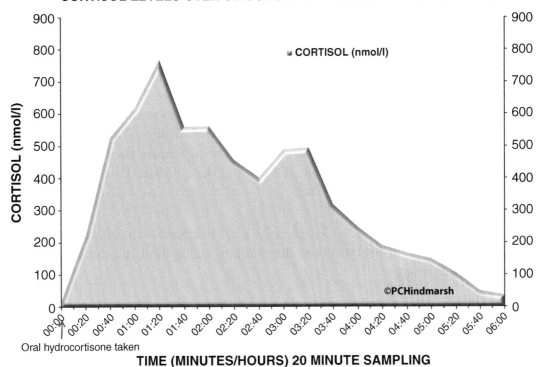

CORTISOL LEVELS OVER 6 HOURS AFTER TAKING HYDROCORTISONE

Oral hydrocortisone taken

TIME (MINUTES/HOURS) 20 MINUTE SAMPLING

Figure 20.1 *Blood profile after taking a high dose of hydrocortisone (tablets) at Time 00:00.*

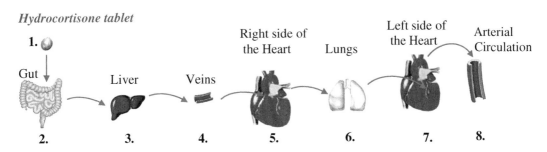

1. Ingestion of oral hydrocortisone tablet.
2. Absorbed in the gut.
3. Carried from the gut to the liver by hepatic portal system.
4. Carried from the liver through the venous (veins) circulation into the right side of the heart.
5. From the right side of the heart carried through the pulmonary arteries to the lungs.
6. From the lungs it is carried back to the left side of the heart.
7. From the left side of the heart it is them pumped out into the aorta.
8. From the aorta it is carried through the arterial circulation.

Figure 20.2 *Steps involved in the uptake of hydrocortisone from the gut and distribution into the blood stream.*

HOW FAST IS THE HYDROCORTISONE REMOVED FROM THE BODY WHAT IS HALF-LIFE?

The situation is further complicated by how fast people clear cortisol from the blood stream. The half-life of a drug is the time it takes to remove half the concentration of drug from the body, in other words, the time it has taken from its maximum peak level to reach half of that maximum peak level, is the half-life. This is an important number because it also tells us how long it will take to remove the drug completely from the blood. It actually comes out at 4.5 times the half-life. This is for any drug not just hydrocortisone.

If we look at the graph in Fig. 20.3 we can see what is termed as the pharmacokinetics which is the study of drug absorption, distribution, metabolism and excretion which is relevant to all drugs.

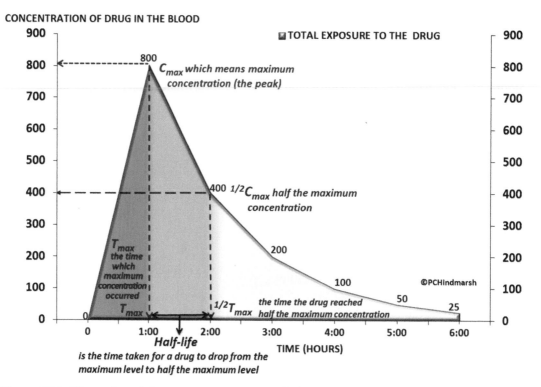

Figure 20.3 *Illustration of the parameters measured after intravenous injection of a drug in this case hydrocortisone.*

Hydrocortisone is also used for its anti-inflammatory properties to treat other conditions such as arthritis, colitis and when used for this purpose, the anti-inflammatory effect lasts longer than the drug stays in the blood stream. This is known as the duration of action. The duration of action for hydrocortisone is approximately 8–12 hours, whereas the drug as cortisol lasts approximately 6 hours depending on the individual half-life.

This happens because glucocorticoids act on cells via their receptor, an area we cover in Chapter 18. When they do this, there is a time lag between the glucocorticoid attaching itself to the cell and having its effect on the DNA machinery in the cell. This produces various target proteins which all have effects in the cell, or perhaps locally. All this takes time and this is termed as the duration of action. Duration of action therefore, includes the time we can actually measure the glucocorticoid in the body, plus the effect on the target cells. For example, the glucose raising effect of cortisol is at maximum about 4–6 hours after the peak cortisol level is achieved, at a time when cortisol levels are falling or are low. Fig. 20.4 illustrates this point.

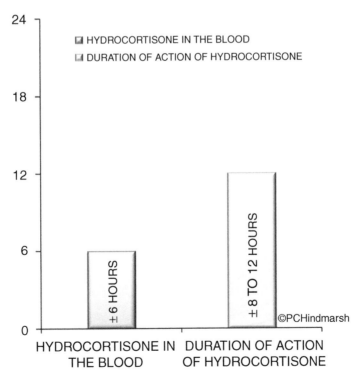

Figure 20.4 *Difference in time between how long cortisol is present in the bloodstream compared to how long it actually acts on the target organs.*

CLEARANCE

The clearance of any drug is the time it takes for the drug to be completely removed from the blood plasma. The half-life has an influence on this because the shorter the half-life, the quicker the clearance will be. Every drug is cleared from the system in around 4.5 half-lives.

To achieve the optimal dosing schedule, you need to have optimal concentration of the drug in the blood plasma for which we use a scientific mathematical formula, which includes both the maximum concentration achieved (C_{max}) and the time it takes to achieve the maximum concentration (T_{max}), to calculate not only the optimal maximum concentration, but also the half-life and clearance. We do this to prevent both short and long term side effects.

Another important factor is that it does not matter what the total maximum concentration of the drug is, i.e. how high the peak is, the half-life does not change. We can see an example of this in the data in Fig. 20.5 where we have used various cortisol levels and show the clearance time from the peak using the half-life.

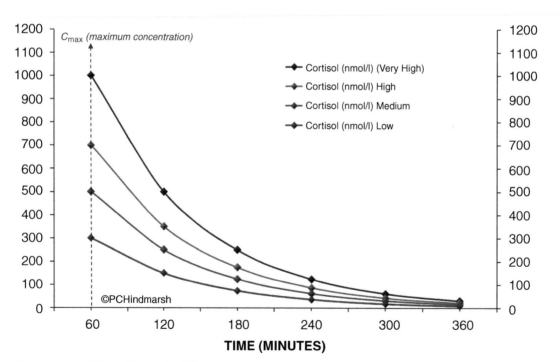

Figure 20.5 *The effect of different starting* C_{max} *concentrations on subsequent cortisol concentrations. Half-life is constant.*

In Fig. 20.5 we can see the different peak levels (C_{max}) and the cortisol measurements which decrease over the 360 minutes (6 hours). The half-life is constant. It is important to note that the highest maximum concentration of 1000 nmol/l does not last much longer in time than the lowest concentration of 300 nmol/l, in fact when we look at the values at 360 minutes the 1000 nmol/l has dropped to 31.5 nmol/l and 300 nmol/l down to 9.37 nmol/l, not all laboratories can measure these very low cortisol levels. Of note, cortisol levels in normal production do not normally fall this low, so even though the 31.5 nmol/l is higher than the 9.37 nmol/l, both these readings are below normal values.

HALF-LIFE OF HYDROCORTISONE

The half-life of cortisol (hydrocortisone) is approximately 80 minutes. This means for example, if in the blood you have at any one time 600 nmol/l of cortisol, then 80 minutes later there would only be 300 nmol/l left. Again there is variation in this (Fig. 20.9).

There are various factors which can influence the half-life of hydrocortisone.

The main site of cortisol metabolism is the liver. The hepatic enzyme found in the liver which is called 11β-hydroxysteroid dehydrogenase type 1 (11β–HSD1) biologically converts inactive cortisone to cortisol (Fig. 20.6).

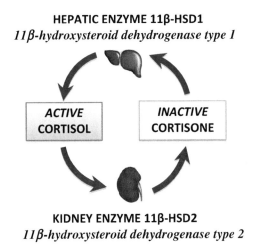

HEPATIC ENZYME 11β-HSD1
11β-hydroxysteroid dehydrogenase type 1

ACTIVE CORTISOL

INACTIVE CORTISONE

KIDNEY ENZYME 11β-HSD2
11β-hydroxysteroid dehydrogenase type 2

Figure 20.6 *Action of 11β-hydroxysteroid dehydrogenase type 1 and type 2.*

Cortisol is the active form and to ensure there is balance, 11β–hydroxysteroid dehydrogenase type 2 converts cortisol to cortisone. This system is known as the cortisol shuttle. Overall, the net effect is that 11-beta HSD1 serves to increase the local concentrations of biologically active cortisol in a given tissue; 11–beta HSD2 serves to decrease local concentrations of biologically active cortisol, particularly in the kidney.

11β–Hydroxysteroid dehydrogenase type 2 is predominantly found in the kidneys, so you can measure the effect of this enzyme in urine collections where we look at the ratio of cortisol to cortisone metabolites. Measuring the activity of the type 1 enzyme is not as easy to do as you either need a tissue sample from the liver, or undertake a cortisone acetate loading test. The latter is difficult to do as cortisone acetate is no longer available.

The results obtained are shown in Fig. 20.7 which shows a rise in cortisol as the cortisone is converted in the liver into cortisol.

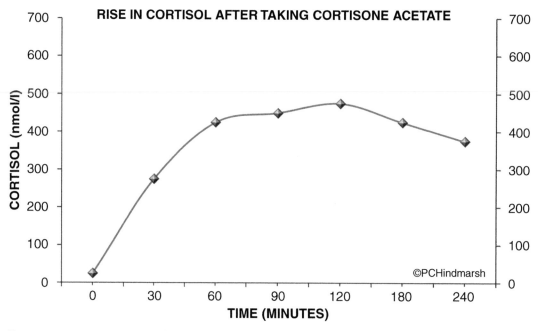

Figure 20.7 *Rise in cortisol after taking oral dose of cortisone acetate. The rise reflects the activity of 11β-hydroxysteroid dehydrogenase type 1 in the liver.*

In addition to 11β-hydroxysteroid dehydrogenase type 1 in the liver, there are other enzymes which metabolise cortisol by modifying the ring structure and then adding on sulphate or glucuronic acid to facilitate excretion in urine.

We can measure these metabolites in the urine (see Chapter 8). Cortisol is also metabolised into 5–alpha tetrahydrocortisol (5–alpha THF) and 5–beta tetrahydrocortisol (5–beta THF), reactions for which 5–alpha reductase and 5–beta reductase are the rate-limiting enzymes, respectively. 5–beta reductase is also the rate-limiting factor in the conversion of cortisone to tetrahydrocortisone (THE). An alteration in 11–beta HSD type 1 has been suggested to play a role in the pathogenesis of obesity, hypertension and insulin resistance known as metabolic syndrome (Fig. 20.8).

Metabolic Syndrome is a constellation of features which arise as a result of a primary defect in the action of insulin on cells. This is known as insulin resistance. To overcome this, the pancreas makes more insulin which then triggers a series of other responses in other tissues, all due to the high insulin levels. These tissues include fat, leading to obesity, the blood vessels leading to high blood pressure and the liver where the balance is shifted towards the production of LDL-cholesterol from HDL-cholesterol. LDL-cholesterol is the cholesterol which is associated with heart attacks.

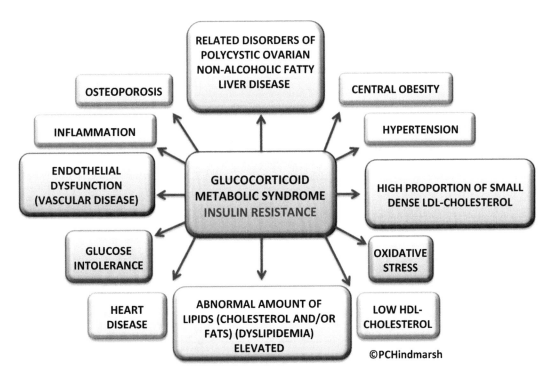

Figure 20.8 *The components of the Metabolic Syndrome. Glucocorticoids, if present in high amounts lead to impaired insulin action and insulin resistance which is the central part of the syndrome.*

Glucocorticoids also raise insulin levels in the blood if the cortisol or steroid level is high for long periods of time. This is why in Fig. 20.8, glucocorticoids producing insulin resistance are at the centre of the Metabolic Syndrome as these are factors which drive the person to develop this problem.

MEDICATION CAN ALSO ALTER THE HALF-LIFE AND CLEARANCE

We have a list of medications which show how they affect hydrocortisone at the end of the chapter (Fig. 20.15). However, as an example, we will discuss the effect of the contraceptive pill on hydrocortisone and anyone who is on glucocorticoid replacement and plans to start taking the contraceptive pill, should discuss this with their endocrinologist before starting.

The contraceptive pill

Estrogen in the oral contraception pill alters the way in which hydrocortisone is handled in the body and means the total amount of cortisol present might increase, so dose adjustments may be needed to cope with the changes (Fig. 20.9).

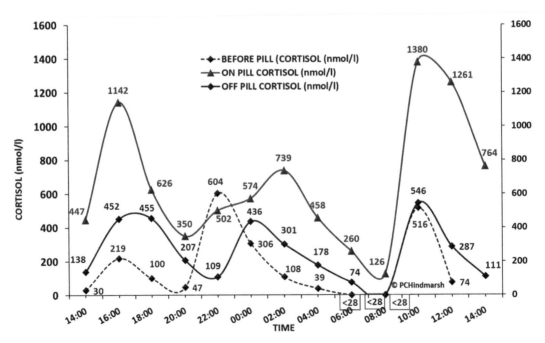

Figure 20.9 *Effect of introducing and then stopping the oral contraceptive pill on cortisol levels. The pill markedly increases the total cortisol measures (red line) compared to values pre (purple dashed line) and post (blue line) taking the oral contraceptive pill.*

CALCULATING DOSES

It is very important to consider all the aforementioned factors when calculating doses and working out dosing schedules.

In Fig. 20.10 we can see the vast variation in the half-life of a study done in 58 individuals on hydrocortisone replacement. None of the individuals were on any known medication which could influence the half-life, yet the half-life data ranged from 225.3 to 40 minutes. The slowest half-life was 225.3 minutes which means hydrocortisone would last a lot longer in this patient and therefore they would probably only need two to three doses of medication a day.

The fastest half-life was 40 minutes and this individual needed six doses a day to achieve reasonable concentrations of cortisol in the blood. The individual also needed higher doses to achieve the optimal concentrations in the blood.

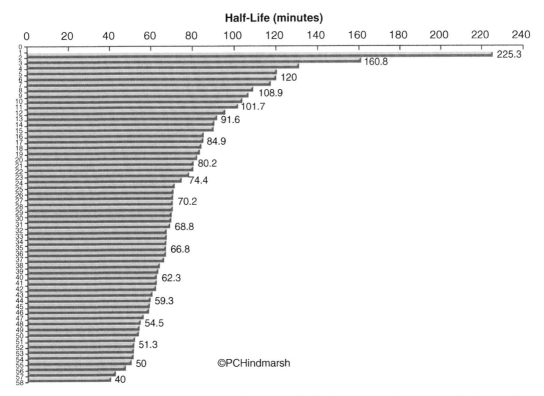

Figure 20.10 *Half-life of cortisol measured in 58 individuals showing large variation from 40 to 225.3 minutes.*

The situation can become very complicated, as you might have people who absorb slowly, but clear either quickly or slowly and people who absorb quickly and clear either quickly or slowly.

So a quick absorber/quick clearer might need very frequent doses, whereas a slow absorber/slow clearer might have good cortisol replacement on twice a day medication. The message is, therapy has to be individualised.

This is reinforced as we have mentioned, by the fact that cortisol is cleared from the body by several mechanisms such as, removal by the kidneys, metabolism in the liver and inactivation to cortisone. All these pathways differ between individuals.

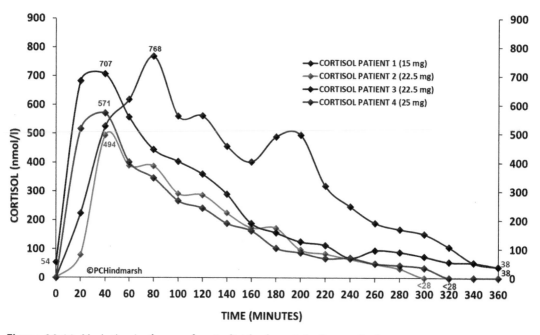

Figure 20.11 *Variation in the way four individuals metabolise cortisol.*

In Fig. 20.11 we can see the variance in how these four individuals metabolise hydrocortisone. Each patient is of a similar age and BMI. They were given a higher dose than their usual dose. Patient 3 (blue line) was the only one to have a measurement of cortisol (54 nmol/l) in the sample taken prior to the oral dose being taken. Blood samples were taken every 20 minutes to measure cortisol.

What is remarkable is Patient 1 who took the lowest dose of 15 mg of hydrocortisone:

1. Reached the highest peak level.
2. Took the longest time to reach this peak (80 minutes).
3. Still had a value of 38 nmol/l after 6 hours (360 minutes).

This patient would be classed as a slow absorber and slow metaboliser.

Patient 2 (green line) and Patient 3 (blue line) both took the same dose, although Patient 3 (blue line) had a value of 54 nmol/l prior to the dose being taken, even if we exclude this from the peak value of 707 nmol/l, the peak from the dose would be 653 nmol/l which is far higher than the peak achieved in Patient 2 (green line) at 494 nmol/l. Both peak around the same time of 40 minutes; however, there is a difference in how they metabolise the cortisol. Patient 2 (green line) has no measurable cortisol at 300 minutes (5 hours after taking the tablet), whereas Patient 3 (blue line) still has a measurement of 38 nmol/l at 360 minutes (6 hours after taking their tablet).

Patient 4 (red line) who took the biggest dose of 25 mg, achieved a lower peak of 571 nmol/l at 40 minutes, than Patient 1 (purple line), who achieved a peak of 768 nmol/l at 80 minutes when taking a dose of 15 mg. The 25 mg dose was also metabolised faster. Patient 4 (red line) was cortisol deficient at 320 minutes compared to the 15 mg dose taken by Patient 1 (purple line), who still had a value of 38 nmol/l at 360 minutes (6 hours).

Understanding the impact of differences in absorption and clearance is important in interpreting 24 hour profiles and getting the dosing schedule right. What has been suggested as a more useful way to describe the way cortisol is handled in the blood, is something called the terminal plasma half-life. Terminal plasma half-life starts to take into account how the drug is absorbed as this will impact, as we have seen, on the peak level and also how long it takes to get to the peak. We are only just starting to understand this idea as the mathematics of it is quite daunting!

Although daunting, we will probably in the future need to think carefully on this. What we described in terms of absorption and half-life are the classic ways that a drug has been assessed. The intravenous study however, and to a certain extent the absorption type of study, are different to what actually happens. For example, in people who can make cortisol and in the intravenous study, cortisol goes straight into the veins and to the heart (step 4 onwards in Fig. 20.2). However, tablet treatment uses the gut and portal blood system that goes to the liver first (all these steps can be seen in Fig. 20.2). This means there will be direct removal of some cortisol by the liver when taking tablets, before cortisol has a chance to get to the organs of the body.

In this situation, what we get in the blood will depend on lots of things, but importantly what the liver does. Quite a large part of clearance is probably determined by heredity influencing on how the genes which regulate the enzymes that handle cortisol, work. In addition, age and gender might influence clearance. We know there is a difference in the pattern of growth hormone secretion between males and females and that these patterns can influence how the liver enzymes work. If you can produce cortisol normally, then these differences probably do not matter as you can always alter the amount of cortisol made which we can see in Figs 21.2 and 21.3 where cortisol values are similar. However, in CAH where fixed doses might be used, this may not be the case and unless you are being checked with 24 hour cortisol profiles, it will not be possible to tell whether there are problems or not. All this is important.

One final point to remember about clearance is that it is also a valuable way to regulate cortisol levels. In people with normal adrenal function, if too much cortisol is produced, the body will clear it more quickly to keep levels unchanged. If the system is saturated, then levels will rise. This allows the body to keep to its set level of sensitivity to the hormone, as the next stage of defence would be to make the tissues less sensitive to cortisol when levels are too high. This may be a very important issue for cortisol replacement, although at present, we do not have a lot of information on this. The situation may be even more complex because it is possible that liver clearance of cortisol and kidney clearance of cortisol may be regulated differently!

Now we want to introduce you to how this all works in clinical practice. When patients have elevated 17OHP, there is a temptation for the doctors to increase the dose of medication. This is quite a natural response but may not actually be the right one.

The reason for this is the way in which the body removes hydrocortisone is quite efficient as we have seen previously when we talked about half-life.

Now imagine two situations which are shown in Fig. 20.12:

1. Firstly, after a standard dose of hydrocortisone of say 10 mg, the maximum blood level of cortisol achieved is 500 nmol/l. Eighty minutes later we expect the blood value to be about 250 nmol/l.

2. Secondly, now imagine that you give an increase in the dose to 12.5 mg. This would increase the peak value to about 600 nmol/l, but 80 minutes later the actual value of cortisol in the blood would only be 300 nmol/l, so from that increase in dose the actual amount of cortisol getting around the circulation and holding out in the circulation, is not great. Indeed, if we take this out to 6 hours, the actual difference at that particular point between the 10 mg dose and the 12.5 mg dose is almost negligible (3 nmol/l in fact!).

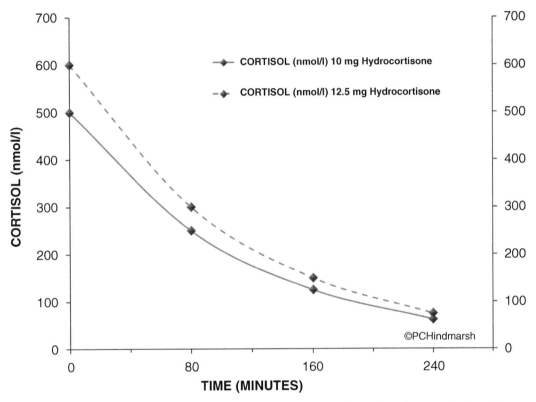

Figure 20.12 *Two doses of hydrocortisone one 25% greater than the other producing different peaks at time zero but similar levels at 240 minutes (4 hours).*

So an important point here is that it is not just a question of increasing the amount of hydrocortisone, it is also important how often it is given.

When people are running out of hydrocortisone too quickly the answer is not to give more but to give it more frequently.

SIDE EFFECTS

We now need to think about how best to monitor hydrocortisone replacement in CAH, but before we get into the real detail of this, it is worth looking at the side effects profile of hydrocortisone, as well as contraindications. The side effects profile applies to prednisolone and dexamethasone equally.

Cautions

In children and adolescents growth retardation is the main concern. High blood pressure can result with the use of high doses and there is also a potential problem with the way glucose is handled by the body.

Osteoporosis may be problem, although in CAH there is little evidence for this in the short term, but in older patients problems have been reported in the 40 years + population. In fact, this may also relate to chronic salt loss rather than glucocorticoids themselves.

Contraindications

It is important to remember that hydrocortisone in CAH is replacement therapy. This means it is safe to receive all vaccinations.

Excess Glucocorticoid

Short Term Therapy	Long Term Therapy
Gastritis	Gastric ulcers
Growth arrest	Short stature
Increase in appetite	Weight gain
Hypercalciuria	Osteoporosis, fractures
Glycosuria	Slipped epiphyses
Immune suppression	Ischemic bone necrosis
Masked symptoms of infection, esp. fever and inflammation	Poor wound healing
Toxic psychoses	Catabolism
Headaches	Cataracts
Hypertension (high blood pressure)	Bruising (capillary fragility)
	Adrenal/pituitary suppression
	Toxic psychosis
	Striae – stretch marks

Figure 20.13 *Complications of high dose glucocorticoid therapy.*

Inadequate Glucocorticoid

Short Term Therapy	Long Term Therapy
Growth acceleration	Short stature as bone maturation advances
Reduced appetite	Weight loss
Low blood sugar	Muscle weakness
Tiredness	Hypotension (low blood pressure)
Collapse	Impaired fertility
Headaches	Adrenal rests or TART
Increased body hair	Skin pigmentation from high ACTH levels

Figure 20.14 *Complications of using too low dose glucocorticoid therapy.*

Drug interactions

Some drugs alter the way hydrocortisone is metabolised in the blood and it is important to always check with your doctor if you are prescribed any of the following drugs listed in the table (Figs 20.13–20.15). The table shows on the left, the particular drug and on the right what effect hydrocortisone will have on the effect of that drug. Some drugs, like the barbiturates or the oral contraceptive pill, upset hydrocortisone metabolism and how much cortisol appears in the blood as a result, so a lot of care is needed when taking these medications together.

ACE Inhibitors	Antagonism of hypotensive effect
Acetazolamide	Increased risk of hypokalaemia
Adrenergic Neurone Blockers	Antagonism of hypotensive effect
Alpha-blockers	Antagonism of hypotensive effect
Aminoglutethimide	Metabolism of glucocorticoids accelerated (reduced effect)
Amphotericin	**Increased risk of hypokalaemia (avoid concomitant use unless glucocorticoids needed to control reactions)**
Angiotensin-II Receptor Antagonists	Antagonism of hypotensive effect
Antidiabetics	Antagonism of hypoglycaemic effect
Aspirin (also Benorilate)	Increased risk of gastro-intestinal bleeding and ulceration Glucocorticoids reduce plasma-salicylate concentration
Barbiturates and Primidone	**Metabolism of glucocorticoids accelerated (reduced effect)**

Beta-blockers	Antagonism of hypotensive effect
Calcium-channel Blockers	Antagonism of hypotensive effect
Carbamazepine	**Accelerated metabolism of glucocorticoids (reduced effect)**
Carbenoxolone	Increased risk of hypokalaemia
Cardiac Glycosides	Increased risk of hypokalaemia
Clonidine	Antagonism of hypotensive effect
Coumarins	**Anticoagulant effect possibly altered**
Diazoxide	Antagonism of hypotensive effect
Diuretics	Antagonism of diuretic effect
Diuretics, Loop	Increased risk of hypokalaemia
Diuretics, Thiazide and related	Increased risk of hypokalaemia
Erythromycin	Erythromycin possibly inhibits metabolism of glucocorticoids
Hydralazine	Antagonism of hypotensive effect
Ketoconazole	Ketoconazole possibly inhibits metabolism of glucocorticoids
Methotrexate	Increased risk of haematological toxicity
Methyldopa	Antagonism of hypotensive effect
Mifepristone	Effect of glucocorticoids (including inhaled glucocorticoids) may be reduced for 3-4 days after mifepristone
Minoxidil	Antagonism of hypotensive effect
Moxonidine	Antagonism of hypotensive effect
NSAIDs	Increased risk of gastro-intestinal bleeding and ulceration
Nitrates	Antagonism of hypotensive effect
Nitroprusside	Antagonism of hypotensive effect
Estrogens	Oral contraceptives increase plasma concentration of glucocorticoids
Phenytoin	**Metabolism of glucocorticoids accelerated (reduced effect)**
Progestogens	Oral contraceptives increase plasma concentration of corticosteroids
Rifamycins	**Accelerated metabolism of glucocorticoids (reduced effect)**
Ritonavir	Plasma concentration possibly increased
Somatropin	Growth promoting effect may be inhibited
Sympathomimetics, Beta$_2$	Increased risk of hypokalaemia with concomitant use of high doses
Theophylline	Increased risk of hypokalaemia
Vaccines	High doses of glucocorticoids impair immune response; avoid use of live vaccines

Figure 20.15 *List of drugs that are known to alter the handling of glucocorticoids or are affected by glucocorticoids.*

CONCLUSIONS

The dose and frequency of hydrocortisone dosing, needs to be altered in individuals depending on the half-life of cortisol in the circulation and the absorption of oral hydrocortisone from the gastrointestinal tract, to avoid over and under dosing and the associated side effects.

FURTHER READING

Charmandari, E., Johnston, A., Brook, C.G.D., Hindmarsh, P.C., 2001. Bioavailability of oral hydrocortisone in patients with congenital adrenal hyperplasia due to 21-hydroxylase deficiency. J. Endocr. 169, 65–70.

Hindmarsh, P.C., Charmandari, E., 2015. Variation in absorption and half-life of hydrocortisone influence plasma cortisol concentrations. Clin. Endocrinol. 82, 557–561.

CHAPTER 21

Dosing and the Circadian Rhythm

GLOSSARY

Circadian rhythm Changes in hormone levels, in this case cortisol, throughout the 24 hour period where values peak in the morning and reach low levels late evening.

Cortisol replacement dose This is worked out in relation to the normal cortisol production rate over 24 hours and takes into account cortisol that is lost through the gut.

Metabolism of cortisol The way cortisol is absorbed, carried around the blood and cleared from the circulation.

Over stacking The phenomenon which happens if the timing of doses is incorrect. Occurs where the dose is taken to too early and builds onto the cortisol remaining from the previous dose, leading to higher cortisol levels than would have been expected from the dose given.

Stacking The addition of a dose upon another dose within a certain time frame, usually the time the drug is in the circulation.

Useful stacking Cortisol is added when cortisol drops to a desired level, which not only prevents levels dropping too low but also allows a smaller amount to be added to give the optimal peak.

DOSING WITH HYDROCORTISONE

Generally speaking, hydrocortisone is the preferred glucocorticoid for replacement therapy of cortisol in congenital adrenal hyperplasia.

Why is hydrocortisone used and not the longer acting steroids?

We have discussed this in Chapter 18. It would seem a great idea to be able to move to taking a single dose of glucocorticoid which would last the whole 24 hour period, or failing that a twice daily regimen. Indeed, in the past as discussed in Chapter 17, we used to use hydrocortisone twice per day but the results from many studies suggested that a 3 times per day administration gave much better overall suppression of 17OHP and cortisol cover which led to less of an increase in body weight, than caused by the very high peaks which occurred with twice a day dosing. Further studies have shown that as hydrocortisone lasts for around 6 hours and there are 24 hours in a day, 4 times a dosing gives an overall better distribution of cortisol over the period.

Congenital Adrenal Hyperplasia. http://dx.doi.org/10.1016/B978-0-12-811483-4.00021-0

251

Dosing 4 times a day allows smaller, more frequent doses which approximate better to the normal cortisol circadian rhythm.

When we consider all the information on how hydrocortisone works in the body and the variance between the half-life, clearance and absorption of the medication, what is clear is that dosing needs to be tailored to the individual and using a blanket formula for all will not give optimal cortisol coverage. Suboptimal distribution of cortisol will lead to both short and long term side effects.

THE BODY'S NORMAL PRODUCTION OF CORTISOL

In Chapter 1 we looked at the circadian rhythm of cortisol. One of the main rules of endocrinology is to replace the missing hormones, as close as possible to the way that the body would naturally produce them. Studying the data obtained by performing 24 hour profiles allows us to start to think about how we might do that.

The graph in Fig. 21.1 shows the average cortisol levels from 28 children and adolescents with samples drawn every 20 minutes for the 24 hour period.

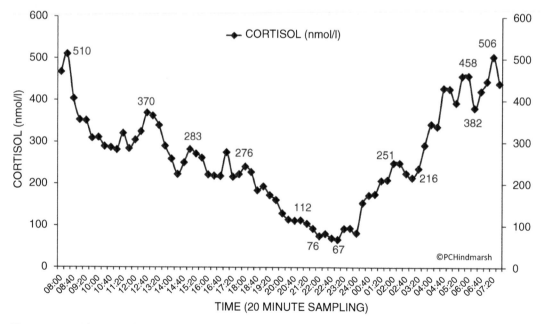

Figure 21.1 *The circadian rhythm of cortisol in the blood.* The data are the average cortisol levels from 28 children with samples drawn every 20 minutes for the 24 hour period. Cortisol is low at 22:00 then rises to a peak in the early hours of the morning returning gradually back to low values in the late evening. Actual values are shown next to some of the data points.

The amount of cortisol can vary to some extent between individuals but the pattern which is the circadian rhythm, remains remarkably reproducible between individuals. There are several important points to note from this profile:

- The body is not without cortisol at any point in time although the values are low at about 10 p.m. (22:00).
- From this very low value in the evening, the amounts in the blood start to rise progressively until they reach a peak in the early hours of the morning between about 6 a.m. and 8 a.m. (06:00–08:00). This is due to the increased drive of ACTH from the pituitary which forms a significant surge from around 3 a.m. (03:00) onwards.
- This increase in cortisol remains during the morning hours and only starts to decline to the low values in the late evening from early afternoon.

If we are to mimic the physiological situation then we would need to take different doses of hydrocortisone throughout the daytime. How often hydrocortisone should be taken is determined by how long it takes to remove cortisol from the blood stream.

We also need to think about whether things differ with age. Do adults have different cortisol levels to children? The graphs in Fig. 21.2 show the circadian rhythm in adult males and females compared to that of boys and girls. What we can see is that the circadian pattern is the same between adults and children. The peak cortisol is achieved at the same time around 7 a.m. (07:00) and the level attained similar. The main difference is when the lowest cortisol level is achieved.

Notice that the cortisol level is never zero. There is always cortisol present.

We have shown the lowest values in the graphs. For boys and girls this occurs between 10:30 p.m. (22:30) and 11:00 p.m. (23:00), whereas for the adults it occurs slightly later at midnight. This is because the children went to bed earlier than the adults. Notice that the rise in cortisol starts earlier in the children compared to the adults as well.

So the patterns and levels do not differ appreciably with age, but are there differences between males and females? Fig. 21.3 looks at this. We can see that the circadian pattern is superimposable between the males and females irrespective of age. There is no real difference between when the peak cortisol occurs between the sexes or the actual peak level and the time of the lowest cortisol value.

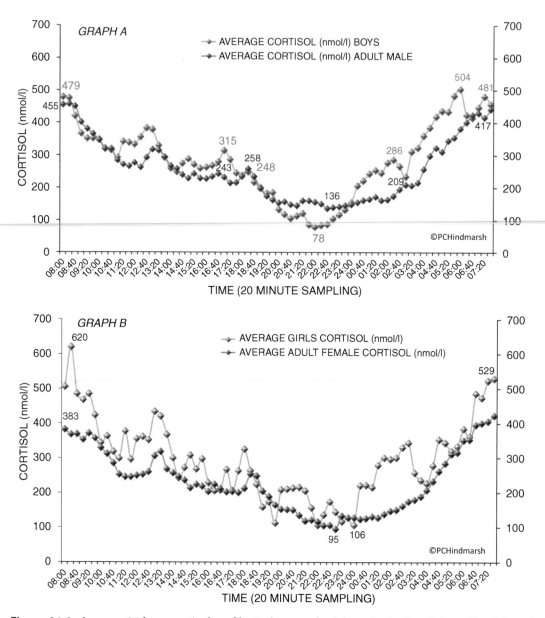

Figure 21.2 *Average 24 hour cortisol profiles in boys and adult males in Graph A and in girls and adult females in Graph B.* Samples were taken at 20 minute intervals during the study. There were 28 children in the study and 80 adults.

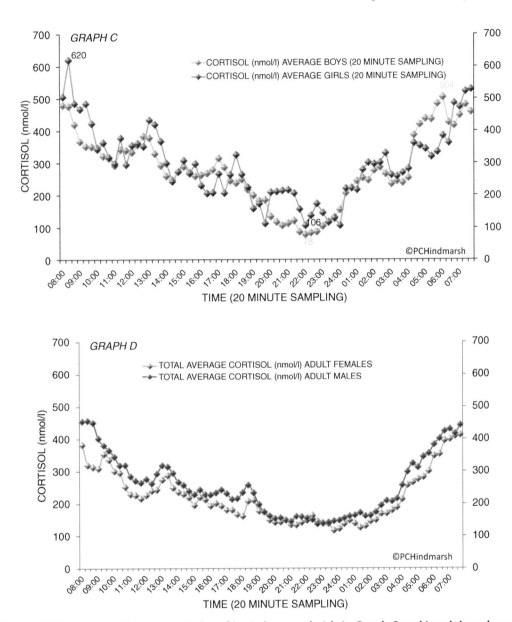

Figure 21.3 *Average 24 hour cortisol profiles in boys and girls in Graph C and in adult males and females in Graph D.* Samples were taken at 20 minute intervals during the study. There were 28 children in the study and 80 adults.

These are very important pieces of information, because it means we can use a standard representation of the circadian rhythm to aim for in males and females and at any age. It also shows us cortisol is always present in the blood stream and rarely goes below 50 nmol/l. These observations now give us good values to aim for when we start to replace with hydrocortisone.

However, we still need to remember absorption and clearance of hydrocortisone which we explained in Chapter 20, are very important factors we need to introduce to attain these cortisol values and best mimic the circadian rhythm.

Do we need any more information? Does measuring 17OHP help in addition to knowing what cortisol levels we are achieving are? This is an important question as many hospitals only measure 17OHP rather than cortisol. 17-Hydroxyprogesterone is only one part of the story as we shall see in the next chapters.

THE DISTRIBUTION OF CORTISOL AND IMPORTANCE FOR DOSING

Circadian dosing

You might hear a lot of discussion at meetings and in medical literature about the idea of circadian dosing. This simply is a way of trying to administer hydrocortisone so it mimics the normal circadian rhythm. Central to this idea, is understanding how cortisol is actually produced and distributed through the 24 hour period.

From measuring cortisol in the blood, we can by using some very clever mathematical formulas, work out what the adrenal glands would have to do to be able to produce this amount of cortisol in the blood at any one time. Using this technique we have been able to determine two important points.

Firstly, the total production rate of cortisol by the adrenal glands is about 8–10 mg/m^2 body surface area/day. We talked about this in Section Two when we were thinking about poor growth and weight gain. This is a rather strange term 'per mg/m^2/day' and what it tells us is that the amount of cortisol produced is signified by the mg (milligrams) (weight), we then standardise this expression in terms of the period (day) and also in terms of a unit of body size (body surface area in square meters; m^2). The body surface area is like taking off all the skin and laying it out flat and seeing how much ground it will cover. Perhaps an odd idea, but one that works well when thinking about drug doses! So this is a very useful number to know about. When using oral medications we have to take into account that some is lost in the gut

(Chapter 20). In fact, when we are thinking of replacement therapy for CAH we are talking about doses between 10 and 12 mg/m^2/day.

There is a slight variation in this and some people only need about 8 mg/m^2/day, yet others might go up to about 16 mg/m^2/day and this is due to their individual clearance which is very variable. Fast clearers will need higher hydrocortisone doses and will need to take doses more frequently than slow clearers.

The importance of this number is that it gives us a rough estimate of the amount of hydrocortisone we might expect an individual to need. The exact amount however, can only be worked out by a careful study of how cortisol is actually delivered into the blood stream by the hydrocortisone and to do this we need to obtain 24 hour profile measurements.

Secondly, we are also able to work out what the cortisol distribution derived from the dose should be between the split times. The actual timing of the doses to achieve these amounts would need to take into account the individual's metabolism of hydrocortisone. We can see the percentage in the given time frames we need to aim to achieve in Fig. 21.4.

Please note this is *only* for oral dosing schedules.

TIME	PERCENTAGE OF DAILY DOSES
00:00	30
06:00	35
12:00	20
18:00	15

Figure 21.4 *The total daily percentage of cortisol which needs to be achieved if using a '4 times per day dosing' schedule.*

This means when thinking about delivering hydrocortisone, we have a total amount you would need to give in mg/m^2/day and also how that should be broken up in terms of the total dose as percentages during the 24 hour period. However, this is the percentage of the cortisol distribution needed in these time frames and to achieve this, you would need to consider the way the individual metabolises hydrocortisone, i.e. clearance and absorption.

Although, from 18:00 to midnight 15% of the total daily dose is needed, the afternoon dose is best given at 16:00 because there is a natural surge of ACTH around this time. This raises cortisol which then peaks around an hour later; again this depends on the individual's handling of hydrocortisone. The cortisol level then slowly declines in the early hours of the evening until midnight, as it would in the body's natural production.

So having thought about the circadian rhythm and how best to match this, we go back to the original question, 'Why is hydrocortisone used and not the longer acting steroids?'

As you will probably have noticed the circadian rhythm studies show:

- Hydrocortisone can best approximate the natural rhythm.
- Prednisolone has a longer glucocorticoid action of approximately 8 hours, so it still needs to be given 3 times a day.
- Dexamethasone has an even longer glucocorticoid action of approximately 12 hours. It could be given twice a day but because it lacks the 'peakiness' of hydrocortisone and prednisolone it becomes extremely difficult to match the times of the day when the peaks and troughs are required. It is very difficult when using dexamethasone to avoid over treatment because of this.

So although you think using a long acting steroid would be better, this is not necessarily the case, as both prednisolone and dexamethasone have a tendency to suppress growth which is why we use hydrocortisone in children. A further advantage is we can measure hydrocortisone as cortisol in the blood but not prednisolone or dexamethasone.

Cortisol stacking—why dose timing is important?

We mentioned this earlier in Chapter 20 when we discussed calculating doses. If the dose of hydrocortisone is given too early or if the person is a slow absorber and takes the dose at a normal 6 hour interval, the cortisol level will be increased which will generate a higher peak than expected as the cortisol will 'stack' onto the amount of cortisol remaining in the blood from the previous dose. In this case we call this 'over stacking' (Fig. 21.5).

This 'over stacking' will lead to over exposure at this point and if timing of doses is not correct, then this over exposure day after day will lead to long term side effects.

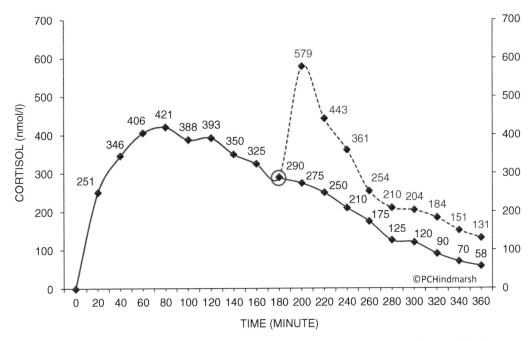

Figure 21.5 *Cortisol over stacking occurs when doses are given too close together and leads to over exposure to cortisol as shown by the dashed line when a dose is given at 180 minutes.*

In this situation what happens is that if a reasonable period of time is not allowed between doses, then one dose becomes superimposed on the other and quite high levels can be attained without the individual realising. At the concentration point shown in the red circle if an extra dose is taken, then high values of 579 nmol/l ensue which might not be expected.

This means doses must be given at fixed times and these times need to be worked out on the basis of time of day and how the individual absorbs the drug and how quickly they remove it from circulation. There is another situation where stacking needs to occur to avoid periods of time when cortisol levels would drop too low, this is known as 'useful stacking'. So if we look at our stacking picture again, but this time look at the point where the cortisol level reaches 90 nmol/l, we can see that unless more hydrocortisone is taken, the person will quickly run out of cortisol.

In this situation stacking is advantageous (useful stacking) because if the individual now takes hydrocortisone the cortisol level will be boosted to 394 nmol/l which gives better coverage and prevents the individual becoming cortisol deficient and suffering side effects such as headaches (Fig. 21.6).

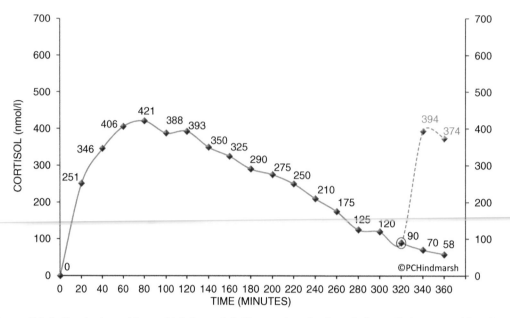

Figure 21.6 *Cortisol stacking which is useful. Here a dose is given before all the cortisol has been removed from the blood so that instead of a low value at 360 minutes good coverage is provided.*

The data from a 24 hour profile helps guide us as to when the best time to stack cortisol and also the level achieved, guides us to what dose we should use to gain optimal cortisol levels. This prevents the very common problem of over and under stacking that tends to occur when doses are not individualised.

So if asking the question, does moving the dose an hour either earlier or later make a difference? The answer would be, yes it makes a big difference!

CONCLUSIONS

The circadian rhythm tells us how we should dose with hydrocortisone. Cortisol distribution is important as it is cortisol which determines the feedback system for the hypothalamo-pituitary-adrenal axis. Getting cortisol right is the key in this whole process.

FURTHER READING

Hindmarsh, P.C., Charmandari, E., 2015. Variation in absorption and half-life of hydrocortisone influence plasma cortisol concentrations. Clin. Endocrinol. 82, 557–561.
Peters, C.J., Hill, N., Dattani, M.T., Charmandari, E., Matthews, D.R., Hindmarsh, P.C., 2013. Deconvolution analysis of 24h serum cortisol profiles informs the amount and distribution of hydrocortisone replacement therapy. Clin. Endocrinol. 78, 347–351.

CHAPTER 22

Cortisol and 17-Hydroxyprogesterone

GLOSSARY

17-Hydroxyprogesterone (17OHP) 17OHP is an intermediary steroid in the formation of cortisol from cholesterol. It is the substrate for the enzyme CYP21 which converts 17OHP to 11-deoxycortisol and also progesterone to deoxycorticosterone. Loss of enzyme function leads to a buildup of 17OHP.

Androstenedione One of the adrenal androgens which is made from dehydroepiandrosterone by the action of the enzyme 3beta-hydroxysteroid dehydrogenase type 2. Level rises in CAH when cortisol replacement is suboptimal.

Feedback loop system A system where a change in a hormone acts back on the central controlling system. In this case, cortisol feeds its level back to the pituitary to adjust ACTH production which in turn will influence 17OHP production from the adrenal. When the adrenal is working normally it would be cortisol which is regulated and this is a closed loop feedback system. When we have to replace cortisol because it is missing this is called an open loop feedback system.

Replacement cortisol Cortisol derived from administered hydrocortisone used to replace the missing cortisol which occurs in CAH.

GENERAL

We now need to think about the relationship between cortisol and 17-hydroxyprogesterone (17OHP). In particular, we need to determine if measuring 17OHP is useful, alongside the cortisol levels attained. This is an important question as many hospitals only measure 17OHP and use this to determine how well cortisol is replaced, rather than actually measuring cortisol. 17OHP is only one part of the story, as we shall see later in Chapter 23 when we come to examine questions we want answered when assessing hydrocortisone treatment.

Before you go to the next chapter, it is worth reading about cortisol and 17OHP, because 17OHP is measured commonly in people with congenital adrenal hyperplasia (CAH) and decisions are often based solely on this measurement. Twenty-four hours profiles have shown that 17OHP levels form only a part of the overall assessment. Understanding what the measure means and the part this steroid hormone plays is

Congenital Adrenal Hyperplasia. http://dx.doi.org/10.1016/B978-0-12-811483-4.00022-2

very important, particularly when appreciating and understanding hydrocortisone dosing.

17-HYDROXYPROGESTERONE

17OHP is a steroid hormone and it is not an androgen (Fig. 22.1). It is present in the blood of everyone whether they have CAH or not. The main difference is how much is actually produced. What it does, is not understood.

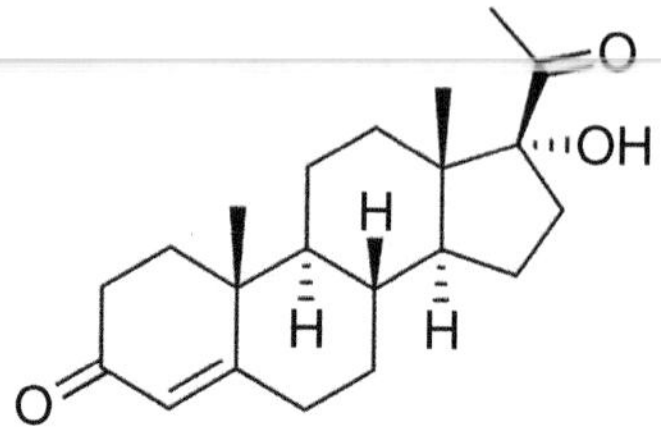

Figure 22.1 *Structure of 17-hydroxyprogesterone (17OHP) a steroid hormone.*

In CAH, we use 17OHP as a marker of how active the adrenal glands are. In other words, it gives us an idea of how much ACTH is produced by the pituitary gland. This is because when there is no or very low cortisol levels in the blood, the 17OHP level rises, except when the adrenal production of 17OHP is compromised by either the adrenal glands being shut down from over treatment with steroids, or in other diseases which affect the adrenal glands such as Addison's disease, or when the adrenal glands are not formed properly such as adrenal hypoplasia congenita.

However, 17OHP cannot be used as a marker on its own in CAH for hydrocortisone replacement. It has to be interpreted with respect to how it is affected by cortisol, i.e. how much hydrocortisone has been given, when it was given, how long the cortisol lasts in the blood and what levels of cortisol were achieved. Further, if 17OHP is low, we do not know if this is because we have the cortisol replacement just right, or perhaps giving too much. It is not easy to distinguish between over treatment and just right on the basis of 17OHP. It is possible to have no cortisol and no measurable 17OHP at the same time. This is due to either the time lag between the effect cortisol has on 17OHP, or that 17OHP production has become totally suppressed (switched off) as a result of a long period of over treatment (Fig. 17.5). Sometimes, the 17OHP measured, could be produced by adrenal rest tissue, or polycystic ovaries (PCOS), both of which are known to produce 17OHP.

This means we have to measure CORTISOL AND 17OHP over a period of time, to make the right treatment adjustments.

FACTORS INFLUENCING 17-HYDROXYPROGESTERONE

17OHP is influenced by a number of factors. It varies even in people without CAH during the 24 hour period. You would expect this, as it is in the pathway to cortisol formation and we know that cortisol and ACTH have a circadian rhythm, so too does 17OHP. However, the variations in 17OHP levels over 24 hours in individuals without CAH, is minimal.

17OHP also varies during the menstrual cycle (Fig. 22.2) which adds more complexity as to how to assess cortisol replacement in CAH. In women without CAH during the early part of the cycle, levels range between 0.6 and 3.0 nmol/l, in midcycle between 3 and 7.7 nmol/l and in the second half of the cycle up to 15 nmol/l. Interestingly, normal 17OHP levels in men without CAH are almost double those seen in woman, during the early part of their cycle.

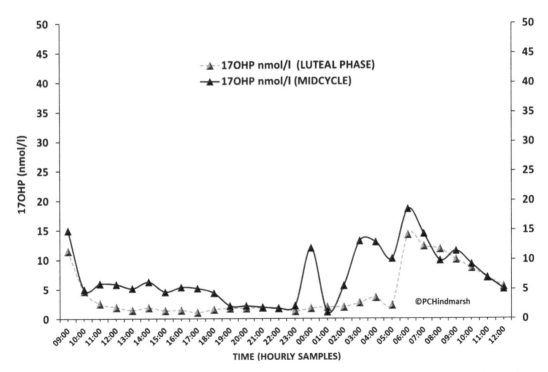

Figure 22.2 *Differences in 17OHP at different stages of the menstrual cycle with higher values midcycle shown in dark purple.*

We also need to be aware that women with PCOS (Fig. 14.3) make more 17OHP than women who do not have PCOS. This 17OHP comes from the ovary not the adrenal glands, so treating it by increasing the dose of hydrocortisone in a person with CAH will not make any difference. All that will happen is the person will put on more weight and exacerbate the problem of PCOS where weight gain is already an issue. As PCOS is more common in women with CAH it is really important to understand this problem. Fig. 22.3 shows the profile data from a person with CAH and PCOS.

Here we see changes in cortisol, androstenedione and 17OHP as well as testosterone and estradiol. The point here is 17OHP and particularly androstenedione (which is discordant with the 17OHP changes) change without any clear relationship with cortisol (ACTH is low) and these (particularly androstenedione), as they track more with estradiol, are ovarian in origin. This demonstrates care needs to be taken in situations such as this in interpreting the 17OHP and androstenedione as the source may not be adrenal and changing the hydrocortisone dose would not be appropriate.

Of note, it has been documented that about 90% of the normal production of 17OHP measured in men without CAH, comes from the testes. What this tells us is we need to be very careful in interpreting 17OHP levels especially if we do not relate them to the main regulator of the system in adrenal disorders, the replacement cortisol.

This is also a problem when adrenal rests are present (Fig. 14.12). Rests are made up of adrenal like cells and will make steroids in response to ACTH. This means in this situation if 17OHP is measured and is raised, it could be coming from the adrenal glands or rest tissue. This is important because increasing hydrocortisone may not deal with the problem. This is because adrenal tissue can express aberrant receptors for luteinising hormone (LH) which means even though ACTH is reduced or suppressed, the normal functioning of the hypothalamo–pituitary–gonad axis will still allow LH to influence rest function.

Another problem which arises from 17OHP's place in the adrenal pathway to cortisol, is that it will respond to stress. How the body deals with stress varies depending on the type of stress and whether it is of short or long duration. Chronic stress, e.g. starvation leads to a persistent activation and resetting of the hypothalamo–pituitary–adrenal axis. Short term stress, particularly pain, leads to a rapid increase in ACTH and cortisol within a matter of 5–10 minutes.

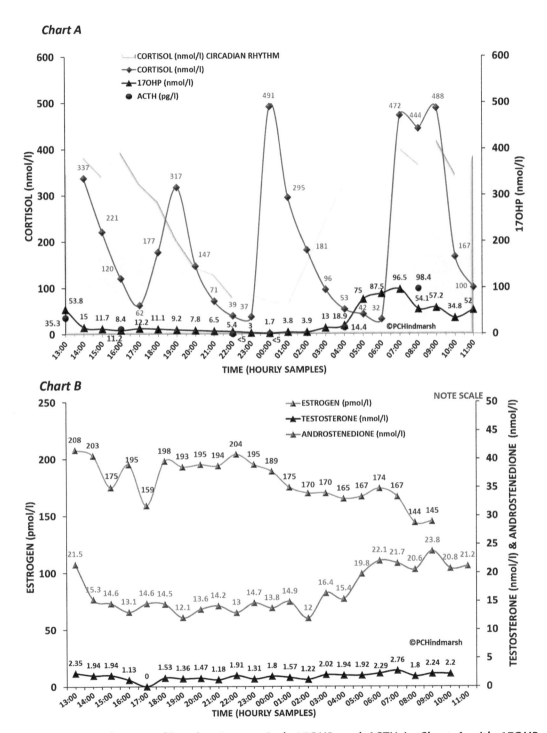

Figure 22.3 *24 hour profiles showing cortisol, 17OHP and ACTH in Chart A with 17OHP starting to rise at 01.00 before there is any increase in ACTH which is 14.4 pg/ml at 04:00.*

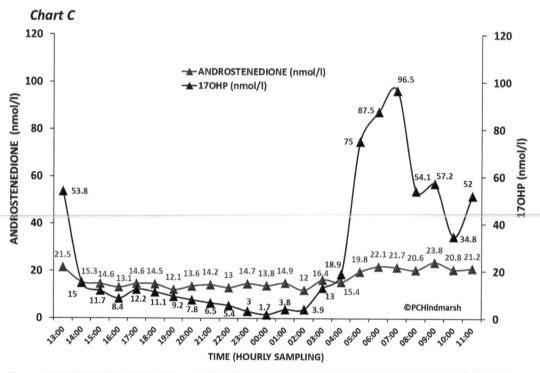

Figure 22.3 (cont.) *In Chart B androstenedione starts to increase from 02:00 as well at a time when estradiol levels are constant. Chart C shows the changes in 17OHP and androstenedione in greater magnification and illustrates the rise taking place independent of ACTH.*

A painful experience, e.g. difficulty when taking a blood sample, is enough to raise cortisol in people with normal adrenal glands. In people with CAH we would not see a rise in cortisol as they cannot make any. Rather, we would see a rise in 17OHP (Fig. 22.4). This is why extreme care has to be taken in interpreting one-off 17OHP blood samples. We discuss this in more detail in Chapter 23. So if getting the blood sample is painful/stressful, then ACTH will rise and will drive 17OHP up. This will give a falsely high value.

It is another reason why we do samples through a cannula as it removes this stress element. We usually put the cannula in place then leave a period of time of an hour to let the system calm down after insertion.

Fig. 22.4 shows this effect. Here there was a very difficult cannulation at the start and the 17OHP is high at 55.4 nmol/l and declines thereafter. The following morning at the same time, the cortisol is exactly the same as the previous day as the person is on a pump but 17OHP is well within the normal range.

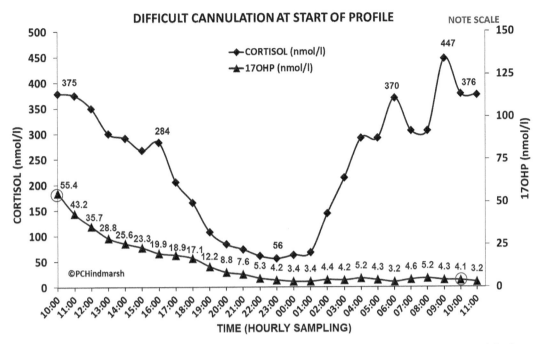

Figure 22.4 *The effect of a difficult cannula insertion on the 17OHP level which is high and declines compared to the following morning when cortisol is the same but 17OHP is normal.*

RELATIONSHIP BETWEEN CORTISOL AND 17-HYDROXYPROGESTERONE

When we start to look at how cortisol and 17OHP interrelate the situation is even more complicated. There is a lag between a change in cortisol in the blood and a corresponding change in 17OHP. The reason for this is as we show in Fig. 20.2, when cortisol appears in the blood it has to go to the heart and then to the organs of the body before it can have an effect.

It produces effects; in this case it alters the pituitary production of ACTH by regulating different genes, particularly in the pituitary the proopiomelanocortin (POMC) gene. (This is the gene that codes for the formation of the precursor of ACTH. This large form of ACTH is then chopped up in the pituitary gland to produce the normal sized ACTH, which is then released into the blood stream.)

ACTH then has to be released into the blood stream and go back to the heart and then out again to the adrenal glands. Even then the journey is not over as ACTH has to then tell the adrenal glands to make more or less cortisol.

Normally, there would be an increase in cortisol production but in CAH, as the adrenal glands cannot produce cortisol, the adrenal glands respond by producing more 17OHP. This process takes time and this is where the lag occurs. Fig. 22.5 shows all the steps!

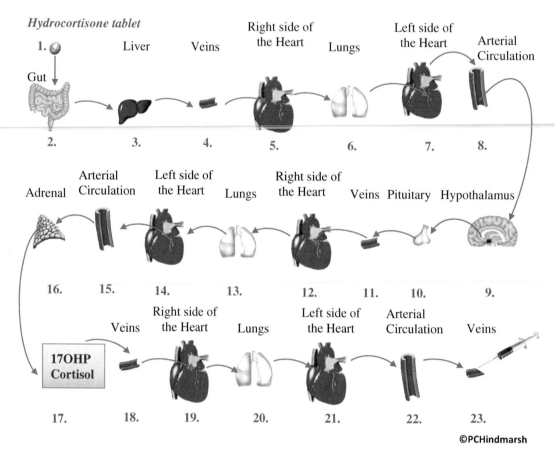

©PCHindmarsh

Figure 22.5 *All the steps needed to get 17OHP into blood and taken as a sample.*

The following explains the steps shown in the diagram (Fig. 22.5):

1. Ingestion of oral hydrocortisone tablet.
2. Absorbed in the gut.
3. Carried from the gut to the liver by hepatic portal system.
4. Carried from the liver through the venous (veins) circulation into the right side of the heart.
5. From the right side of the heart carried through the pulmonary arteries to the lungs.

6. From the lungs it is carried back to the left side of the heart.

7. From the left side of the heart it is them pumped out into the aorta.

8. From the aorta it is carried through the arterial circulation.

9. Arrives at the hypothalamus and causes reduction in corticotrophin hormone production.

10. Less corticotropin releasing hormone means that pituitary gland processes less POMC from the POMC gene and this leads to fall in ACTH release into the veins leading out of the pituitary area.

11. Veins carry ACTH message to heart.

12. From the right side of the heart carried through the pulmonary arteries to the lungs.

13. From the lungs it is carried back to the left side of the heart.

14. From the left side of the heart it is then pumped out into the aorta.

15. From the aorta it is carried through the arterial circulation.

16. Gets to the adrenal glands and reduced message says make less 17OHP.

17. Less 17OHP is now released from adrenal glands.

18. 17OHP now enters veins leaving adrenal glands and heads for the heart.

19. From the right side of the heart carried through the pulmonary arteries to the lungs.

20. From the lungs it is carried back to the left side of the heart.

21. From the left side of the heart it is then pumped out into the aorta.

22. From the aorta it is carried through the arterial circulation.

23. The cortisol from the hydrocortisone is then carried through the veins to the body's organs and it is during this transportation phase, that a blood sample is taken from the vein.

This becomes very evident when we give an intravenous bolus of hydrocortisone and measure the effect it has on 17OHP. Fig. 22.6 shows an intravenous bolus of hydrocortisone and the effects the high cortisol levels achieved have on 17OHP.

In Fig. 22.6 the intravenous hydrocortisone bolus study has been undertaken in the morning. The person was asked to miss their morning dose, so there was as little cortisol as possible in the blood stream at the start of the clearance study. This results in there being no cortisol feedback on the pituitary production of ACTH, which rises and is reflected in the 17OHP levels which also rise slowly.

The intravenous bolus of hydrocortisone produces a rise in cortisol very quickly and to an extremely high level. 17OHP does not change however, if anything continues to rise even though the cortisol levels are high. It is not until we get out to 80 minutes after the injection that we start to see changes in 17OHP and the levels start to decrease.

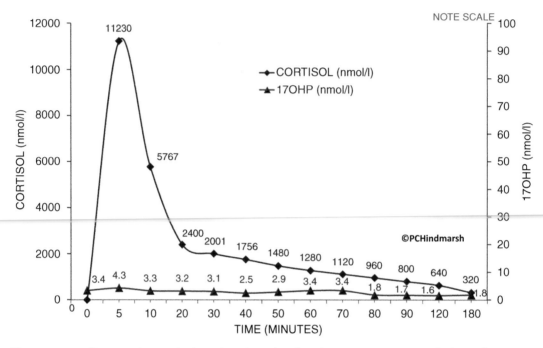

Figure 22.6 *Changes in cortisol and 17OHP levels after an intravenous bolus of 100 mg hydrocortisone.*

A similar but slightly slower situation takes place after taking a hydrocortisone tablet. Cortisol peaks around 1–2 hours after taking a dose and this reduces ACTH production by the pituitary gland. This takes time for the change in ACTH to occur and then even more time before the adrenal glands reduce the production of 17OHP. This switch off takes approximately 1–2 hours after the cortisol has peaked.

As an example, Fig. 22.7, after oral hydrocortisone has been ingested, cortisol peaks approximately 1 hour later. Remembering cortisol has to instruct ACTH in the pituitary to dampen down its production, we can see the time it takes before the adrenal glands switches off the production of 17OHP and for the 17OHP levels to start to fall.

Notice that once 17OHP starts to fall following the cortisol peak, it remains low until cortisol levels start to fall. It looks almost as if cortisol levels have to get below about 50–75 nmol/l before 17OHP starts to rise again.

This adds to the complexity of sampling to determine control. Not only do we need to capture peak cortisol and the pre dose values for 17OHP and cortisol, but we now need to take extra samples after the cortisol peak to determine the true effect on

17OHP. This argues for detailed profiles along the lines we undertake with regular 1–2 hourly blood sampling. This level of detail is required to be able to make the decisions on the dosing schedule both in terms of amount and frequency.

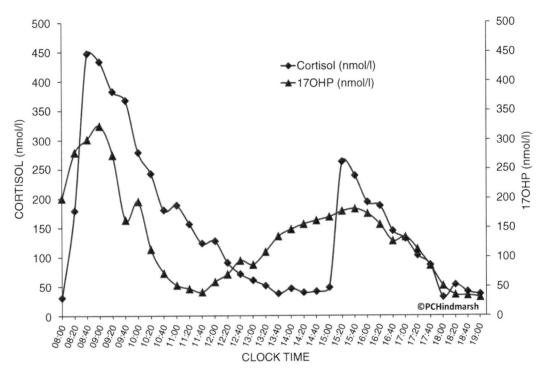

Figure 22.7 *Relationship between cortisol resulting from taking an oral tablet of hydrocortisone in blue and 17OHP in purple. As cortisol levels rise 17OHP begins to fall and the lowest 17OHP levels occur about 1–2 hours after the cortisol peak.*

CONCLUSIONS

17OHP follows the amount of cortisol given. Cortisol ultimately controls 17OHP production through the feedback on ACTH which instructs and normalises 17OHP. This means when cortisol replacement doses are optimal, both 17OHP and adrenal androgens levels will follow, unless 17OHP production is not from the adrenal glands.

FURTHER READING

Charmandari, E., Matthews, D.R., Johnston, A., Brook, C.G., Hindmarsh, P.C., 2001. Serum cortisol and 17-hydroxyprogesterone interrelation in classic 21-hydroxylase deficiency: is current replacement therapy satisfactory? J. Clin. Endocrinol. Metab. 86, 4679–4685.
Strott, C.A., Yoshimi, T., Lipsett, M.B., 1969. Plasma progesterone and 17-hydroxyprogesterone in normal men and children with congenital adrenal hyperplasia. J. Clin. Invest. 48, 930–939.

CHAPTER 23

Using Profiles to Assess Cortisol Replacement

GLOSSARY

Cannula insertion This is when a plastic tube is inserted into a vein so that samples can be taken regularly over 24 hours. It can occasionally be painful which raises 17OHP. To overcome this problem, we prefer to insert the cannula an hour or two before starting a profile. We also attain a crossover of time in sampling, so common start and end results can be closely compared.

Over stacking The phenomenon which happens if the timing of doses is incorrect. Occurs where the dose is taken too early and builds onto the cortisol remaining from the previous dose, leading to higher cortisol levels than would have been expected from the dose given.

GENERAL

As we have mentioned, we are looking at many factors when we study the results we get from 24 hour profiles. To determine more precisely the amount of hydrocortisone which is required, we need quite detailed information, not just on how much cortisol is actually delivered from the tablet into the blood stream, but also what effect cortisol has on the other hormones, such as 17-hydroxyprogesterone (17OHP). The 17OHP acts as a marker of how well we are decreasing the pituitary drive through ACTH to the adrenal glands.

Everyone's production of cortisol varies. To assess optimal individualised dosing schedules when treating CAH, we use both the cortisol and 17OHP levels to determine whether the dose of hydrocortisone is correct.

The cortisol levels tell us:

1. How much cortisol from the hydrocortisone dose is achieved.
2. How long cortisol from the hydrocortisone lasts in the blood.
3. The point at which the next dose needs to be taken, based on when cortisol drops to a certain level which varies throughout the 24 hour period (the best time to stack the dose (Fig. 21.6).
4. How closely we are achieving normal production (circadian rhythm).

Congenital Adrenal Hyperplasia. http://dx.doi.org/10.1016/B978-0-12-811483-4.00023-4

The 17OHP level is used as a marker to guide us as to how much cortisol the individual needs. However, it is not as simple as that. We need to look at both the cortisol and 17OHP over a 24 hour period because as discussed in Chapter 22, many things can influence 17OHP. Painful or difficult blood draws (Fig. 22.4) as well as the lag between cortisol and 17OHP levels are important factors (Fig. 22.7).

There is also the situation when the adrenal glands are enlarged and produce high levels of 17OHP, which would mean as the adrenals shrink back to a normal size, less cortisol is needed. If too much cortisol is given over a long period, the adrenal glands shrink and 17OHP production is 'switched off' and even when there is no cortisol in the blood for many hours, 17OHP remains dormant. This would give a false picture and would indicate over treatment. There is in fact, both over and under treatment (Fig. 23.1).

The only way to fine tune dosing is by looking in detail at both cortisol and 17OHP levels over 24 hours. This way we can prevent both the long and short term side effects.

WHAT WE NEED TO CONSIDER

Is there adequate cortisol at the appropriate times of the day? We can tell this by looking at the circadian rhythm as well as the 17OHP level. Remember, you cannot judge by looking at 17OHP only, as this will not show how much cortisol there is in the blood stream and as discussed previously, 17OHP production can be totally switched off after prolonged periods of overtreatment as the adrenal glands shrink and become dormant (Figs 17.5 and 23.1).

The most important thing is to think about what we are trying to achieve and this means considering the following points:

- What is missing in CAH is *cortisol*.
- What we are replacing is *cortisol* using hydrocortisone.
- What we need to know first and foremost is what *cortisol* replacement looks like?

So when we are looking at the data a profile provides and considering the dosing schedule, we are interested in the following:

1. Is cortisol distribution the best it can be over the 24 hour period?
2. Are there periods where cortisol *over* stacking (Fig. 21.6) is occurring when a dose is taken too early?
3. Are the cortisol peaks too high or too low and occurring at the right times of the day?

4. Is the dose providing adequate cortisol cover? Is the dose lasting long enough and are there periods where cortisol levels drop too low or where there is no cortisol in the blood stream?

5. What effect is cortisol having on 17OHP? Are the 17OHP levels too high, which means more cortisol is needed, or are the 17OHP levels too low, which means the dose needs to be adjusted by lowering or moving the time the dose needs to be taken.

In this chapter, we illustrate several examples of 24 hour profiles where we have superimposed the normal circadian rhythm with a twice daily dosing with hydrocortisone (Fig. 23.1), then with 3 times a day dosing of hydrocortisone (Figs 23.2 and 23.3) and finally 4 times a day dosing of hydrocortisone (Figs 23.4 and 23.5).

24 HOUR PROFILE—2 TIMES PER DAY DOSING WITH HYDROCORTISONE

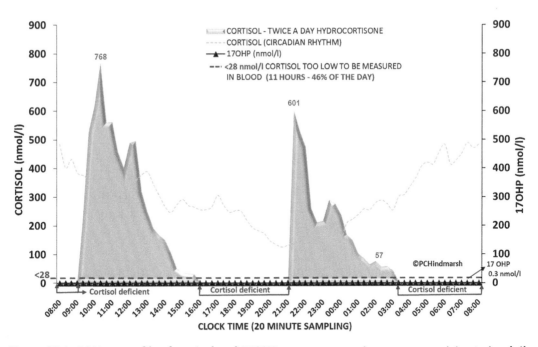

Figure 23.1 *24 Hour profile of cortisol and 17OHP measurements in a person receiving twice daily hydrocortisone. Note the high cortisol peaks with complete suppression of 17OHP. Samples taken at 20 minute intervals.*

When we use twice daily dosing, there are long periods where the cortisol measurements are so low that it cannot be measured in the blood, which indicates under treatment. The doses are so spread out that cortisol stacking does not occur.

Cortisol stacking cannot occur on a twice daily regimen unless of course, the doses are taken one after the other or at late breakfast and early lunch.

When we consider hydrocortisone lasts on average between 4 and 6 hours (depending on the individual's half-life and clearance of hydrocortisone (Fig. 20.10), twice daily dosing would equate to approximately 11–12 hours of cortisol replacement, which is only half the 24 hour period.

In Fig. 23.1 there are very high peaks of cortisol in the morning and evening. Only the morning peak is aligned to the circadian rhythm, although it is occurring too late and the level achieved, 768 nmol/l, is excessively high, well above the normal range. The evening peak of 601 nmol/l is also excessively high and comes at a time when normal cortisol production is present, but low.

The cortisol lasts for reasonable periods of time probably because the person is a slow metaboliser. There are periods of time when there is simply no cortisol present when there should be, as well as periods where the cortisol levels drop too low. We can see that in the afternoon from 14:00 onwards, the cortisol levels are very low when there should be a good amount. Again, in the early hours of the morning the cortisol levels drop very low from around 01:00 and there is no cortisol from 03:00. The person yo-yos between under and over treatment in the same day.

The high peaks have completely suppressed 17OHP. This is very evident in the early hours of the morning, when there is a natural surge of ACTH around 04:00 and the adrenal glands would normally make cortisol in response to the rise in ACTH, but as we can see there is no measurable cortisol and no change in 17OHP (<0.3 nmol/l).

If you used 17OHP as a marker to judge the cortisol replacement, then you would say this individual was over treated. However, looking at the cortisol levels it is very evident there is both over and under treatment; in fact there is no cortisol in the system for 11 hours (47%) of the 24 hour period.

24 HOUR PROFILE—3 TIMES PER DAY DOSING WITH HYDROCORTISONE

When taking three doses of hydrocortisone a day, there are still periods where the cortisol level is much lower than it should be; however, the peaks of cortisol are not as high as with twice a day dosing. As we know, on average hydrocortisone only lasts as cortisol in the blood for 6 hours at the most and as there are 24 hours in a day, when we calculate the time period three doses cover, it only equates to 18 hours! We have seen how variable the individual half-life can be (Fig. 20.11) and this has become very apparent when studying the vast number of profiles we have undertaken with patients on three doses of hydrocortisone a day.

Many people who take three doses of hydrocortisone a day and who have not had cortisol profiles, have been told their 'CAH is well controlled' with cortisol replacement based solely on 17OHP measurements which are within the normal range. This does not tell us whether cortisol is adequately replaced or correctly distributed through the 24 hour period, as there may be periods where they have no cortisol, too low cortisol, or in fact too much cortisol. We will now look at two different examples of this.

Example One

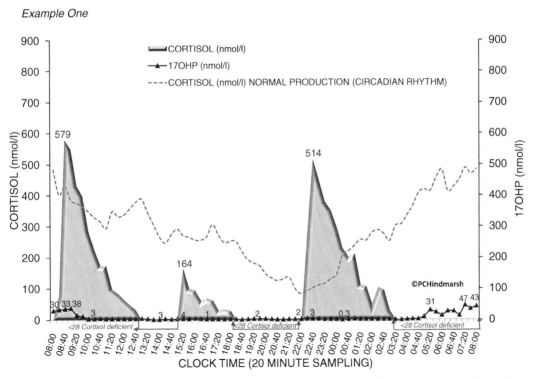

Figure 23.2 *24 Hour profile of cortisol and 17OHP measurements in a person receiving thrice daily hydrocortisone.* Note the better cortisol peaks with less suppression of 17OHP. Samples taken at 20 minute intervals.

The cortisol levels look better than in the previous profile (Fig. 23.1) but they do not mimic the circadian rhythm. The morning peak is good, but we can see that the morning dose does not last until the next dose and in fact from 13:00 until the afternoon dose is taken at 15:00, there is no cortisol measurable in the blood stream! Looking only at 17OHP during this period and as the 17OHP levels remain constantly low, this would indicate good 'control' even when there is no cortisol present! However, when considering both the cortisol and 17OHP levels, it would indicate the morning dose is peaking too high.

To correct this we would make an adjustment to the morning dose, although the morning peak of cortisol does not seem excessively high, its effect on 17OHP levels indicates that the morning dose could be lowered slightly. Despite there being no cortisol between 13:00 and 15:00 and none from 18:00 to 22:00 and also taking into account the delayed effect the cortisol has on 17OHP, the 17OHP levels do not rise significantly.

We should add in a dose at noon (similar amount to the dose that was given in the afternoon at 15:00). The noon dose would then 'stack on' the cortisol remaining from the morning dose which would raise the cortisol levels appropriately, as the circadian rhythm indicates the body naturally has a good level of cortisol at this time.

With the additional dose taken at noon, the afternoon dose time should then be moved to 16:00 to give good cortisol levels in the early evening which would slowly decline until the late night dose is taken.

The evening dose is again taken at the wrong time and needs to be moved later, to midnight. This would give a dosing schedule which will deliver cortisol levels more in line with the circadian rhythm.

Based on the results of the data obtained from this profile, we can see this person seems to have a fairly fast metabolism and would be better suited to four or five smaller doses throughout the 24 hour period. The doses and times should be worked out on the half-life and then fine tuned by another profile.

The high evening peak of 514 nmol/l does not suppress the early morning rise in 17OHP. In CAH, a large dose of hydrocortisone is often given at night to try to suppress the natural surge of ACTH which occurs in the early hours of the morning. This has been called reverse circadian dosing. However, these high levels of cortisol at a time when cortisol is naturally low will produce side effects and will not suppress the ACTH surge as the cortisol will not last long enough to suppress the ACTH surge. We can see evidence of this surge as 17OHP starts to increase around 05:00, after remaining at very low levels despite there being no cortisol in the blood stream from around 03:00. This means the evening dose needs to be given later than 22:00.

We now look at another example of three doses a day (Fig. 23.3).

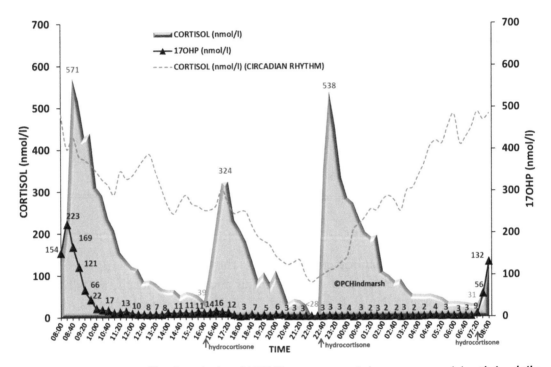

Figure 23.3 *24 Hour profile of cortisol and 17OHP measurements in a person receiving thrice daily hydrocortisone. Note the high cortisol peaks morning and evening with spikes of 17OHP in the morning. Samples taken at 20 minute intervals.*

These results show a much better distribution of cortisol over 24 hours than the data shown in the previous two profiles (Figs 23.1 and 23.2), as there is much less time where there is no cortisol present in the blood. However, the cortisol levels drop too low early in the afternoon and remain low until the 16:00 dose is taken. These very low levels of cortisol also occur in the early hours of the morning and this is at a time when the body's normal cortisol production is high.

Although stacking occurs when both the morning and afternoon doses are taken, on both occasions the stacking occurs later than it should, as we can see that the cortisol levels drop lower than they ought. To overcome this, the doses could be taken earlier and the amount adjusted, as less hydrocortisone would be required to buildup the cortisol level to where it should be. The peaks in the morning and in the evening are both over 500 nmol/l. The morning peak is good, perhaps slightly high and the dose could be taken earlier at 06:00. This would mean the next dose should to be taken around midday which would give good cortisol levels until the 16:00 dose. This dose would probably need to be lowered as it would 'stack' appropriately on the remaining cortisol from the dose that was introduced at 12:00. We can see the dose taken at 22:00 gives a very high peak of cortisol at a time when the cortisol levels are naturally at their lowest. To overcome this, the dose could be reduced and given later, as 17OHP still rises in the early morning but is not as suppressed as the twice daily approach seen in Fig. 23.1. Note, that if the measurement of 17OHP was taken pre dose, it would show 9 nmol/l at 07:20. This is because the effect from the high dose taken at 22:00 on 17OHP has started to wear off and we can clearly see that it still rises higher despite the morning dose being taken. This illustrates the delay in the action of cortisol on 17OHP (Fig. 22.7), so the blood spot or test measuring the 17OHP pre dose would give a false picture of what was really happening.

24 HOUR PROFILE—4 TIMES PER DAY DOSING WITH HYDROCORTISONE

Although taking tablets cannot exactly mimic the circadian pattern, we find that many people achieve better cortisol distribution and 17OHP levels, by taking their dose split into 4 times a day as shown in Fig. 23.4. This gives smaller peaks of cortisol and better distribution throughout the day. We find that children under the age of 5 years and adolescents do better with a 4 times per day treatment schedule.

Now we look carefully at the data from someone who is taking hydrocortisone 4 times a day Fig. 23.4. We can see that this gives very good cortisol coverage over the 24 hour period, but can still see that a few fine adjustments could be made.

The peak from the 08:00 dose seems a bit high, but 17OHP is not suppressed so it is probably satisfactory for this person. The cortisol level at 15:00 is too low and this could be corrected by moving this dose to 14:00. This would not only mean that a lower dose could be used when given at 14:00 as there would be a better cortisol level in the blood for the dose to stack on, it would also prevent the low cortisol level of 36 nmol/l occurring. The cortisol peak is high for the time of the day, so moving and reducing the dose will give better cortisol levels without causing side effects.

Example One

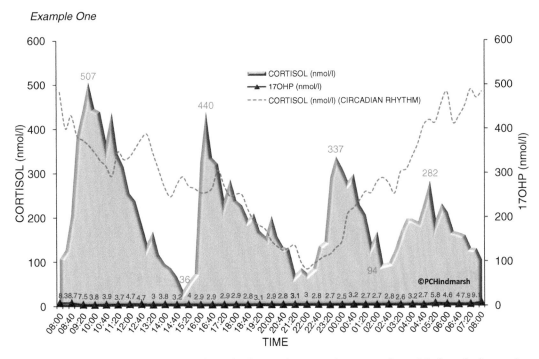

Figure 23.4 *Profile from person taking hydrocortisone 4 times per day with fourth dose taken at 02:00.*

It is evident that the 22:00 dose gives a high peak, so this dose could be slightly reduced and the dose taken at 02:00 slightly increased. The stacking taking place is useful as it is keeping cortisol at good levels; however, the timings of the stacking need to be adjusted.

The 17OHP levels are very good and lowering the dose at 22:00 and then by increasing the dose at 02:00 in the morning, 17OHP at 08:00 is 8.3 nmol/l on day 1 and 9.1 nmol/l on day 2, will come down to under 5 nmol/ which is in the normal range.

It is interesting to note that this individual had a normal BMI and normal cortisol clearance (half-life 81.8 minutes). Blood glucose was 4.8 mmol/l with a normal insulin of 12.3 mU/l. Androstenedione was also well within the normal range as was the ACTH level at 08:00. This individual was postpubertal.

We now look at another example of four doses a day (Fig. 23.5).

Example Two

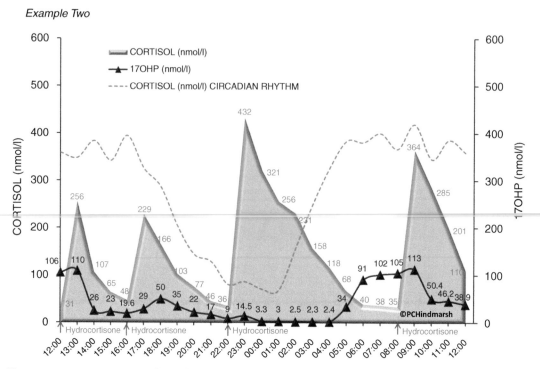

Figure 23.5 *24 Hour profile of cortisol and 17OHP measurements in a person receiving hydrocortisone 4 times per day.*

In this profile cortisol distribution is better than the 2 and 3 times per day dosing schedules. Note the profile starts at midday. We start by looking at the morning dose which is taken too late at 08:00. It should be taken as early as possible and preferably at 06:00. The morning cortisol peak (364 nmol/l) is low, so the morning dose needs increasing. The 17OHP confirms this, as it is rising from 05:00. However, the decision based on morning 17OHP only, would have been to increase the evening dose to bring down the morning 17OHP but looking at the cortisol we can see that would be incorrect.

The cortisol peak after the lunchtime dose is also low, but if we move the dose to an earlier time (10:00) then we can capitalise on stacking to get a good peak at this time. Before we do this, it would be better to check with a profile to determine the effects of the morning dose change. This person has a very fast clearance and would be better on a 5 times per day dosing schedule. The next dose would then have to be at 14:00, with a further smaller dose to be taken at 18:00 to take them through the evening. The evening dose needs to be moved to midnight or 01:00. Again, care will be needed if dose changes are to be made to avoid over stacking.

These examples illustrate how complex it is to individualise dosing because of the variation in half-life between people. This emphasises the importance of 24 hour profiles as you cannot just apply blanket formulae without incurring side effects as described in adult studies with CAH.

A 17OHP WITHIN THE NORMAL RANGE DOES NOT INDICATE OVERTREATMENT

It is important to remember that everyone needs differing amounts of cortisol to bring 17OHP levels into the normal range. Profiles help us tailor doses individually in terms of the right amount and the correct time. This helps minimise side effects.

So if we look back at the twice per day profile (Fig. 23.1) it is not the 'control' of the 17OHP level that matters. Too many clinical staff focus only on 17OHP, rather than considering how the cortisol replacement looks. We really need to look at how well cortisol is replaced and the way it is distributed throughout the 24 hours. As can be seen, there are several hours of the 24 hour period, where individuals may be totally without cortisol, so effectively under treated. During these periods glucose could drop low and the person could suffer from headaches, tiredness and feel generally unwell.

When we start to look and think about how the situation is interacting with the pituitary using 17OHP as a marker, then we also see quite a different picture. We see periods of time when 17OHP is very well suppressed and we would be quite proud of achieving that. However, we can also see in these periods when cortisol is not present, 17OHP rises.

CRITICAL NATURE OF DOSE TIMING

What we have done so far is to look at how best we can mimic the circadian rhythm. One of the clear messages is that timing of doses is extremely important. As hydrocortisone lasts about 6 hours in the blood, a 3 or 4 times per day treatment plan is ideally what is required. We have also shown how important it is to get the distribution of cortisol right. This becomes very apparent when we look at what is a common practice by adult endocrinologists which is to not give any further hydrocortisone after 18:00 (6 p.m.).

This has been suggested to help with going to sleep, although there is no evidence for this and there is no actual difference in the number of patients between those who do get off to sleep alright and those that do not, even when this plan is followed. In fact, adequate cortisol during the night is important for processing and storing information acquired by the brain during the day. This is discussed in more detail in Chapter 15.

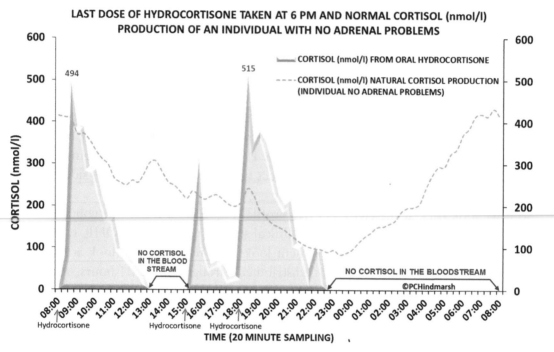

Figure 23.6 *Cortisol levels in the blood when the last dose of hydrocortisone is given at 18:00 compared to the normal circadian rhythm.*

When the last dose is given at 18:00 (Fig. 23.6), cortisol cover overnight is zero which places the person at risk of nocturnal hypoglycaemia, other symptoms and side effects of cortisol deficiency, as well as being left vulnerable to experiencing an adrenal crisis, especially in illness. The ACTH surge will be evident for most of the night and this probably explains why people with Addison's disease in particular, have hyperpigmentation problems and over time it might lead to the development of TART.

If the person had CAH, the ACTH drive would force up the adrenal androgens and there would be an increased risk of all the effects of androgen exposure. A similar situation arises if doses are missed leaving the person under treated with cortisol.

VARIATION IN DOSE DURING THE 24 HOUR PERIOD

One final point to make, is we should not assume that if we give a dose in the morning and again in the evening, the same cortisol levels will result. Fig. 23.7 shows an example of this.

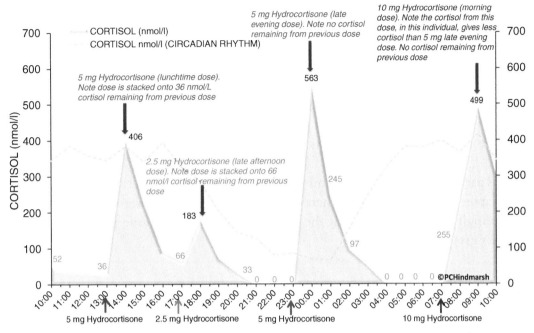

Figure 23.7 *24 Hour cortisol profile where hydrocortisone has been given 4 times per day. At 13:00 and 23:00 the same dose of hydrocortisone (5 mg) was given but the peak cortisol levels attained are different.*

What we can see in Fig. 23.7 is a difference in the peak cortisol despite the same dose being given. The dose at 23:00 reaches a peak close to 600 nmol/l whereas the 13:00 dose gets to just over 400 nmol/l. The reason for this is not well understood, but probably relates to differences in the handling of hydrocortisone by the body at different times of the day. The main message is we should not assume that a drug is handled the same at different times of the day and the only way to be sure is to check all doses using profiles.

REVERSE CIRCADIAN DOSING

You may have read or heard about this. The idea is that giving the highest dose of hydrocortisone at night would suppress the ACTH surge in the early hours of the morning. This is what is called reverse circadian dosing. Now that you have read this chapter and looked at the figures you will realise that this will not work. Have another read of the half-life section in Chapter 20 and look at Fig. 20.3. All that will happen is there will be very high cortisol levels which are perfectly illustrated in Fig. 23.5 at 22:00. No matter how high this value reaches, it will not make the hydrocortisone last any longer in time, this is because of the maths of half-life. It will have no impact on the early rise of ACTH and will cause short and long term side effects. You will remember we said that if we had a level of cortisol of say 500 nmol/l at midnight, then 80 minutes later (the average half-life of cortisol) the value would be 250 nmol/l and after 4 hours at 04:00 the level would be 62.5 nmol/l. Even if we doubled the midnight level to 1000 nmol/l, it would only reach a level of 125 nmol/l at 04:00. These high levels of cortisol when cortisol is naturally low, will produce side effects and not achieve what we want which is to suppress the early morning ACTH surge.

This is particularly important in children. Growth hormone secretion as we mentioned in Chapter 6 occurs at night. If there is a high level of cortisol present in the early part of the night then this will blunt the amount of growth hormone produced and lead to poor growth.

CONCLUSIONS

Thinking about the correct hydrocortisone dose is not simply about how much hydrocortisone is being delivered, but represents a careful interaction and balancing act between the cortisol delivered, the effects on 17OHP as well as other potential symptoms which could occur if cortisol is missing, such as headaches, tiredness and low blood glucose. To this, we also need to add the points we discussed in previous chapters, namely the importance of clearance and absorption.

Timing of doses is very important to avoid cortisol over stacking or periods where there is no cortisol, so if the question is asked, 'does it make a difference if we move the dose back an hour, or forward an hour?' the answer is yes. If we are also monitoring CAH only on pre dose 17OHP blood spots, the blood spot results will give no indication on how much cortisol there is in the blood at that point, and cortisol is the hormone we are replacing!

FURTHER READING

Charmandari, E., Matthews, D.R., Johnston, A., Brook, C.G.D., Hindmarsh, P.C., 2001. Serum cortisol and 17 hydroxyprogesterone interrelation in classic 21-hydroxylase deficiency: is current replacement therapy satisfactory? J. Clin. Endocrinol. Metab. 86, 4679–4685.

CHAPTER 24

Monitoring Hydrocortisone Therapy

GLOSSARY

Acne A skin condition characterised by red pimples on the skin, especially on the face, due to inflamed or infected sebaceous glands.

Adrenal rests The presence of adrenal tissue in the testes. This tissue responds to ACTH stimulation leading to an increase in size. The rests are hard and irregular in shape and can be mistaken for testicular cancers. These can occur wherever there are adrenal cells but mainly in testes and rarely ovaries. These are often referred to as Testicular Adrenal Rest Tissue or TART.

Aliasing A mathematical phenomenon where there is mismatch between what is actually happening to a hormone in the blood stream and what is measured. Usually happens when there are long sampling intervals where levels are underestimated.

Androstenedione One of the adrenal androgens which is made from dehydroepiandrosterone by the action of the enzyme 3beta-hydroxysteroid dehydrogenase type 2. Level rises in CAH when cortisol replacement is suboptimal.

Cataracts Condition in which the lens of the eye becomes progressively opaque, resulting in blurred vision.

Coronary heart disease Blockage of the blood vessels supplying the heart muscle which leads to chest pain on exercise and risk of sudden death.

Cortisol The major glucocorticoid in humans. Made in the adrenal glands. Cortisol regulates over two thirds of human genes. Cortisol regulates blood glucose, muscle function, the body's response to infection, fat distribution and brain thought processes.

Diabetes Raised blood glucose due to lack of insulin (type 1) or impaired insulin action (type 2).

Dizziness Symptoms are often associated with mineralocorticoid deficiency and occur in conjunction with low blood pressure. Noted especially on standing up quickly from a sitting position.

Gastritis Inflammation of the lining of the stomach which can lead on to an ulcer.

Glycosuria Loss of glucose into the urine which occurs when blood glucose levels go above 10 mmol/l.

Growth acceleration Increase in height usually expressed over a period of 1 year. Usually associated with an increased exposure to adrenal androgens or sex steroids. Often indicative of under replacement with hydrocortisone.

Growth arrest Complete cessation of growth in height. Often occurs with prednisolone or dexamethasone use.

Congenital Adrenal Hyperplasia. http://dx.doi.org/10.1016/B978-0-12-811483-4.00024-6

Growth retardation Decrease in growth rate usually expressed over a period of 1 year and sometimes actual arrest of growth. Usually associated with over replacement of hydrocortisone.

Half-life The time taken for the level of a drug or hormone in the blood, to fall by half the value.

Hirsutism Excessive body hair in men and women where body hair is normally minimal or absent, for example, appearance of facial hair in a female.

Hydrocortisone Synthetic form of cortisol.

Hypercalciuria Increase excretion of calcium in the urine.

Hypertension A blood pressure reading greater than 95th centile for age and height.

Infertility Defined as the failure to achieve a clinical pregnancy after 12 months or more of regular unprotected sexual intercourse. In CAH this may arise in males, because of reduced sperm production due to the presence of adrenal rests, or in females, due to polycystic ovarian syndrome.

Ischemic bone necrosis Situation where blood supply to bone is interrupted leading to death of some bone cells.

Metabolic syndrome The collection of obesity, hyperlipidaemia, hypertension, raised insulin, type 2 diabetes which is associated with increased risk of heart disease and stroke.

Obesity Abnormal or excessive fat accumulation which may impair health. Usually estimated by body mass index (person's weight in kilograms divided by the square of their height in meters). For adults, obesity is a BMI greater than or equal to 30.

Osteoporosis A marked reduction of mineral in bone which weakens the bone structure thereby increasing the risk of fracture.

Polycystic ovaries This is a particular appearance where the ovaries are enlarged and filled with dense stroma in the middle, with lots of small cysts around the periphery of the ovary.

Short term memory loss Classic effect of glucocorticoids. Recall of recent events or recently learnt facts is impaired.

Side effects Side effects, both short term and long term, resulting from suboptimal cortisol replacement. Short term side effects which occur within the first few years are growth acceleration, growth retardation, weight gain, short term memory loss, dizziness, headaches, hirsutism and acne. Long term side effects develop over many years and may not become apparent until later in life, such as infertility, adrenal rests, polycystic ovaries, short term memory loss, osteoporosis, obesity, diabetes, metabolic syndrome, coronary heart disease and hypertension.

Slipped epiphyses Condition where the cartilage on the hipbone becomes loosened and displaced. Produces a limp and requires urgent surgical assessment.

Testosterone Male sex hormone mainly produced by testes but can on occasion be produced by the adrenal glands when cortisol replacement is very poor.

Toxic psychosis Altered mental state with confusion, hallucinations e.g. strange voices and thought disorder.

Weight gain In paediatrics this is represented by an increase in weight during childhood, of more than 2.5–3 kg/year. In CAH this can be a result of over treatment with hydrocortisone.

GENERAL

Monitoring therapy is a critical part of CAH care. Both over and under dosing with hydrocortisone leads to many problems and these are summarised in Chapter 20. The most important point about the treatment of CAH, is we are replacing the hormone that is missing, namely cortisol, and we are doing this with cortisol in the form of hydrocortisone tablets and therefore a measure of our replacement should be cortisol in the blood.

If we get cortisol right then the other measures used such as 17-hydroxyprogesterone (17OHP) and androstenedione (A4) should fall into line as we have shown in Chapter 22, where we discuss the relationship between 17OHP and cortisol. We need to know how much cortisol is in the blood to avoid periods of time when levels are too high or too low. 17OHP tells us how the pituitary is responding to cortisol so is a useful measure *in addition* to cortisol.

Historically, the measurement of 17OHP has been used as the marker for assessing 'control' in CAH, rather than assessing cortisol replacement, which is the missing steroid and being replaced with glucocorticoid therapy. In the treatment of diabetes, we think about insulin replacement rather than just 'controlling it', in the case of CAH, with cortisol, we replace the hormone as close to the normal pattern of production as possible. We know that in diabetes if we do this, we will get excellent results and we would expect the same in CAH.

So cortisol replacement is the primary issue.

We will look at 17OHP and A4 and how they interact with cortisol later in the chapter, as people often consider these as 'control measurements' rather than considering cortisol which is being replaced. We do not think this is the correct way as endocrinology is all about replacing the hormone which is missing, as close to how it works in the normal situation.

Firstly, we will look at why we need to test blood levels.

DO I NEED TO HAVE BLOOD TESTS AND HOW OFTEN SHOULD THESE BE TAKEN?

There are many ways of measuring cortisol and 17OHP. These include taking blood samples, collecting saliva or measuring the breakdown products in the urine. Each of these has advantages and disadvantages.

The saliva method is easy to carry out but the relationship between the measures in the saliva and what is actually happening close to the dosing schedule, is far from clear. The reason for this is only free cortisol is measured in saliva and to measure free cortisol, the amount of cortisol in the blood has to exceed the binding of cortisol to the binding protein, cortisol binding globulin. This means only high peaks of cortisol will be measured. Although it can be a guide, it is probably not precise enough to allow for subtle dosing changes. There are further problems with saliva measures, as cortisol is broken down to cortisone in the salivary glands, so how much cortisol appears will depend on how active that enzyme is. In addition, you have to be very careful in sample collection as things such as coffee or acidity can affect values. In particular, a thorough mouthwash is required following taking hydrocortisone tablets A good volume of saliva is needed. If ill and dehydrated it might not be possible to produce enough saliva. This will also be a problem for very young children and babies.

Urine measures are also attractive, but they are more difficult to interpret because urine is often collected over very long periods of time and so the precise relationship to the time a dose of hydrocortisone was taken, as an example is difficult to define. In addition, urine measurement can only average the effect over a period of several hours and that is not what we want when we are thinking about the close interaction between cortisol, 17OHP and the amount of hydrocortisone given. Finally, we are often measuring breakdown products of the steroids in the urine, so these are reflecting not just what is going on in the blood but they will also be influenced by how efficiently the liver is working. This means the measures may not be directly related to what is going on in the blood.

This leaves us with blood tests, which we know are not very popular with many people but they do allow us to establish a very close relationship between cortisol, 17OHP and hydrocortisone. Several hospitals use blood spots, which are relatively easy to obtain by finger pricking but suffer from the limitations in the amount which can be obtained over a 24 hour period and also, there are some concerns over how much cortisol in particular and 17OHP is actually measured in the spot (Fig. 8.3). In addition, unless the spots are collected with good coverage of the filter paper area, problems can occur with analysis. As the blood spots only measure 17OHP this gives no indication of cortisol in the blood at that time, which as we said previously, is what we are substituting with hydrocortisone. A normal or within range 17OHP measurement pre dose does not necessarily mean that the cortisol replacement is optimal, or indeed that there is cortisol in the blood when the blood spot is taken. A very low measurement of 17OHP does not mean there is too much cortisol in the blood at that time because of the lag effects we have talked about in Chapter 22. So, these blood spots, even if taken pre dose for several days, will only show a snapshot of the 17OHP measures at that moment in time.

More detailed blood profiles, which can be done in a hospital by taking blood samples every 1–2 hours, with an extra sample around the dose time, give a much better picture of what is happening and helps establish the close relationship between cortisol, 17OHP and hydrocortisone. This enables us to pinpoint the precise point at which changes to the dose or frequency of hydrocortisone administration can be made. The profiles also allow us to gain an idea of how high cortisol peaks, as well as how low it drops and for how long.

The number of samples which need to be taken needs careful consideration. There is no place at all for just taking random samples, because that does not help us understand what changes are needed to the hydrocortisone dose. Instead, careful matching of the blood test to the time the hydrocortisone dose is given, is required. We know that if you take samples anything less frequently than 2 hourly, then the overall estimate of how much hydrocortisone is being delivered and how much cortisol in the blood results, deteriorates.

A pre and 2 hour post dose blood sampling sounds attractive, but it is better overall to extend this so we can determine, not only the relationship after the dose, but also how long that dose actually lasts and whether there are periods of time not covered with cortisol in the blood. So we prefer regular 2 hourly samples and more recently, we have moved to hourly sampling to better define the amount of cortisol in the blood and the relationship with 17OHP.

The timing of samples is very important. If samples are taken too infrequently, then information on the true peaks and how long cortisol is in the blood, is lost as the information is not captured. Equally, too many samples are unhelpful. You can work out the sampling frequency by knowing the half-life. If the half-life is 60 minutes, then sampling every 120 minutes means underestimations will take place as cortisol could well disappear over that time interval. Sampling less than 60 minutes, is unlikely to give much more information. In fact, with an average half-life of 80 minutes, hourly sampling is more appropriate. Fig. 24.1 shows the patterns observed over a 6 hour period if sampling is undertaken every 20, 60 or 120 minutes. Hourly sampling gives good approximation to what is actually happening, whereas 2 hourly loses detail and underestimates the findings.

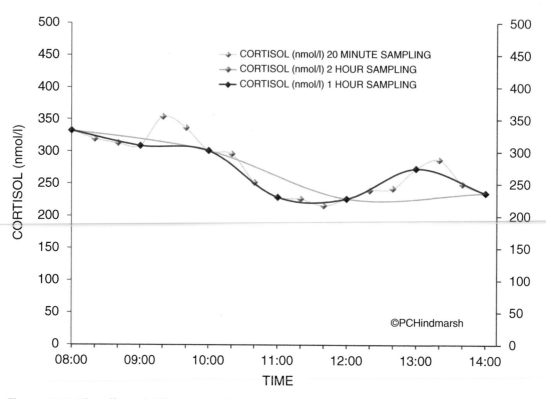

Figure 24.1 *The effect of different sampling intervals on the data obtained.* *20 minute sampling defines actually what is happening. 60 minute sampling approximates this but 120 minute sampling leads to less well defined peaks in particular.*

So with this in mind, we are going to start with Fig. 24.2 which is the classic profile obtained from a blood test measurement of 17OHP. We will start with trying to understand what can be learned from one blood test per day. Then we will build on this, to show the increased detail and wealth of information which we can get from detailed 1–2 hourly profiles of cortisol and 17OHP and compare these data to those from one-off or random samples.

SINGLE BLOOD TEST

Here we have 17OHP measured without considering the cortisol (Fig. 24.2).

The data are plotted in the 24 hour format. As you can see, the only information we have is that 17OHP at 13:00 is 4 nmol/l. We cannot tell where we are with the result as we do not know how this relates to the hydrocortisone taken and the cortisol level.

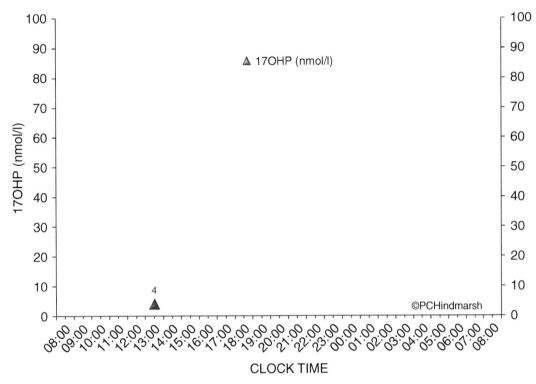

Figure 24.2 *17-hydroxyprogesterone (17OHP) measurement taken from a person after a clinic appointment at 13:00.*

In most centres, this information is used to adjust doses, along with growth and bone age measurements. Both these latter measurements will only highlight problems after they have occurred and will not give the information needed or what cortisol distribution is like over the 24 hour period.

We could say, based on this 17OHP result, that we are doing well and no changes are required. However, we have no idea of the exact time the tablet was taken in relation to the dose, it might have been taken earlier or later than usual, nor do we have any idea of the cortisol level or what is happening for the rest of the day, to 17OHP or cortisol. This is of course an extreme point but it serves to indicate the importance of getting the sampling right.

BLOOD SPOTS (17OHP MEASUREMENTS DONE AT HOME PRE DOSE)

Now we look in a bit more detail at the results of pre dose blood spots which are done before each dose of hydrocortisone is taken (Fig. 24.3).

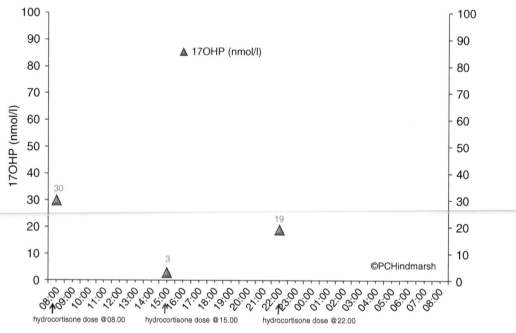

Figure 24.3 *17OHP measurements taken by using blood spots before each dose of hydrocortisone.*

This is the information we would get from the data which might not show the peaks and troughs of 17OHP or cortisol. If we were to join these dots we do not see a true picture of what is happening to 17OHP (Fig. 24.4).

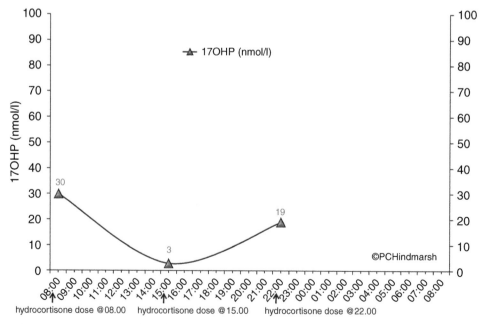

Figure 24.4 *Pattern we would get from the 17OHP blood spot results over the 24 hours.*

The problem with this, is that it is not possible to be sure what needs to be changed. For example, increasing the evening dose will not help the 22:00 17OHP level as it is rising as the 15:00 dose wears off. In addition, altering the 22:00 dose is unlikely to make much difference to the early morning sample as the duration of action of hydrocortisone is such that the system will not be suppressed much after 03:00. Looking at the afternoon result in the graph indicates cortisol replacement may be satisfactory.

What is not clear, is how this is achieved. Is the hydrocortisone dose just right or perhaps too high? Is the timing of the doses correct, as they could easily have run out of hydrocortisone earlier and about to escape from 'control'?

What we are going to show now in Fig. 24.5 is what happens if we add these measurements to what is actually happening. The graph shows 17OHP in a complete profile. What we can now see is this patient is experiencing periods when 17OHP looks good and periods when 17OHP looks less optimal.

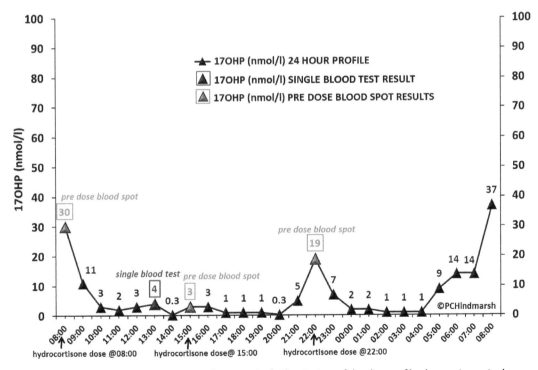

Figure 24.5 *17OHP levels over the 24 hour period. The timing of the doses of hydrocortisone is shown. In addition the data of the single blood test from Fig. 24.1 (orange) and the pre dose blood spot blood spot data (green) from Fig. 24.2 are shown.*

However, we have not answered the question as to what is going on with the most important measure, cortisol. Because cortisol is what we are supposed to be replacing, how are we doing with that?

Fig. 24.6 shows us what is happening when we superimpose the cortisol and 17OHP measurements taken over the 24 hour period.

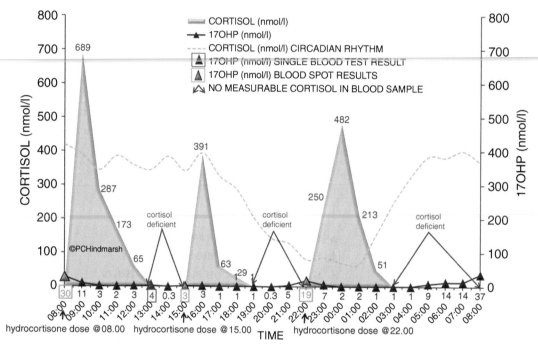

Figure 24.6 *17OHP and cortisol levels superimposed with the original 17OHP blood spots (in green squares) and the single blood sample (orange square). Hydrocortisone is given as thrice daily schedule.*

When we put all the data together, we get a very different picture. Here we have high peaks of cortisol, but it is not lasting until the next dose. This is often apparent when children feel tired or get headaches at lunchtime, as in this case, there is no cortisol present in the blood stream. In fact, when we look at the one–off blood test taken at 13:00, the 17OHP is 4 nmol/l which is within the normal range and the blood spot taken pre dose at 15:00, the 17OHP is 3 nmol/l which again, is within the normal range. However, when we look at the cortisol levels at both 13:00 and 15:00 there is no measurable cortisol in the blood.

Even though 17OHP really looks good, it is cortisol which matters at this time from the symptoms standpoint. When you look at the normal production of cortisol in both adults and children (Chapter 21), there is a good level of cortisol in the blood at this time of the day and although one might say *'control is good'*, that is *only* from the 17OHP standpoint. Remember, we are replacing cortisol and not simply treating the 17OHP. What has happened, is that the very high peak of cortisol has really suppressed 17OHP production and despite there being no cortisol, the next sample shows an even lower level of 17OHP; in fact some labs would not be able to measure this very low level of 0.3 nmol/l. Again, we see this lag between the cortisol and 17OHP levels particularly overnight and in response to the hydrocortisone dose at 08:00.

In the late evening, the peak cortisol post the evening dose is higher than we would like. Cortisol is missing at times and is likely to cause symptoms, so we need to ensure we have got cortisol right and only by measuring cortisol, will we be able to determine this. Both long and short term side effects arise from under or over replacement of cortisol and a common problem is weight gain. If we adjust doses based on 17OHP only without measuring cortisol and increase a dose to bring down 17OHP levels into normal range, symptoms will still occur. The higher dose of hydrocortisone will only give an increased peak of cortisol and will not last longer in the blood stream. Often patients who do not have a full 24 hour profile will be told that their symptoms and side effects have nothing to do with their steroid dose as this is only a replacement dose, but may well have periods of over and under treatment. These data show why a full profile is informative as the balance between over/under treatment with cortisol can only be determined this way.

Another problem with a single sample is how it is taken. Blood samples can be stressful and this can alter the result achieved. The reason for this is ACTH is released in this type of stressful situation and this can happen even when adequate cortisol is present. This means if getting the blood sample is stressful, then ACTH will rise and that will drive 17OHP up. This will give a falsely high value. It is another reason why we do samples through a cannula as it removes this stress element. We go into this in more detail in Chapter 22.

WHY LOOKING AT THE CORTISOL LEVELS OVER THE FULL 24 HOUR PERIOD IS IMPORTANT

We have looked at how single 17OHP spots or blood tests do not show a full picture and we will now illustrate how important it is to look in detail at cortisol over the 24 hours (Fig. 24.6). This patient is on three doses of 7.5 mg of hydrocortisone a day and without looking at the cortisol in full detail, it would be easy to assume that each of these doses would generate the same amount of cortisol and we can also see from these data, how important it is to get the dose timing correct to prevent 'over stacking'.

DAY CURVES

It is tempting to compromise and undertake what is called a day curve. These are popular with adult endocrinologists, although mostly undertaken for cortisol replacement in other adrenal conditions where there are no other markers to measure. The problem with them is they do not cover enough time to be able to make accurate changes to the dosing schedule.

Often, the samples are taken at 2 or 4 hourly intervals which makes it even more difficult to advise on dose alterations as the gap between events is too long. Fig. 24.7 illustrates this point.

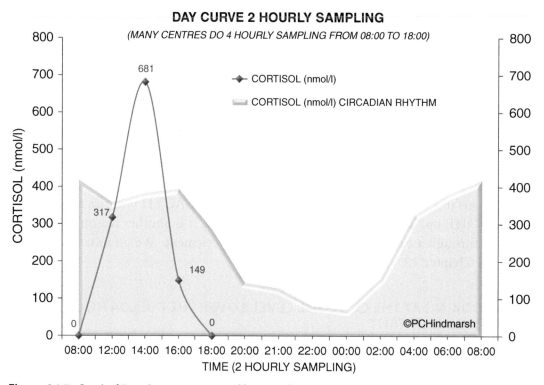

Figure 24.7 Cortisol Day Curve constructed by sampling at 2 hourly intervals.

The first observation on this graph is the very high cortisol peak of 681 nmol/l which would lead you to think the morning dose is too high. We can see at 18:00 there is no cortisol left in the blood to measure and we actually have no idea when the next dose is to be taken and how long it will last in the system.

However, when we add in the data from a full 24 hour profile as shown in Fig. 24.8, we get a totally different view of the distribution of cortisol.

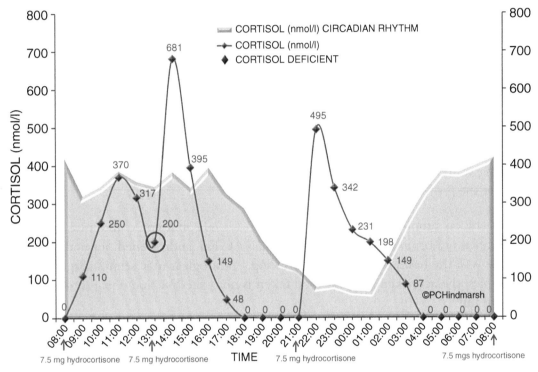

Figure 24.8 *The actual profile from which Fig. 24.7 was constructed.*

Now we see the following:

- The 13:00 dose shows an example of cortisol stacking leading to the very high peak at 14:00 (although another dose could be taken at this time, there is no consideration of the cortisol already in the blood, so the dose is stacked on top resulting in the very high peak). From the data shown in Fig. 24.7 it would be tempting to reduce the morning dose to reduce the 681 nmol/l level but this would be wrong as it is the 13:00 dose which needs adjusting.
- The patient is cortisol deficient from 18:00 until the next dose at 21:00 and we can see from the circadian rhythm, there should be cortisol in the system at this time.

- The 21:00 dose is taken too early to give early morning cover.
- The patient is without cover from 04:00 until the next dose is taken at 08:00, this being at a time when cortisol should be at the highest level in the system.
- The morning peak is happening too late in the morning at 11:00.
- The absorption and peak of the dose taken at 08:00 and 21:00 from the same dosage of hydrocortisone, is different.
- The patient is without any cortisol for a total period of 8 hours which is 33% of the 24 hour period. This occurring on a daily basis will lead to long term side effects, as well as making the patient vulnerable to hypoglycaemia and adrenal crisis in illness.

This is all very important information you do not get from the day curve (Fig. 24.9).

SO HOW DO YOU MAKE A PROFILE?

So it does seem like a good idea to get these profiles constructed, so how do we do it? What we do is to place an intravenous cannula under local anaesthetic cream, in a vein, so that lots of small samples can be taken every 1–2 hours. If the cannula is working well, there is no pain. We usually put the cannula in about an hour before we start the profile to overcome any stress effect.

In these blood samples we measure cortisol and 17OHP, but you could measure lots of other different hormones on the sample such as ACTH, androstenedione and measures of how well the testes or ovaries are working. Although it may seem a large number of samples, the actual amount of blood taken is not excessive and equates to about an egg cup full!

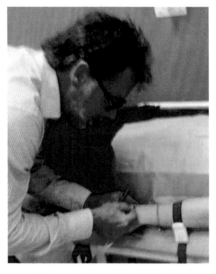

Figure 24.9 *Sampling during a profile.*

As we have stressed it is important not to work with one-off blood tests. It is essential to know the cortisol value, 17OHP, the time the tablet was taken as without considering all this vital information, you could get false information suggesting poor 'control' because you hit an odd occasion when 17OHP is high or low.

A common example of this is when a sample is taken or blood spot is done pre morning dose and the hydrocortisone which was given the previous evening is out of the system, causing the 17OHP value to be high. Then massive morning doses are deemed to be needed to bring the 17OHP level down. This can be seen in the graph in Fig. 24.10.

Notice also, the effect of the evening dose which has a high peak at 22.00 but at this point 17OHP was low anyway. This is because the huge doses have markedly reduced 17OHP. In the early hours of the morning there is a natural surge of ACTH to instruct the adrenal glands to increase cortisol production. In CAH, the adrenal glands cannot make cortisol therefore 17OHP levels (which you are trying to suppress especially at this time), rise as a result. However, the hydrocortisone from the evening dose is wearing off so ACTH levels will keep rising until the morning dose is taken.

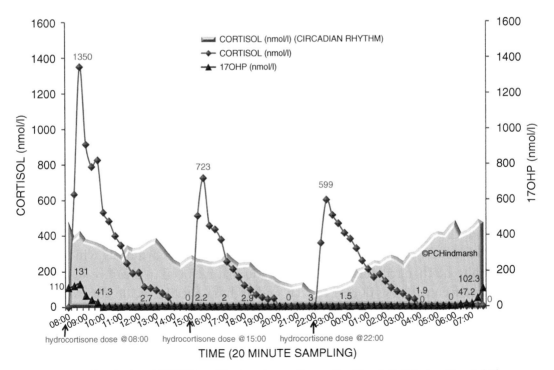

Figure 24.10 *Cortisol and 17OHP profile showing as the cortisol levels fall during the night because hydrocortisone does not last for more than 6 hours the 17OHP rises. Pre morning dose 17OHP will always be high unless the night hydrocortisone dose is given after midnight.*

In some practices, patients are told to take the largest dose at night, this will give a very high peak which temporarily switches off 17OHP and androgen production for the early morning period. However, due to the pharmacokinetics of hydrocortisone, the dose will not last longer and the patient will be without cortisol for a period of time and the high peak will most certainly cause side effects. This is often called reverse circadian dosing and is not effective

This information indicates the best way to deal with this problem is to take hydrocortisone as late as possible at night, preferably as late as 01:00! The data also show us incidentally, that hydrocortisone lasts in this individual for a long time, so it is likely this person is a slow metaboliser.

This is how we create profiles and what we are looking for when we start to analyse them. In Chapter 23, we went into a lot of detail about how we gauge cortisol replacement and what different treatment schedules deliver, so it might be worth rereading the chapter now, so that you understand how profiles are made. What we will do now is to critically evaluate other one-off measures of CAH management.

CAN WE USE A SINGLE MEASURE LIKE ANDROSTENEDIONE OR TESTOSTERONE?

It would be really good if there were only a single measure we could use to tell us how well we were doing. As tempting as this may sound, it is unlikely this will ever be achieved. The reason is the system we are looking at is dynamic, changing during the day and night and we also give frequent doses of hydrocortisone. If we had one single measure it might tell us that something needs changing, but what exactly needs to be changed is not clear?

The situation is similar to that we see in diabetes. Here we have a single measure called glycated haemoglobin or HbA1c. This measure tells us the average amount of glucose that the person has been exposed to over 3 months. It is an important overall measure of insulin replacement therapy. However, it does not tell us which insulin dose needs to be changed during the day. To do that we need to measure actual blood glucose on a frequent basis during the day and night rather like we do cortisol profiles.

In many reports it has been suggested that androstenedione or testosterone can be used as a marker and that you only need one blood sample. This is not the case for two reasons. We can ignore testosterone, as the adrenal production of testosterone does not take place until the adrenal glands become over stimulated by ACTH. It is therefore, a marker of extremely poor cortisol replacement. Once the adrenal glands start to shrink as 'control' is re-established after careful adjustments to the distribution and amount of hydrocortisone, 17OHP and androgen levels will begin to normalise and testosterone from the adrenal glands will disappear. Testosterone will look better even though optimum replacement has not been attained.

Because of this, testosterone is not a very sensitive marker for cortisol replacement. Furthermore, in males, during puberty and adulthood testosterone comes from the testes, so any measure of it would be difficult to interpret – is it testicular or adrenal testosterone? In woman, where polycystic ovaries are common, is the testosterone coming from them?

When considering androstenedione, we know that it is not constant in the blood but varies. Fig. 24.11 shows how androstenedione in the blood varies in a person without adrenal problems throughout the 24 hour period and follows a pattern very similar to that of the cortisol circadian rhythm.

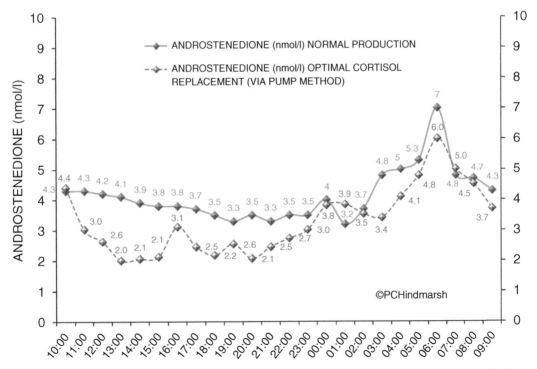

Figure 24.11 *Average androstenedione levels through the 24 hour period in normal individuals in green (solid line) and in a person receiving hydrocortisone using a pump system in turquoise (dashed line). Note the peak in people without adrenal problems and how the pump matches this change.*

In addition, the relationship between androstenedione and 17OHP is such that as 17OHP increases so does androstenedione (Fig. 24.12).

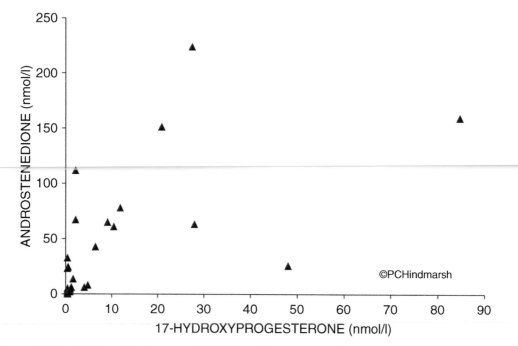

Figure 24.12 *Relationship between 17-OHP and androstenedione is positive so that as one increases so does the other.*

Note, however, that for any given 17OHP level there can be a wide range of androstenedione values. If we now look at the relationship between 24 hour mean cortisol and androstenedione we see a different picture (Fig. 24.13).

In this situation, androstenedione does not relate that well to cortisol. In other words, you have to keep increasing 24 hour mean cortisol to a value of about 150 nmol/l then suddenly the androstenedione drops. This means androstenedione can show if it is high, that there is not enough cortisol present, but when it comes into range it is not possible to be sure what the cortisol level is, as it could be anything between 150 and 350 nmol/l or indeed, as the graph shows in some cases less than 150 nmol/l. In addition, even if we have this one–off measure and it shows the person needs more cortisol, it does not tell us when more cortisol is needed. Only a cortisol profile with 17OHP measures can show us that.

In addition, we also know that the mean 24 hour cortisol levels in normal individuals range between 200 and 600 nmol/l. This means if we simply went for androstenedione suppression using an average 24 hour cortisol measurement of 150 nmol/l, we would still be under replacing with cortisol and therefore symptoms of under replacement would occur.

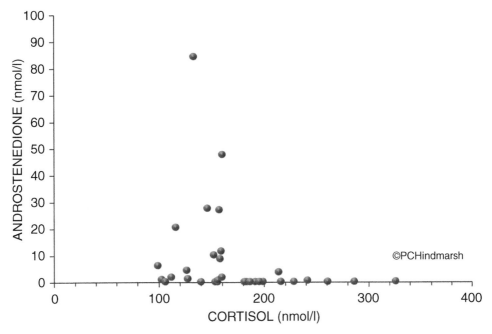

Figure 24.13 *Relationship between 24 hour mean cortisol and androstenedione. As cortisol increases there is step down in androstenedione that is quite sudden.*

When 17OHP and androgen levels are high, the adrenal glands enlarge due to increased ACTH drive (Fig. 22.14). This allows them to produce androstenedione more easily. To get on top of this situation, ACTH needs to be switched off to allow the adrenal glands to reduce in size and the androstenedione levels fall.

Once the adrenal glands are reduced in size, less hydrocortisone is required. Profiles help us to get this right as we aim to get cortisol replacement right because once this is achieved, then 17OHP and androstenedione will be 'controlled', in other words, be brought to normal values. Not only will they be normalised, but cortisol replacement will also be optimal for the individual.

If doses are too high, the adrenal glands can shrink and become inactive. The production of 17OHP (Fig. 17.5) and androstenedione is totally switched off and in some instances, even if there is no cortisol for more than 24 hours, the adrenal glands remain dormant and may need to be stimulated by giving synacthen, to 'wake them up'.

It is imperative that cortisol is the target hormone for replacement therapy, otherwise if androstenedione is the target, 'control' will be achieved from the androgen standpoint. However, the patient is likely to be still cortisol insufficient (Fig. 24.14).

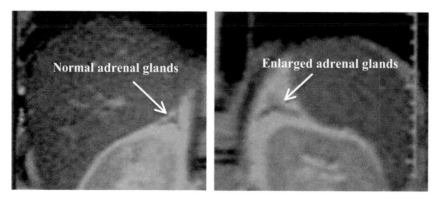

Figure 24.14 *Normal adrenal scan on the left to an enlarged adrenal glands on the right obtained during a period of poor cortisol replacement. Scans at same magnification.*

Finally, just as 17OHP is not affected immediately by hydrocortisone, androstenedione does not change rapidly either. Fig. 24.15 shows how the effects of high circulating levels of cortisol from a bolus of hydrocortisone do not impact much initially on androstenedione and 17OHP levels.

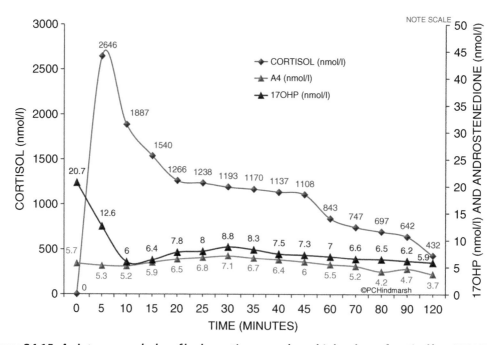

Figure 24.15 *An intravenous bolus of hydrocortisone produces high values of cortisol but 17OHP and androstenedione (A4) are unaffected until 120 minutes after the injection when they start to change.*

CONCLUSIONS

Hydrocortisone is the preferred glucocorticoid for cortisol replacement. Initially, the dose can be worked out in terms of body size, then adjusted depending upon the results of blood profiles. Glucocorticoids have a number of side effects associated with them and important drug interactions such as the oral contraceptive pill. Detailed blood monitoring is the way to minimise these side effects.

24 hour profiles help us decide how much hydrocortisone to give and how frequently. When high peaks are achieved a reduction in dose might be needed. If the hydrocortisone is not lasting as long as expected then more frequent doses will be required. 17OHP is responsive to cortisol but there is a lag between the cortisol peak and the subsequent 17OHP trough.

> *Getting cortisol replacement right is the key. Once this is optimised the rest (17OHP and adrenal androgen measures) will follow!*

FURTHER READING

Hindmarsh, P.C., 2009. Management of the child with congenital adrenal hyperplasia. Best Pract. Res. Clin. Endocrinol. Metab. 23, 193–208.

Krone, N., Webb, E.A., Hindmarsh, P.C., 2015. Keeping the pressure on mineralocorticoid replacement in congenital adrenal hyperplasia. Clin. Endocrinol. 82, 478–480.

CHAPTER 25

Other Hormones and Their Roles

GLOSSARY

Androstenedione One of the adrenal androgens which is made from dehydroepiandrosterone by the action of the enzyme 3beta-hydroxysteroid dehydrogenase type 2. Level rises in CAH when cortisol replacement is suboptimal.

Estradiol Female sex hormone produced in the ovary.

Follicle-stimulating hormone (FSH) Hormone produced by the pituitary gland which is involved in sperm formation from the testes in males. In females, along with luteinising hormone, it is involved in egg selection and production of estradiol.

Hypothalamo-pituitary-adrenal axis The system which controls cortisol production and release. The hypothalamus is the control centre coordinating cortisol feedback and hosting the clocks which determine the circadian rhythm. A message, corticotropin releasing factor instructs the pituitary to release adrenocorticotropin hormone (ACTH) which causes cortisol release from the adrenal glands. The system amplifies production so that the amount of cortisol produced is far higher than expected from the amount of ACTH produced.

Luteinising hormone (LH) Hormone produced by the pituitary gland which generates testosterone from the testes in males. In females, along with follicle-stimulating hormone, it is involved in egg selection and production of estradiol.

Testosterone Male sex hormone mainly produced by testes but can on occasion be produced by the adrenal glands when cortisol replacement is very poor.

GENERAL

We have discussed in detail how looking at cortisol levels achieved which are derived from the synthetic form of cortisol, hydrocortisone, along with 17OHP levels over a 24 hour period allow us to fine tune and individualise dosing. There are many other hormones we can study which gives us a more accurate knowledge of other aspects of CAH.

ADRENOCORTICOTROPIN HORMONE

ACTH is a polypeptide tropic hormone which is produced and secreted by the anterior pituitary gland (Fig. 1.2) and it stimulates the secretion of glucocorticoid steroid hormones from adrenal cortex cells, especially in the zona fasciculata of the adrenal glands. It is the key regulator of cortisol production. When cortisol levels rise,

ACTH levels normally fall and when cortisol levels fall, ACTH levels normally rise. In CAH there is no or very little production of cortisol, so ACTH levels rise as the pituitary gland keeps instructing the adrenal glands to make cortisol.

ACTH is difficult to measure in that samples need to get to the laboratory very quickly and have to be transported on ice. We usually take a measurement of ACTH at midnight (00:00) and 4 a.m. (04:00) or 6 a.m. (06:00) if 17OHP levels are high, to check whether the pituitary gland is producing ACTH in an uncontrolled way. Very high ACTH can result from under treatment with hydrocortisone and is responsible for the brown pigmentation called hyperpigmentation, or sometimes referred to as ACTH patches and these are often seen when replacement is poor (Fig. 16.4). Persistently high ACTH levels can also lead to TART formation.

The other reason ACTH is difficult to measure, or rather interpret is the half–life is very short, somewhere in the region of 4 minutes. This means lots of samples, every 5 minutes, are really needed if we wanted to know what is actually happening. This is one reason why it is useful to have 17OHP as a proxy marker of what is happening to ACTH.

Fig. 25.1 illustrates what a 24 hour profile measuring ACTH in a person without any medical conditions looks like. During this profile blood samples were taken at 20 minute intervals so was an underestimate of what was actually happening.

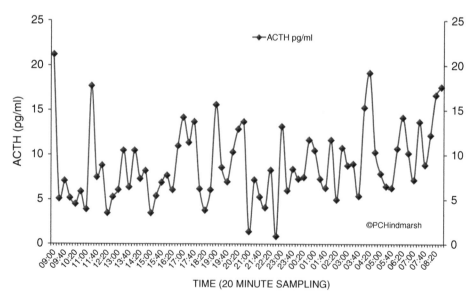

Figure 25.1 *24 Hour ACTH profile in a young adult. Secretion takes place in pulses with a gradual increase upwards from 22:00 onwards. Note spike activity at 11:00 and 16:00 which may reflect pre meal signal to increase blood glucose.*

Although the samples are not as frequent as we would like, the rise in ACTH overnight can be seen. We can also pick out bursts of activity just before lunch and in the late afternoon. These are accompanied by cortisol spikes as well and probably reflect the ACTH drive to increase cortisol and blood glucose, as the body at these times will be entering a fasting state as no food will have been consumed from breakfast or lunch.

SEX STEROIDS—ESTRADIOL AND TESTOSTERONE

Estradiol

Using profiles also enables us to carefully evaluate the sex steroids over the 24 hour period. During prepuberty, there is no LH and FSH present to drive production of estradiol or testosterone (Fig. 7.2). However, in early puberty the system becomes more active and LH and FSH are produced during the night/early morning period (Fig. 7.3). but not during the day. It is not until late puberty and adulthood that sex steroids can be measured during the day and night (Fig. 7.4).

The situation becomes more complex in females with the onset of periods as estradiol levels vary not only during the day and night, but also during the monthly cycle as can be seen in Fig. 25.2.

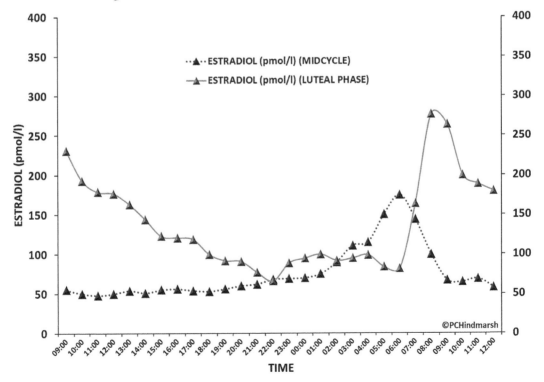

Figure 25.2 *24 Hour profile of estradiol during the menstrual cycle.*

Here we can see that the amount of estradiol produced is quite different, so it is important to be able to interpret any estradiol measures in light of the stage of the cycle. Notice, that irrespective of the stage of the cycle the early morning surge can be measured. The difference resides in the magnitude of the surge and how long the higher values last for.

In polycystic ovary syndrome the ovaries continue to make estradiol, but the cycle of estradiol and progesterone which gives the menstrual bleed, is disrupted leading to irregular and/or infrequent bleeds. Using this approach of comparing the 24 hour 17OHP, androstenedione, cortisol and estradiol allows us to start working out where the hormones are actually coming from.

So if androstenedione is high, but 17OHP and cortisol are where we want them to be, then the likely source of the androstenedione is the ovary which would be what we would expect if polycystic ovaries were present (Fig. 22.3).

Testosterone

When we look at the sex steroids, just as with 17OHP and cortisol, a one-off measurement does not give us the whole picture. This is particularly the case with testosterone as both the adrenals and testes in males, can produce testosterone if all is not right in CAH. We are going to use testosterone as an example here. Fig. 25.3 shows the average testosterone and cortisol levels taken from 29 profiles done on 4 healthy adult males.

Fig. 25.3 shows that testosterone rises early in the morning to reach a peak around 06:00. When we are thinking about CAH, we would expect if we get cortisol replacement right, 17OHP will follow as will the adrenal androgens. So when we have got it right, any testosterone we measure will be from the testes in males.

As discussed in Chapter 24 using a one-off blood sample can give a false picture as to what is happening for the rest of the day.

Elevated testosterone levels can also come from the adrenal glands or polycystic ovaries and even when tested in conjunction with androstenedione, a one-off blood test result may give an incorrect idea of what is going on.

Fig. 25.4 shows the result of a one-off blood test taken at 08:00 to measure the testosterone level of a male with SWCAH.

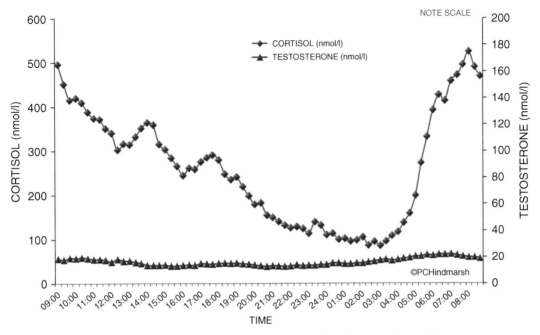

Figure 25.3 *Average 24 hour cortisol and testosterone levels from 29 profiles undertaken on 4 healthy adult men over a 12 month period.*

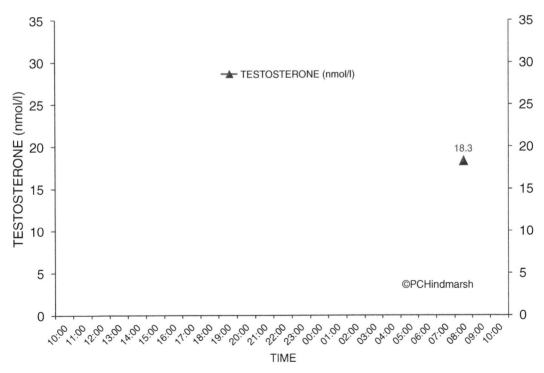

Figure 25.4 *A single testosterone measurements which although viewed as normal for time of day does not tell us what is taking place during the rest of the 24 hour period.*

This one-off measurement looks quite good and if we compare it to the data from the studies in normal individuals, it is actually within normal range, as the average value at that time of day was 20 nmol/l. But is it? In actual fact, androstenedione was high as was 17OHP, which would indicate the testosterone is probably coming mainly from the adrenal glands, rather than just the testes.

We need all this extra information to interpret the result. If we actually look at what was happening throughout the 24 hour period in Fig. 25.5, then we see a different picture.

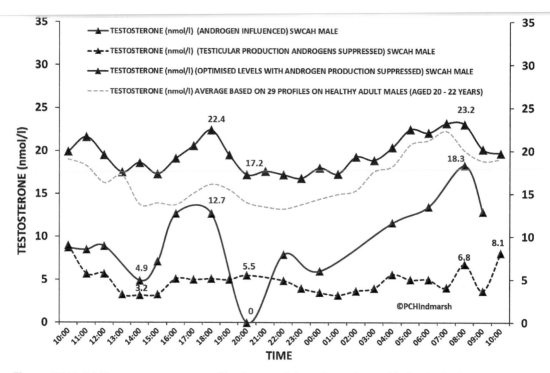

Figure 25.5 *24 Hour testosterone profiles in an adult male patient with SWCAH when treatment was suboptimal (red line). Optimal cortisol replacement with no excess androgen production (brown dashed line) and when stabilised on standard replacement therapy (dark blue line). The average value for young males is shown as the dotted line.*

In fact, the 18.3 nmol/l is the best testosterone level achieved and overall the results are considerably lower than the testosterone values in the young males without CAH for most of the 24 hour period (Fig. 25.5 dotted light blue line).

Fig. 25.5 illustrates further important points. Initially, the patient's cortisol replacement was suboptimal and resulted in elevated androgen levels. The testosterone although measurable, was not generated just from the testes but also had an adrenal component. Introducing hydrocortisone in a dose that reduced 17OHP and shrank the adrenal glands, led to a drop in testosterone to quite low values as the adrenal contribution to circulating testosterone was reduced. Simply returning to conventional dosing based on attaining a normal cortisol profile was then associated with an improvement in testosterone. At the same time, 17OHP and androstenedione were normal so the change in testosterone represented the recovery of the testes to produce normal amounts of testosterone, which follow exactly the amount and pattern seen in young adults without CAH.

ANDROSTENEDIONE

Androstenedione is made in the adrenal glands as well as the testes and ovaries. In females, androstenedione is converted to provide around half of all testosterone and almost all of the body's estrone, a form of estrogen. Although the testes produce large amounts of androstenedione in males, they secrete little of this into the blood and instead, rapidly convert it into testosterone within the testes. The adrenal glands also produce androstenedione in men, but this contribution is minimal compared to the contribution from the testes. In this chapter, we are going to consider the androstenedione made predominantly by the adrenal glands in CAH. This is also covered in Chapter 1.

Androstenedione has a circadian rhythm (Fig. 24.11). Again, looking at a one-off androstenedione level does not show the real picture (Fig. 25.6). If this patient had a blood sample taken to measure androstenedione level at 10:00, the result of 9.9 (nmol/l) would suggest that levels over the 24 hours would all be acceptable.

However, when we plot in the rest of the 24 hour measurements (Fig. 25.7) we can see the variation during this period. If the sample had been taken an hour later it would have shown an elevated value of 28.2 nmol/l and at 20:00 the level drops very low to 1 nmol/l.

The measurement the next morning at 07:00 shows a rise to 40 nmol/l. So over the 24 hour period, there is considerable variation and depending on when we take a single sample, we would say over treated, under treated or just right!

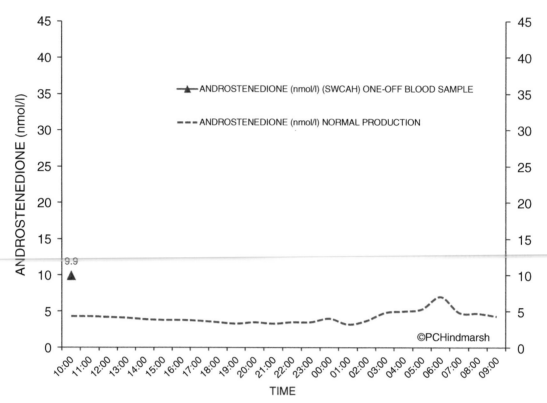

Figure 25.6 *24 Hour profile of androstenedione in individuals without CAH and a single measure made in a patient with CAH.*

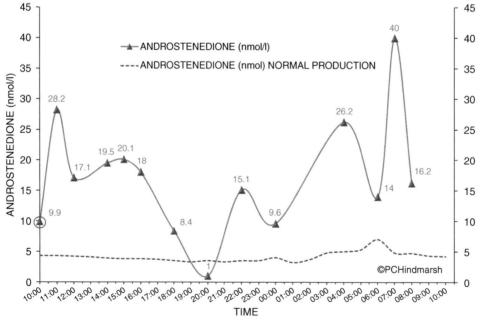

Figure 25.7 *24 Hour profile of androstenedione in an individual with CAH illustrating the single value from Fig. 25.6 and the values subsequently. Dashed line shows the circadian rhythm of androstenedione.*

In the next example (Fig. 25.8) we look at the results of a blood test taken at 13:00 where both the 17OHP and androstenedione level were measured.

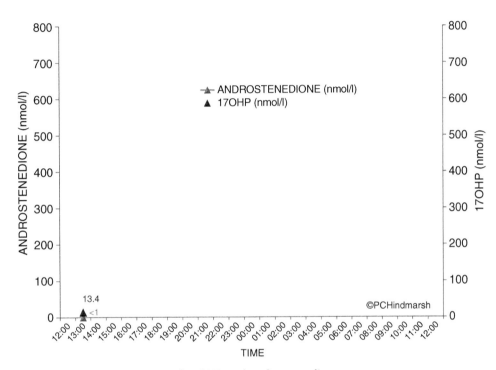

Figure 25.8 *Single measurement of 17OHP and androstenedione.*

Fig. 25.8 shows there is no measurable androstenedione in the blood stream which would suggest over treatment; however, when we look at 17OHP at the same time, 13:00, the result is 13.4 nmol/l.

This is slightly elevated for the measurement range at this time of day so this might be put down to the effect of the blood test.

Looking at the full androstenedione profile in Fig. 25.9 along with cortisol, we get a different picture on what needs to be adjusted. For the whole day there is no measurable androstenedione which would most certainly point to over treatment with cortisol. What does the cortisol look like?

When the cortisol levels are plotted, we can see there are actually periods where there is no cortisol present in the blood stream. In fact, at 13:00 this is the case despite there being no measurable androstenedione and although there is a slightly elevated 17OHP there is no cortisol present in the blood stream.

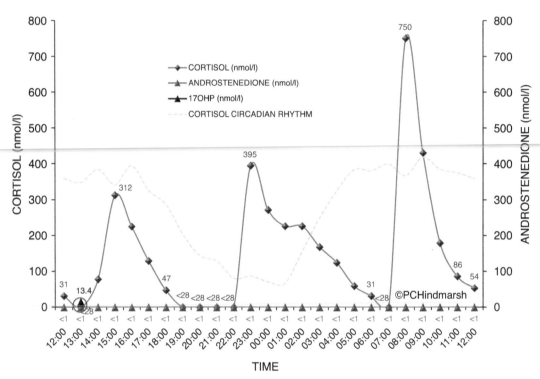

Figure 25.9 *24 Hour profile of androstenedione and cortisol along with the one-off 17OHP measurement at 13:00 and the normal cortisol circadian rhythm.*

If in Fig. 25.9 we did not have the cortisol to guide us, we might conclude this patient is over treated but the cortisol shows us distribution is wrong. There are 4 hours where there is no cortisol present and a very high peak of 750 nmol/l from the morning dose, therefore this patient is both over and under treated.

So again, we learn the importance of collating data namely cortisol, 17OHP and androstenedione.

These hormones are all interlinked, androstenedione and 17OHP are all driven by how much cortisol is present to feedback onto the pituitary. Just like 17OHP, there is a lag in androstenedione as shown in Fig. 25.10, where the high cortisol peak does not influence androstenedione until about 60 minutes later.

Of note, is that when the adrenal glands are large they produce androstenedione quite easily. Once they start to shrink, the androstenedione production falls to normal but 17OHP often takes a longer period of time before it too is back into the normal range. So again, how we interpret profile data, depends on dose and frequency of hydrocortisone administration, along with prior knowledge of how well CAH has been treated in the past and the likely size of the adrenal glands at the time the profile is undertaken.

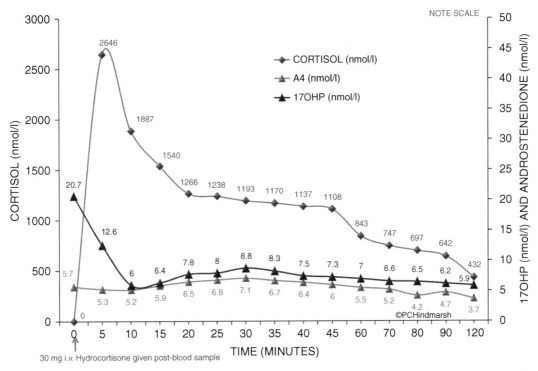

Figure 25.10 *Effect of an intravenous bolus of hydrocortisone on androstenedione. Note the high cortisol peak and the lowering of androstenedione does not start to take place until some 60 minutes after the peak and is still not switched off at 120 minutes.*

LUTEINISING AND FOLLICLE-STIMULATING HORMONES

Luteinising hormone

Luteinising hormone (LH) is produced by the pituitary gland under the direction of the hypothalamus. In males, LH drives the testes to make testosterone whereas in females, there is a balance with follicle-stimulating hormone (FSH) to make estradiol and progesterone. Production is low in prepubertal children, then increases overnight at first in early puberty and by the end of puberty it takes place during the day and night (Fig. 25.11) (see Chapter 7).

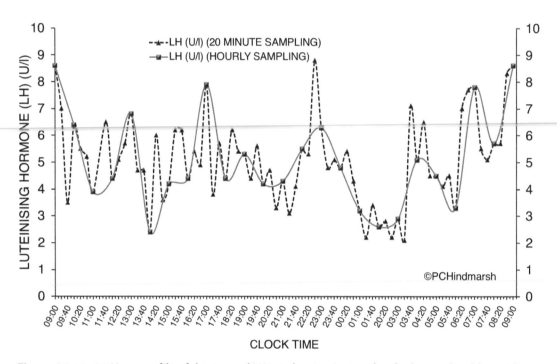

Figure 25.11 *24 Hour profile of the normal LH production in a male who has no health problems. The 20 minute sampling was undertaken in a clinical trial and shows the bursts of LH and superimposed on the solid lighter blue line shows what the results would look like if the samples were taken hourly which gives enough information to know that this male has normal production of LH.*

The reason we undertake an LH profile is that it gives us an idea of activity in the hypothalamo-pituitary-gonadal axis. If cortisol replacement is not optimal, then the elevated adrenal androgens will suppress the LH, while androstenedione and testosterone will be measurable. Once the cortisol replacement is optimised, the adrenal androgen production will be suppressed and the LH will rise.

This is shown in Fig. 25.12. We can use this approach also to determine whether someone is entering into puberty or not.

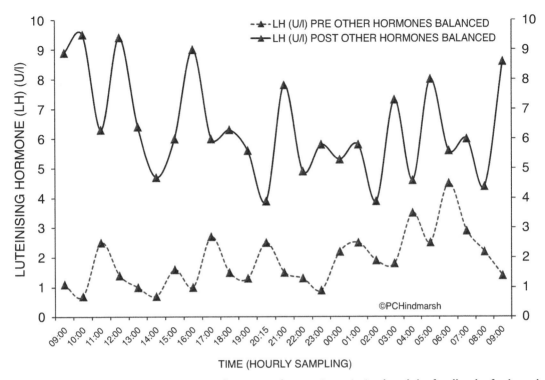

Figure 25.12 *Change in LH as CAH replacement therapy is optimised and the feedback of adrenal androgens is suppressed. LH pulses are heightened.*

FOLLICLE-STIMULATING HORMONE

FSH is secreted from the same cell in the pituitary as LH. The amount of LH or FSH produced depends on the frequency of the gonadotropin releasing hormone pulses hitting the pituitary cells.

Fast bursts lead to more LH being produced, whereas slow bursts lead to more FSH produced. In males, FSH instructs the Sertoli cells to mature sperm cells, whereas in females there is a complex interaction with LH to produce estradiol and to help select the egg during each menstrual cycle.

Fig. 25.13 shows a profile of FSH and Fig. 25.14 shows again what happens in a person with CAH when cortisol replacement is improved, resulting in better FSH secretion due to the reduced feedback effect of the adrenal androgens on the gonadotropin producing cells in the pituitary.

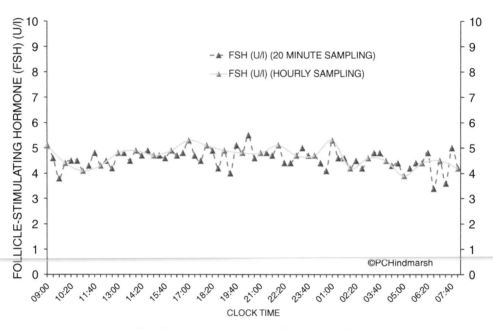

Figure 25.13 *24 Hour profile of FSH in a male who has no health problems. The 20 minute sampling was undertaken in a clinical trial and shows the bursts of FSH and superimposed on the solid lighter turquoise line shows what the results would like if the samples were taken hourly which gives enough information to know that this male has normal production of FSH.*

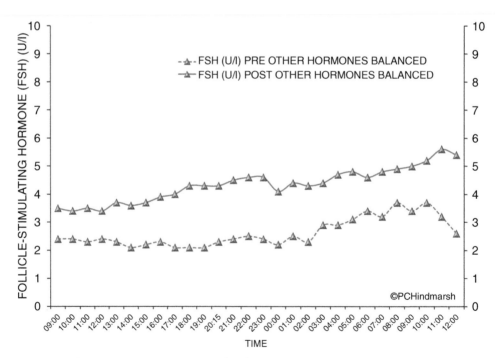

Figure 25.14 *Change in FSH as congenital adrenal hyperplasia (CAH) replacement therapy is optimised and the feedback of adrenal androgens is suppressed. FSH pulses are not as well defined as LH as the FSH half-life is greater than LH but heightened levels can be noted.*

GROWTH HORMONE

Growth hormone (GH) is also secreted in bursts from the pituitary. It is produced mainly at night, but technically does not have a circadian rhythm like cortisol. There are various tests which can be carried out during the day for GH, but a 24 hour profile can also be undertaken. During the day, GH levels are very low with bursts confined mainly to the night time.

If there are concerns about growth in someone with CAH we add GH to our set of test measurements. Usually, what we see during the night are three bursts of GH rising to values at least above 12 mU/l (Fig. 25.15). These values are lower in adults who make less GH.

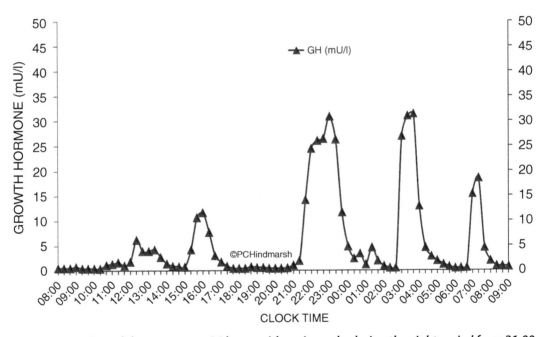

Figure 25.15 *Growth hormone over 24 hours with main peaks during the night period from 21:00 through to 07:00 in a young peripubertal person.*

BLOOD GLUCOSE

Blood glucose can be measured during a 24 hour profile profile as well. This can be very useful in determining whether there are periods of time when the blood glucose becomes low. Low blood glucose might be expected at times when the circulating cortisol level is also low. A critical period of time is at 04:00 (4 a.m.) when there is very little cortisol present if a person is on hydrocortisone, especially if the evening dose of hydrocortisone is given early in the evening, rather than at midnight or as late as possible. Fig. 25.16 shows the blood glucose over the 24 hour period. Notice that it does not change very much and is kept within a very narrow target range of 3.5–7.0 mmol/l. A blood glucose profile is very useful at times, to check whether there are unexpected periods of hypoglycaemia which might mean changes are needed to the distribution of hydrocortisone. There is a tendency for low blood glucose to occur in the early hours of the morning in people deficient in cortisol, (particularly when unwell) and this is the reason that we advocate More@4 during periods when the person is unwell (see Chapter 29, Stress Dosing).

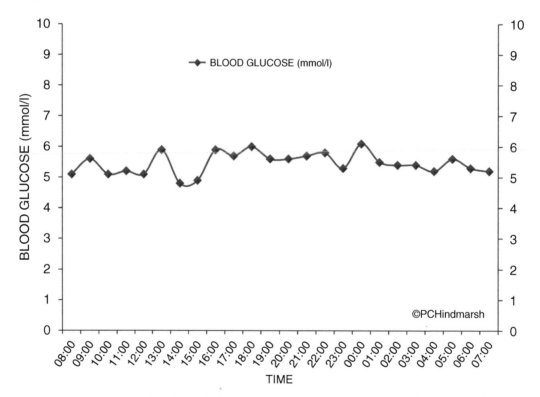

Figure 25.16 *24 Hour profile of blood glucose in a person with CAH and good cortisol replacement showing that it is tightly regulated between 3.5 and 7.0 mmol/l.*

OTHER IMPORTANT MEASUREMENTS UNDERTAKEN DURING 24 HOUR PROFILES

We can also measure other levels during a profile.

Glucose, insulin and fasting lipids

Glucose, insulin and cholesterol (part of a lipid profile) are taken as fasting samples early in the morning. We measure these samples to check for diabetes and fat problems. Fatty substances in the blood are known as lipids, and cholesterol is one type of lipid. Cholesterol is transported to cells around your body by lipoproteins in a similar way that cortisol is. Low-density lipoproteins can lead to a buildup of cholesterol in the artery walls and lead to disease, whereas high-density lipoproteins are good as they are not associated with disease. Triglycerides are another type of lipid and are used by the body to provide energy. However, unused triglycerides are stored in fatty tissues and if there are high levels of this lipid in the blood, it also means an increased risk of heart problems. Have a look at Chapter 12 where we look at glucose and insulin.

Plasma renin activity

This tells us how well we are replacing aldosterone with fludrocortisone. If the plasma renin activity (PRA) level is elevated, this indicates the dose of fludrocortisone may need increasing. A low PRA level indicates the dose of fludrocortisone may need decreasing. We take samples recumbent (after resting all night and before the patient is up and about in the morning) and then another one several hours later when the patient is active and been walking around. If the result from the standing sample is higher than the recumbent one by a value of 5 pmol/l/hour, then this suggests that the fludrocortisone dose is too low, as normally the rise in renin on standing should be less than 5 pmol/l/hour. At the same time to support the renin measurement, we undertake standing and resting blood pressure measurements, as this also helps determine how well we are doing with the fludrocortisone therapy.

Likewise, we measure sodium and potassium using a single blood sample and we talk about this in the chapter on fludrocortisone (Chapter 32).

Calcium

We can also measure calcium but this is not a good measure of bone health we need a DEXA scan for that (Chapter 13).

FURTHER READING

Gardner, D., Shoback, D., 2011. Basic and Clinical Endocrinology, ninth ed. McGrawHill, New York.

CHAPTER 26

Missing a Dose of Hydrocortisone

GLOSSARY

Cortisol deficient No cortisol measurable in the blood. Serious situation which unless treated leads to adrenal crisis.

Hypoglycaemia Symptoms and signs which occur when blood glucose falls below 3.5 mmol/l. The first signs of shakiness and sweating usually appear when the blood glucose reaches 3.2 mmol/l.

Missing dose This can happen at any stage especially the lunchtime/afternoon dose as this is a busy time of the day. Good way to remember is to use an alarm on watch or phone set to go off at tablet time. Timed boxes which pharmacists provide are also very useful.

GENERAL

Inevitably, there will be an occasion when a dose is forgotten or remembered several hours after the dose should have been taken. In this chapter we will show using 24 hour profiles, the effect of this and what we suggest you do, as soon as you remember or realise that the dose has been missed. As always, it is best to check with your endocrinologist for their advice.

In CAH there are two problems which occur when missing a dose. Firstly, the individual will be left totally cortisol deficient until the next dose is taken. Secondly, this will affect the ACTH levels and then the 17-hydroxyprogesterone (17OHP) levels, both will become elevated.

CORTISOL

Doses are usually administered at the point where cortisol levels are already low from the previous dose and will stack on the remaining cortisol, to keep the supply of cortisol in the blood at a good level. If the dose is missed, this leaves the individual at risk of low blood glucose levels and all the other symptoms of low cortisol.

It has often been reported parents realise that the dose has been forgotten by their child's behaviour and we have had many reports of patients themselves saying they either suffer a headache, feel very lethargic and some patients have reported they feel very angry.

Congenital Adrenal Hyperplasia. http://dx.doi.org/10.1016/B978-0-12-811483-4.00026-X

We are going to work through what happens when a dose is missed, using examples at different times of the day when a person is receiving 3 or 4 times per day hydrocortisone. We will give two examples of each to illustrate various points.

The following suggestions are a general guide based on the data we have acquired over many years of doing 24 hour profiles, measuring and studying in detail cortisol replacement as well as the relationship between cortisol and 17OHP. Again, always check with your endocrinologist.

MISSING A DOSE WHEN TAKING HYDROCORTISONE 3 TIMES A DAY

Missing the morning dose

We are going to start with a person who takes hydrocortisone 3 times a day. In the first example (Fig. 26.1) we will show what happens when the morning dose is missed. These are two examples of actual profiles with the morning dose removed to illustrate the period of time each patient is left without any cortisol in the blood, if the morning dose is not taken.

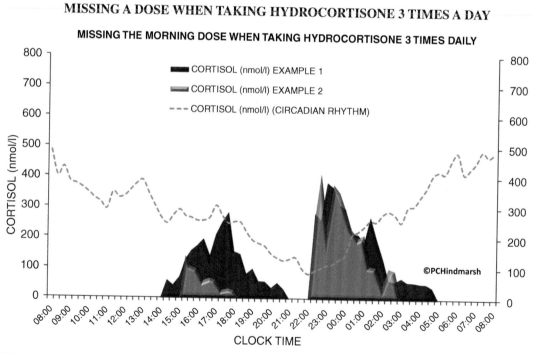

Figure 26.1 *Effect of missing the morning dose in two patients receiving hydrocortisone 3 times per day.*

Fig. 26.1 shows the effect of missing the morning dose of hydrocortisone in two patients on 3 doses of hydrocortisone per day. If we look at the normal production (light blue dashed line), the levels of cortisol are at the highest in the morning and this will lead to symptoms such as low blood glucose, dizziness, headaches, lethargy, and all other symptoms that are associated with low blood glucose.

Example 1 (dark blue)

This patient's usual dosing times are morning dose at 08:00 (8 a.m.), afternoon dose at 14:00 (2 p.m.) and evening dose at 22:00 (10 p.m.). When the morning dose is missed as we can see in Fig. 26.1, there is no cortisol from 08:00 (8 a.m.) until 14:00 (2 p.m.) which leaves them totally cortisol deficient for 6 hours.

When we look at the time when the evening dose runs low we can see that by 05:00 (5 a.m.) cortisol cannot be measured in the blood. In total, this means from 05:00 (5 a.m.) until 14:00 (2 p.m.) which totals 9 hours (37% of the 24 hour period) there is no cortisol. When you look at the circadian rhythm at this time of the day, cortisol production is at its highest.

What to do

Take the missed dose as soon as you remember.

- If you remember the missed dose at any time before 13:00, take the morning dose immediately and then your normal afternoon dose. Although this means you will have a high peak of cortisol from 'over stacking', the 17OHP will have risen significantly and this high cortisol peak should bring the level down as well as boost the blood glucose.
- If you remember to take the dose up to an hour before the next dose is due, i.e. between 13:00 and 14:00, then take the normal morning dose as soon as you remember and take half of the usual afternoon dose at the time that dose is due.

Example 2 (light blue)

In example 2 the patient's usual morning dose is taken at 08:00 (8 a.m.) and the next dose is taken in the afternoon at 15:00 (3 p.m.). Looking at the data, we can see the previous night dose would run out around 03:00 (3 a.m.). So if the morning dose was missed, this would leave the patient without any cortisol in the system from 03:00 (3 a.m.) until the next dose is taken at 15:00 (3 p.m.), leaving the patient for a total of 12 hours without any measurable cortisol in the blood.

We can also see that the afternoon dose is out of the system by 18:00 and the evening dose is taken at 22:00 (10 p.m.), which increases the total amount of time that the patient is without cortisol by another 4 hours, to an overall total of 16 hours which is 67% of the day.

What to do

As soon as you remember the dose has been missed take the morning dose.

- If you remember the dose before 14:00 (2 p.m.), take the morning dose and then at 15:00 (3 p.m.) take the afternoon dose as usual.
- If you remember the dose any time after 14:00 (2 p.m.), take the morning dose and then at 15:00 (3 p.m.) take half the usual afternoon dose.

Missing the afternoon dose

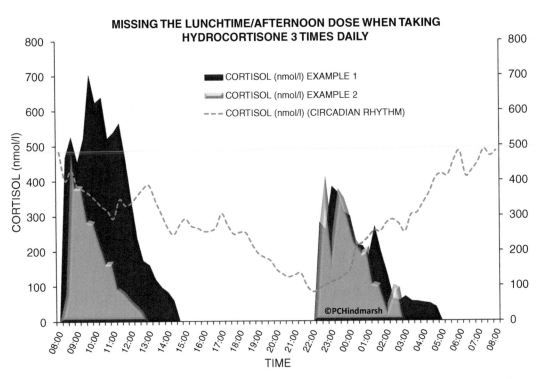

Figure 26.2 *Effect of missing the afternoon dose in two patients receiving hydrocortisone 3 times per day.*

Example 1 (dark blue)

This patient usually takes the afternoon dose at 14:00 (2 p.m.). The data in Fig. 26.2 show there is a low level of cortisol in the blood before the 14:00 (2 p.m.) dose is taken and the dose 'stacks on' the remaining cortisol. This 'useful stacking' obtains good afternoon cortisol levels (Fig. 26.3). However, when the

14:00 (2 p.m.) dose is missed there is no measurable cortisol in the blood from prior to 15:00 (3 p.m.), until the evening dose is taken at 22:00 (10 p.m.).

When we look at the circadian rhythm at this time, we can see that although the cortisol starts to decline in the early evening, there is now no cortisol present for just over 7 hours.

There is a natural surge of ACTH at around 16:00 (4 p.m.) which would give a rise in cortisol around this time. This would precipitate a further rise in the 17OHP level which would already be elevated from the lack of cortisol in the afternoon.

What to do
Take the missed afternoon dose as soon as you remember.

- If you remember the dose before 17:00 (5 p.m.) take the normal afternoon dose.
- If you remember the dose after 17:00 (5 p.m.), then take half the afternoon dose and take the evening dose as late as possible.

Example 2 (light blue)

This patient usually takes their afternoon dose at 15:00 (3 p.m.), however, as you can see the cortisol delivered from the morning dose of hydrocortisone runs out around 13:00 (1 p.m.). The patient has no cortisol for 2 hours prior to when the afternoon dose is taken. If the afternoon dose is forgotten and the next dose is taken at 22:00 (10 p.m.), the patient will be without cortisol for a total of 9 hours! If you consider the further period of time in the early hours of the morning where there is no cortisol in the system from 03:00 (3 a.m.) until 08:00 (8 a.m.), over the 24 hour period the patient would be without cortisol for a total of 14 hours, more than half a day!

What to do
Take the missed afternoon dose as soon as you remember.

- If you remember the dose before 17:00 take the normal afternoon dose.
- If you remember the dose after 17:00, then take half the afternoon dose and take the evening dose as late as possible.

Missing the evening dose

Forgetting to take any dose of hydrocortisone is unfortunate, however, when you miss the evening dose which we advocate to be taken as late as possible, this can upset the system to a large extent. Adults usually take their last dose of the day before they go to bed and many parents will give their child the evening dose as late as midnight. If this is forgotten, it is unlikely that anyone will realise that the dose has been missed due to being asleep. This can lead to low blood glucose levels and if the child should become ill during the night they are at serious risk! Do remember we advocate that everyone, no matter what their age, who is on hydrocortisone tablets, takes double dose (equal to twice the usual morning dose) at 04:00 (4 a.m.) in illness. Remember, this is in addition, to the double morning dose, which still needs be taken at the usual time.

In the early morning around 04:00 (4 a.m.), the body has its biggest surge of ACTH. This happens in every human being, except of course those whose body does not make ACTH and they are usually patients who have had brain surgery and their pituitary gland has been removed. In CAH the ACTH levels rise high to instruct the adrenal glands to make cortisol and the adrenal glands then go into overdrive trying to produce cortisol!

The adrenal glands respond by making an excess amount of 17OHP as well as excess androgens. In conditions such as Addison's disease, the high production of ACTH occurs but the excess production of other hormones does not happen because the adrenal glands have been compromised. However, in both conditions the ACTH levels rise and stay high until a dose of hydrocortisone is taken.

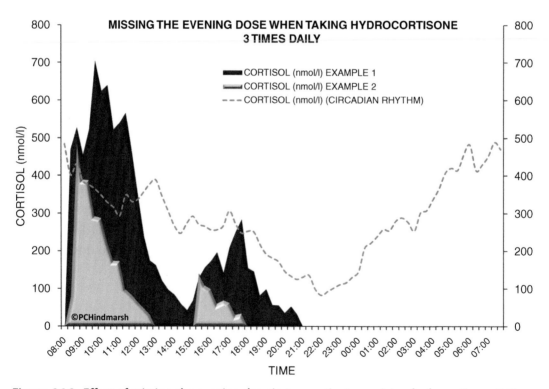

Figure 26.3 *Effect of missing the evening dose in two patients receiving hydrocortisone 3 times per day.*

The data in Fig. 26.3 illustrate two examples of what happens when the evening dose is forgotten.

Example 1 (dark blue)

The patient usually takes their dose of hydrocortisone at 22:00 (10 p.m.). We can see the cortisol from the afternoon dose of hydrocortisone has run out by 21:00 (9 p.m.). Although this is the time when cortisol levels are at their lowest, it is important to note there is always still some cortisol in the blood (Fig. 21.1).

Missing the evening dose for this patient means they are without any cortisol from 21:00 (9 p.m.) until the next morning dose is taken at 08:00 (8 a.m.), which actually leaves the patient totally cortisol deficient for 11 hours.

What to do

- Double the morning dose as soon as you wake in the morning to dampen down ACTH and 17OHP as well as boost blood glucose. Have a sweet drink at the same time as taking the missing dose.
- If you should wake at any time and remember, then take the evening dose even if this is up to an hour before your morning dose is due. Then take the morning dose as usual.

Example 2 (light blue)

This patient also takes the evening dose at 22:00 (10 p.m.). However, if we look at what the afternoon dose achieves we can see that the cortisol is out of the system by 18:00 (6 p.m.). So in fact, missing the evening dose will result in this patient having no cortisol in the blood from 18:00 (6 p.m.) until the morning dose is taken at 08:00 (8 a.m.), totalling a period of 14 hours.

This period combined with the insufficient cortisol cover in the late afternoon would mean this patient is without cortisol for a total of 16 hours (67%) of the 24 hour period.

What to do

- Double the morning dose as soon as you wake in the morning to dampen down ACTH and 17OHP as well as boost blood glucose. Have a sweet drink at the same time as taking the missing dose.
- If you should wake at any time and remember, then take the evening dose even if this is up to an hour before your morning dose is due. Then take the morning dose as usual.

MISSING DOSES WHEN TAKING HYDROCORTISONE 4 TIMES PER DAY

Missing the morning dose

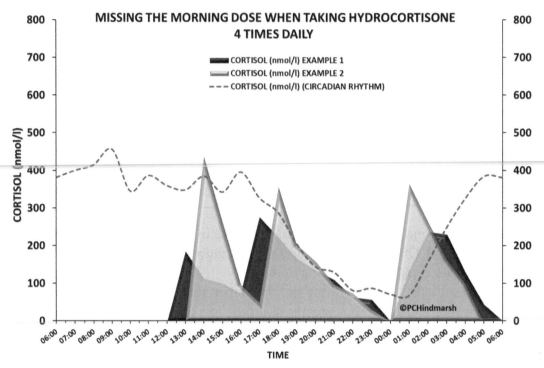

Figure 26.4 *Effect of missing the morning dose in two patients receiving hydrocortisone 4 times per day.*

Example 1 (dark blue)

This patient's usual dosing times are morning dose at 06:00, lunchtime dose at 12:00, afternoon dose at 16:00 and evening dose at midnight (00:00). When the morning dose is missed (Fig. 26.4), we can see there is no cortisol from 06:00 until 12:00, leaving them totally cortisol deficient for 6 hours. This period covers the crucial window when cortisol should be present in high amounts in the morning. This will lead to symptoms of low cortisol.

What to do

If you have missed the morning dose and your next dose would be at 12:00.

- Regardless of the time take the morning dose.
- If you remember and the next dose is due in 1 hour, take the normal morning dose straight away and for the next dose only take half the dose at the usual time.

Example 2 (light blue)

This patient takes their morning dose at 06:00, lunchtime dose at 13:00, afternoon dose at 17:00 and an evening dose at midnight (00:00). When the morning dose is missed (Fig. 26.4), we can see there is no cortisol from $06:00$ until $13:00$, leaving the patient totally cortisol deficient for 7 hours. We can also see that the evening dose has run out by $05:00$, so in fact this patient has no cortisol in the blood for a total of 8 hours. Again, this period covers the crucial window when cortisol should be present in high amounts, in the morning. This will lead to symptoms.

What to do

If you have missed the morning dose and your next dose would be at $13:00$.

- Regardless of the time take the morning dose.
- If you remember and the next dose is due within 1 hour, then take the normal morning dose straight away and for the next dose, only take half the dose at the usual time.

Missing the lunchtime dose

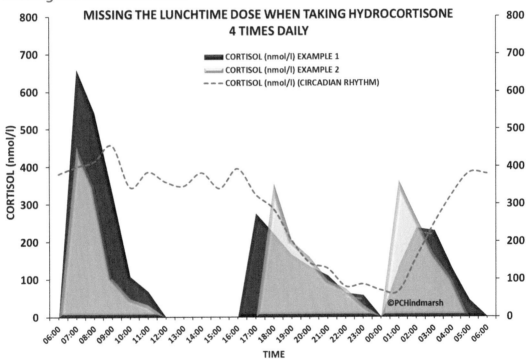

Figure 26.5 *Effect of missing the lunchtime dose in two patients receiving hydrocortisone 4 times per day.*

Example 1 (dark blue)

Here we see quite a gap between the morning dose wearing off at $12:00$ and the $16:00$ dose kicking in. There is a period of 4 hours with no cortisol. Again, we would expect to see symptoms of this as there is still a lot of cortisol present normally at this time. This is particularly the case in children at school who often feel tired in the afternoon if they miss the lunchtime dose (Fig. 26.5).

What to do

If you have missed the 12:00 dose:

- If it is before 15:00, take the normal lunchtime dose.
- If you remember after 15:00, then take half the 12:00 dose and the 16:00 dose as usual.

Example 2 (light blue)

In Example 2 we can see the morning dose has run out by 12:00. If the lunchtime dose which is normally taken at 13:00 is missed (Fig. 26.5), we can see there is no cortisol from 12:00 until 17:00, leaving the patient totally cortisol deficient for 8 hours.

The situation is similar to that seen in Example 1. As we say this can cause symptoms for many late afternoon, particularly if the person does sports after school when they may be unable to finish the games due to lack of energy.

What to do

If you have missed the 13:00 dose:

- If you remember before 16:00, take the normal lunchtime dose.
- If you remember after 16:00, then take half the 13:00 dose and the 17:00 dose as usual.

Missing the afternoon dose

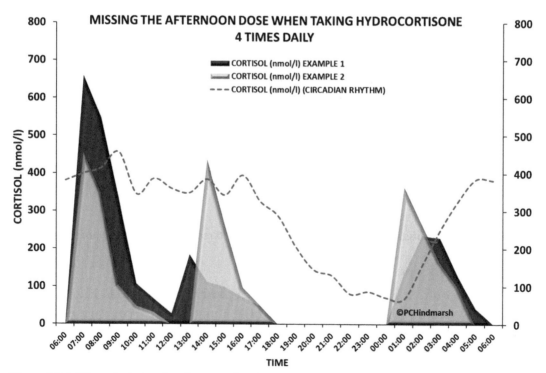

Figure 26.6 *Effect of missing the afternoon dose in two patients receiving hydrocortisone 4 times per day.*

Example 1 (dark blue)

Missing the late afternoon dose leads to lack of cover in the evening. Although cortisol is low at this stage, normally there is always some present. Even lack of this lower amount of cortisol leads to fatigue at the end of the day and often people have to, or feel the need to, go to bed early (Fig. 26.6).

What to do

If you have missed the 16:00 dose:

- If you remember before 20:00, then take the normal 16:00 dose.
- If you remember after 20:00, then take half the 16:00 dose and the late evening dose (normal amount) at midnight.

Example 2 (light blue)

The situation is the same for Example 2.

It is important point to note, that although these patients take their lunchtime tablet at different times and the cortisol peaks achieved from their lunchtime dose are different, they both run out of cortisol at the same time in the evening (18:00). This is a good example of the importance of clearance in determining how much cortisol is present.

What to do

If you have missed the 17:00 dose:

- If you remember before 20:00, then take the normal 17:00 dose.
- If you remember after 20:00, then take half the 17:00 dose and the late evening dose (normal amount) at midnight.

Missing the evening dose

Missing the evening dose even when dosing with four doses of hydrocortisone a day, leaves the patient without cortisol at a time when the natural production starts to rise slowly from midnight. This means the surge of ACTH, which reaches a maximum around 04:00, will increase and remain high until the next dose of hydrocortisone is taken. Blood glucose will drop and if illness occurs during this period, there is a risk of an adrenal crisis occurring. Note that these profiles start at 06:00 (Fig. 26.7).

Example 1 (dark blue)

Here we see the late afternoon dose has worn off by midnight leaving the person without cortisol overnight. Normally, we would be expecting rising cortisol values building up to the peak in the early hours of the morning. This is a problem particularly in babies and young children because if they become ill overnight, there is no cortisol to help fight infection. In addition, their glucose stores will be low and glucose levels will fall. To help with this, for anyone, it is good to have a sweet drink at the same time as taking the missing dose.

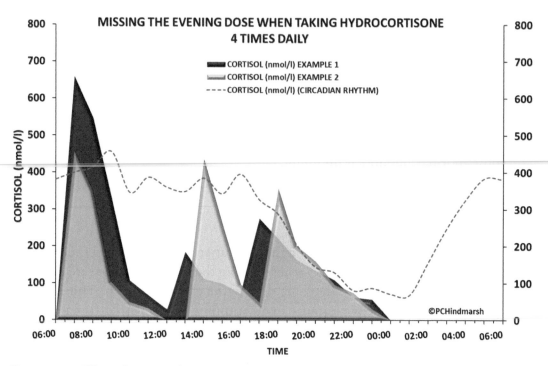

Figure 26.7 *Effect of missing the evening dose in two patients receiving hydrocortisone 4 times per day.*

What to do

If you have missed the evening dose:

- You must take double the morning dose as soon as you wake in the morning to dampen down ACTH and 17OHP and to boost blood glucose. Have a sweet drink at the same time as taking the missing dose.
- If you should wake at any time and remember then take the evening dose even if this is up to an hour before your morning dose is due, then take the morning dose as usual.

Example 2 (light blue)

Again we see the loss of cortisol overnight. This will lead to high ACTH driving the adrenal glands. In CAH there will be an increase in 17OHP and androgens. In Addison's, the rise in ACTH will lead to increased pigmentation if this happens on a regular basis, particularly if the last dose is taken too early at 18:00.

What to do

If you have missed the night time dose:

- You must take double the morning dose as soon as you wake in the morning to dampen down ACTH and 17OHP and to boost the blood glucose. Have a sweet drink at the same time as taking the missing dose.
- If you should wake at any time and remember, then take the evening dose even if this is up to an hour before your morning dose is due, then take the morning dose as usual.

SUMMARY

Here is what to do then if you have forgotten your hydrocortisone tablet.

3 TIMES A DAY DOSING

If you have missed the morning dose and your next dose would be the afternoon dose:

- Regardless of the time take the morning dose.
- If you remember and the next dose (afternoon dose) is due in 1 hour, then take the normal morning dose straight away and for the afternoon dose only take half the dose at the usual time.

Return to normal dosing schedule.

If you have missed the afternoon dose:

- If you remember before 17:00, take the normal lunchtime dose as there is a surge of ACTH at 16:00.
- If you remember after 17:00, then take half the lunchtime dose and the evening dose as late as is possible.

Return to normal dosing schedule.

If you have missed the evening dose:

- You should take double the morning dose as soon as you wake in the morning to dampen down ACTH and 17OHP as well as boost the blood glucose. Have a sweet drink at the same time as taking the missing dose.
- If you should wake at any time and remember then take the evening dose even if this is up to an hour before your morning dose is due, then take the morning dose as usual.

Return to normal dosing schedule.

4 TIMES A DAY DOSING

If you have missed the morning dose and your next dose would be at 12:00 or lunchtime.

- Regardless of the time take the morning dose and then take your 12:00 or lunchtime dose as usual.
- If you remember and the 12:00 or lunchtime dose is due in 1 hour, then take the normal morning dose straight away and for the 12:00 or lunchtime dose only take half the dose at the usual time.

Return to normal dosing schedule.

If you have missed the 12:00 or lunchtime dose:

- If you remember up to two hours after your 12:00 or lunchtime dose is due, then take the normal 12:00 or lunchtime dose. Take your afternoon dose as usual.
- If you remember 2 hours past the time when your 12:00 lunchtime dose was due, then take half the lunchtime dose and the afternoon dose as usual.

Return to normal dosing schedule.

If you have missed the afternoon dose (usually at 16:00):

- If you remember before 20:00, then take the normal afternoon dose and the evening dose (normal amount) as usual.
- If you remember after 20:00, then take half the afternoon dose and the evening dose (normal amount) at midnight.

Return to normal dosing schedule the next day

If you have missed the evening dose:

- You should take double the morning dose as soon as you wake in the morning to get the ACTH and 17OHP back down again and to boost the blood glucose. Have a sweet drink at the same time as taking the missing dose.
- If you should wake at any time and remember then take the evening dose even if this is up to an hour before your morning dose is due, then take the morning dose as usual.

Return to normal dosing schedule.

FLUDROCORTISONE

If you miss the fludrocortisone dose then it is important to replace as well. Although, you will not feel much different physically, the body will start to lose sodium and water and you will dehydrate.

If you take the full fludrocortisone in the morning:

- Take half the morning dose when you remember and then take another half morning dose in the evening.

If you take the full fludrocortisone in the evening:

- If it is before 16:00, then take half the evening dose when you remember and then take the evening dose as usual.
- If it is after 16:00, then take quarter of the evening dose and take the normal evening dose at midnight.

Never double the fludrocortisone dose

If by mistake you do take a double fludrocortisone dose, then cut down on salt intake for that day and increase your water intake for the next 24 hours.

If you are in a hot country, then either increase your intake of salt with salty foods such as crisps, or salt tablets.

CONCLUSIONS

We do recommend not missing doses regularly, as inevitably this will lead to periods of under treatment and if the missed dose is not replaced carefully as mentioned earlier, cortisol 'over stacking' will occur and lead to over treatment. This will not cause problems on a one-off occasion, but if it is a regular event then you will start to see the side effects of too much cortisol.

The other problem is that as soon as the cortisol drops too low to measure, ACTH rises to instruct the adrenal glands that the body needs cortisol urgently. The adrenal glands start to produce 17OHP in response to the ACTH and the ACTH level also becomes elevated. If this happens on a regular basis, because the dose or dose timing is not correct, or the individual regularly misses a dose, the adrenal glands will grow (adrenal 'hyperplasia' – meaning increase in size of the adrenal glands) and the individual will need an overall increase in dose for a period of time to shrink the adrenal glands back to normal size. It is often said at this point when doctors assess the treatment of the condition based on the 17OHP, that hydrocortisone is no longer working and a stronger glucocorticoid is needed. The androstenedione measure will be very high. What is needed are slightly higher doses of hydrocortisone to be used over a short period of time (approximately 1 to 2 months), first ensuring of course, that the dosing frequency is correct. This higher dosing is needed to switch off the ACTH drive to the adrenal glands, which reduces their size and with the reduction in size, comes the return to normal of the 17OHP and androstenedione levels. Once this is achieved the dose can be carefully titrated down using 24 hour profiles to guide the process.

Finally, although it is tempting to sleep in at weekends and take tablets later, it is important not to do this, but to set the alarm for the normal time to take the tablets and then go back to sleep once they are taken. Unfortunately, normal cortisol production does not change over weekends!

FURTHER READING

Lönnebo, A., Grahnén, A., Karlsson, M.O., 2007. An integrated model for the effect of budesonide on ACTH and cortisol in healthy volunteers. Br. J. Clin. Pharmacol. 64 (2), 125–132, Available from: http://www.ncbi.nlm.nih.gov/pmc/articles/PMC2000622/?report=reader.

CHAPTER 27

Intravenous, Intramuscular and Other Forms of Hydrocortisone

GLOSSARY

Cortisol binding globulin A protein made by the liver which attaches itself to cortisol and carries it around the body. This is known as bound cortisol. 90–95% of cortisol is bound in this way with 5% in the free state. The free cortisol is the biologically active cortisol. In blood tests we measure bound and free cortisol and this is called total cortisol.

Hydrocortisone Synthetic form of cortisol.

Hydrocortisone muco-adhesive buccal tablets These tablets which used to be known as Corlan Pellets are made for mouth ulcers. Although they come in a handy 2.5 mg coated tablet, they do not deliver cortisol in the same manner as hydrocortisone tablets. They are not licenced for use in replacement adrenal therapy and there have been reports of patients vomiting them whole, 80 minute after ingestion.

Intravenous bolus injection Injection of dose of hydrocortisone directly into a vein. Used in emergency situations in hospital and before and/or during operations. Also used to measure clearance of cortisol.

Pump method Using a diabetic pump to infuse hydrocortisone continuously, using the Peter Hindmarsh formula to calculate rates which incorporates the individual's metabolism, allowing the delivery of cortisol to precisely mimic the circadian rhythm. The pump has a bolus function as well as functions to deliver double and triple doses.

GENERAL

So far we have talked about giving hydrocortisone as an oral tablet. We have done this deliberately, as this is the way it is given as part of treatment and what most people are familiar with. In this chapter we look at other forms of hydrocortisone. Intravenous hydrocortisone is often used in hospitals in emergency situations or on intensive care or in preparation for surgery.

Many readers will be familiar with the idea of giving intramuscular hydrocortisone as it is currently taught for emergency injections at home or at school. We cover emergency injections in more detail in Chapter 30.

Congenital Adrenal Hyperplasia. http://dx.doi.org/10.1016/B978-0-12-811483-4.00027-1

There are other forms of hydrocortisone available, such as hydrocortisone suppositories as well as Hydrocortisone Muco-Adhesive Buccal Tablets for mouth ulcers, formally known as Corlan Pellets. These will be discussed as well.

INTRAVENOUS AND INTRAMUSCULAR HYDROCORTISONE

Preparations of hydrocortisone

In the United Kingdom there are two preparations of hydrocortisone which can be used for intravenous use. These are Solu-Cortef and Hydrocortisone Sodium Phosphate. Hydrocortisone Sodium Phosphate was previously known as Efcortesol.

Hydrocortisone sodium phosphate 100 mg/ml and 500 mg/5 ml solution for injection (previously known as Efcortesol)

Hydrocortisone Sodium Phosphate is a ready made liquid preparation that has a shelf life of usually, 24 months [Fig. 27.1A(c)]. Hydrocortisone Sodium Phosphate is popular as an emergency injection although it is a thick liquid which makes it harder to inject. Patients can have reactions to Hydrocortisone Sodium Phosphate with one patient who was severely allergic to one of the excipients (Fig. 27.1B). However, it is convenient although sometimes the glass vials are difficult to snap open, so we suggest using an Ampsnap [Fig. 27.1A(d)] which is a plastic cap that fits over the glass top of the ampoule, which helps you to snap it open easily and safely.

Solu-Cortef

Solu-Cortef [Fig. 27.1A(a)] is a freeze dried powder which comes with a separate vial of water for injections. For the quick, safe opening of the glass vial we also recommend using an Ampsnap. Solu-Cortef has a shelf life of 60 months. The sterile water for injection [Fig. 27.1A(a)] is made specifically for this purpose and dissolves the powder very quickly. Once mixed the hydrocortisone can then be given as a bolus, an intravenous infusion or as an emergency injection.

In other parts of the world Solu-Cortef also comes as ACT-O-VIAL which is an automated solution generator using a self mixing system [Fig. 27.1A(b)].

We use Solu-Cortef because it contains less excipients (Fig. 27.1B) and all our clearance studies are done using Solu-Cortef. For pump use, we recommend using Solu-Cortef only, as Hydrocortisone Sodium Phosphate due to its consistency, can pool under the skin causing lumps and skin irritation.

(A) Types of hydrocortisone for intravenous and injection use

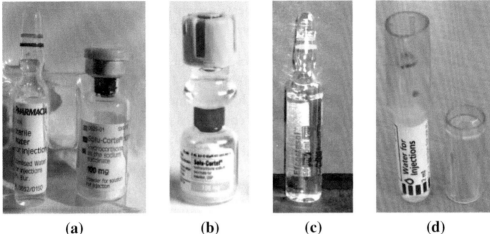

| (a) | (b) | (c) | (d) |

(a) **Solu-Cortef with water for injections.**

(b) **ACT-O-VIAL®.**

(c) **Efcortesol recently rebranded as Hydrocortisone Solution for Injections (Hydrocortisone Sodium Phosphate).**

(d) **Ampsnap for opening ampoules safely**

(B) List of excipients

SOLU-CORTEF	HYDROCORTISONE SODIUM PHOSPHATE
Sodium Biphosphate Sodium Phosphate	Disodium Edetate Disodium Hydrogen Phosphate, Anhydrous Sodium Acid Phosphate Sodium Formaldehyde Bisulphite Monohydrate Phosphoric Acid (10% solution) Water for injections

Medicines Information MHRA Government UK

Figure 27.1 *(A) Different preparations of hydrocortisone, and (B) excipients of Solu-Cortef and Hydrocortisone Sodium Phosphate.*

Infusion of hydrocortisone

A bolus injection given intravenously or intramuscularly is very good for an immediate effect. However if seriously ill, having major surgery or unable to keep oral medication down and further hydrocortisone is required, it is better to give the hydrocortisone as an infusion.

This is done in the hospital using an infusion pump which delivers the hydrocortisone continuously and directly into the vein. Otherwise, what happens with bolus injections is cortisol seesaws between very high and very low values over a 6 hour period.

Fig. 27.2 illustrates how the infusion of hydrocortisone and the bolus look as cortisol in the blood stream when administered. Here, the bolus given through the vein (intravenously) gives very high levels which then come down very quickly and after 5–6 hours there is very little in the way of cortisol left in the bloodstream.

An infusion produces a steady level which can be varied and is exactly what is needed, for example during and after surgery. The problem with infusion is it takes a few hours to achieve a steady state, so it is often best to start with a bolus injection to cover the first few hours before the infusion achieves its steady level.

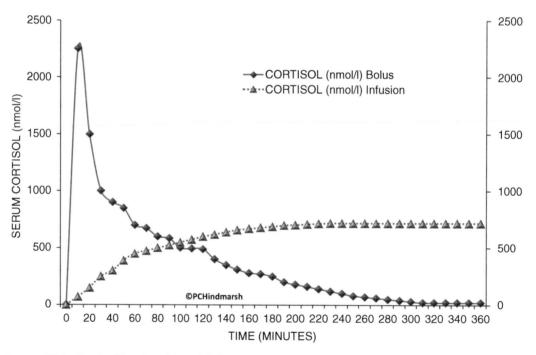

Figure 27.2 *Cortisol levels achieved following intravenous hydrocortisone given as a bolus and as an infusion. The bolus achieves a very high peak which only lasts 5–6 hours. The infusion achieves steady levels after an initial delay.*

Intravenous injection of hydrocortisone

As we can see in Fig. 27.2 the cortisol achieved from the intravenous injection peaks very quickly. This is because it does not have to go through the gut as shown in Fig. 27.3 steps 1 – 3 and part of step 4 are deleted to illustrate this.

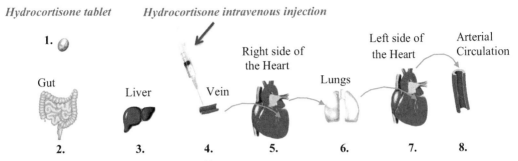

Hydrocortisone tablet   *Hydrocortisone intravenous injection*

1.

Gut

Liver   Vein   Right side of the Heart   Lungs   Left side of the Heart   Arterial Circulation

2.   3.   4.   5.   6.   7.   8.

1. ~~Ingestion of oral hydrocortisone tablet.~~
2. ~~Absorbed in the gut.~~
3. ~~Carried from the gut to the liver by hepatic portal system.~~
4. ~~Carried from the liver.~~ Carried through the venous (veins) circulation into the right side of the heart.
5. From the right side of the heart carried through the pulmonary arteries to the lungs.
6. From the lungs it is carried back to the left side of the heart.
7. From the left side of the heart it is them pumped out into the aorta.
8. From the aorta it is carried through the arterial circulation.

Figure 27.3 *How intravenous hydrocortisone bypasses the steps that an oral tablet goes through.*

HOW DO CORTISOL LEVELS COMPARE WITH THE DIFFERENT PREPARATIONS?

Fig. 27.4 shows what happens when hydrocortisone is given to the same person in different ways.

An intravenous bolus injection of 30 mg gives a rapid peak of over 2500 nmol/l which comes right down after 90 minutes to about 1000 nmol/l. This is because cortisol is rapidly cleared from the body through the urine as the saturation of the cortisol binding globulin protein is exceeded. The intramuscular injection also peaks quite quickly, but at a lower level just short of 1500 nmol/l and the subcutaneous bolus via a pump is not too dissimilar to the intramuscular injection. We go into more detail on the pump bolus in Chapter 28. The oral dose takes longer to reach a peak (60 minutes compared to the 30–35 minutes of the other routes).

What is interesting to know is what happens to the cortisol over a longer period of time than the 100 minutes and this is illustrated in another example in Fig. 27.5 where we look at the cortisol level after 2.5 hours (150 minutes).

We can see that by 11:00 there is not much difference between cortisol levels from the intravenous and intramuscular injections, even though the intravenous bolus reached levels almost double those seen after the intramuscular injection. In fact, the oral route did well too and gave a respectable peak of some 500 nmol/l albeit delayed compared to the other more direct routes.

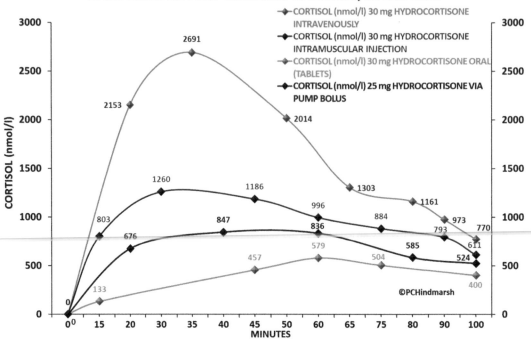

Figure 27.4 *Cortisol levels achieved when 25–30 mg hydrocortisone is given intravenously, intramuscularly, subcutaneously via a pump bolus and as an oral tablet to the same person.*

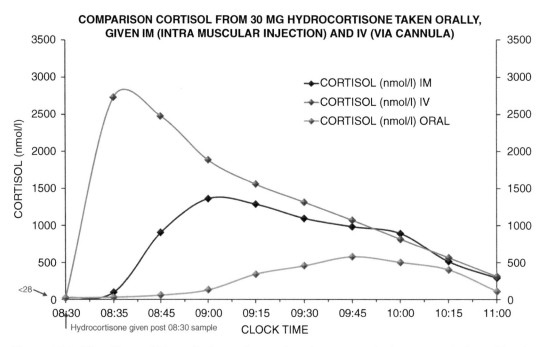

Figure 27.5 *The effects of 30 mg hydrocortisone given intravenously, intramuscularly and by the oral route over a time course of 2.5 hours.*

These effects show that in emergency situations as long as the blood circulation is good, the intramuscular route is as good as the intravenous route.

It is important to note that either route serves only for a short period of time and probably no more than 4 hours, so medical assessment is needed within this time frame.

HYDROCORTISONE SUPPOSITORIES

Hydrocortisone also comes as suppositories. Although initially designed as a treatment for inflammatory bowel conditions, it has been suggested that the rectal route could be used in emergency situations rather than resorting to an intramuscular injection.

Both foams and suppositories have been studied. With the foam, only a very small part of the rectal dose (100 mg) was absorbed which means that for emergency use this preparation is not to be used.

Suppositories fared better but again are variable. One further problem is that the bowel bacteria can break down hydrocortisone so it is not clear what might be absorbed.

Overall it is best to use an intramuscular injection in emergencies.

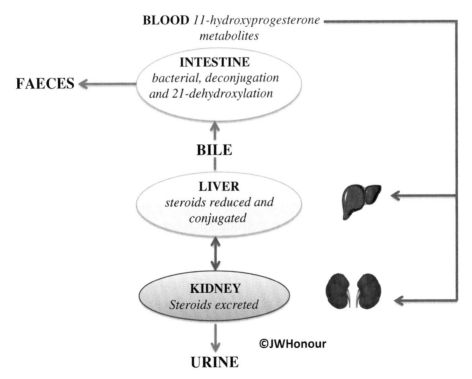

Figure 27.6 *How cortisol is handled by the bacteria in the gut. Cortisol can be metabolised in several ways leading to different products which can be absorbed into the blood stream.*

Fig. 27.6 summarises what can happen to cortisol. In the gut, breakdown by gut bacteria leads to a number of products that are either excreted in the faeces or some can be absorbed into the blood stream. Cortisol is metabolised in the liver and the breakdown products are either excreted into bile which then goes back into the gut (the enterohepatic circulation), or they are taken to the kidney and passed out in the urine. The way that bacteria in the gut metabolise cortisol varies depending which part of the gut that the steroid is in. As most cortisol from hydrocortisone is absorbed in the upper gut, the sequence in Fig. 27.6 applies. In the lower gut/rectum different steroid conversion products are likely.

BUCCAL HYDROCORTISONE

Muco-adhesive buccal tablets of hydrocortisone are available. These were originally called Corlan Pellets. They had the attraction of coming in 2.5 mg tablets which for young children meant that the standard 10 mg hydrocortisone tablets did not need to be cut up. However, the design of the pellet is such that it releases hydrocortisone slowly and it is unclear what happens if the pellet is ingested.

We have seen a marked difference in the distribution and absorption of cortisol attained from these tablets when swallowed. There are reports that these have been vomited up several hours after they have been taken and also passed out in the stool. These tablets are manufactured for mouth ulcers.

Muco-adhesive buccal tablets of hydrocortisone have not been clinically trialled and are not licenced for cortisol replacement therapy. This medication should not be prescribed for cortisol replacement.

There are further drug developments taking place, for example a slow release preparation. Although an attractive concept, it will still be important to ensure that absorption, half-life and clearance is considered when prescribing this, along with the difference in the way hydrocortisone is handled at night. These factors will not change in an individual (Chapter 20). It will still be important not to judge replacement on 17OHP only, but to have cortisol measurements taken to ensure the peak from the slow release is not too high, or indeed too low and that it is occurring at the right time. Our extensive experience in replacing cortisol using the pump system (Chapter 28), where we are able to titrate the dose, has shown that these factors are so important to avoid long term side effects from occurring. Ensuring good cortisol replacement is vital no matter which method or preparation is used.

CONCLUSIONS

Oral hydrocortisone tablets are the mainstay for the treatment of CAH. The other preparation the buccal tablets should not be used for cortisol replacement. Intravenous hydrocortisone can be used in emergency situations and prior to anaesthesia. Where a procedure lasts longer than 90 minutes, it is probably better to follow the intravenous bolus with an infusion of hydrocortisone.

Both intramuscular and intravenous hydrocortisone produce good levels of cortisol. However, these levels only last for about 4 hours so it is important they are repeated. It also means that if an intramuscular injection of hydrocortisone is given in an emergency situation, the person is assessed within 4 hours, as otherwise cortisol will start falling and the person may become unwell again.

FURTHER READING

Efcortesol (hydrocortisone sodium phosphate). Available from: http://www.mhra.gov.uk/home/groups/spcpil/documents/spcpil/con1439527866285.pdf spc-doc_PL 20072-0229.pdf

Honour, J.W., 2015. Historical perspective: gut dysbiosis and hypertension. Physiol. Genomics. 47, 17–23.

Solu-Cortef. Available from: http://www.mhra.gov.uk/home/groups/spcpil/documents/spcpil/con1424668027278.pdf spc-doc_PL 00057-1050.pdf

CHAPTER 28

The Pump Method for Achieving a Normal Circadian Cortisol Replacement

GLOSSARY

Basal rates The rates on a pump that deliver cortisol. These can be changed every half hour if needed but by varying the rates a circadian pattern can be accumulated. Increases as low as 0.025 mg per hour can be given.

Bolus function A feature on a pump that allows a bolus of subcutaneous hydrocortisone to be delivered rather like an emergency injection of hydrocortisone.

Circadian rhythm Changes in hormone levels, in this case cortisol, throughout the 24 hour period where values peak in the morning and reach low levels late evening.

Clearance How fast or slow the body removes a drug from the circulation.

Double or triple rates pattern A pump function available to deliver double and triple rates in illness, a bolus should be given when switching to either the double or triple rate.

Professor Peter Hindmarsh formula Formula based on scientific and complex mathematical calculations incorporating the pharmacokinetics of hydrocortisone and the individual's metabolism. Using this method Professor Peter Hindmarsh was the first in the world to successfully mimic the circadian rhythm of cortisol in adrenal insufficiency and in congenital adrenal hyperplasia, successively normalising 17OHP and ACTH levels.

24 hour cortisol and 17OHP profiles Measures of cortisol and 17OHP in the blood over a full 24 hour period. These are created by taking blood samples through a cannula, at regular intervals, the frequency is determined by age of the patient, however for pump therapy sampling must be hourly.

17-Hydroxyprogesterone (17OHP) 17OHP is an intermediary steroid in the formation of cortisol from cholesterol. It is the substrate for the enzyme CYP21 which converts 17OHP to 11-deoxycortisol and also progesterone to deoxycorticosterone. Loss of enzyme function leads to a buildup of 17OHP.

GENERAL

We have presented a fair amount of information about the circadian rhythm of cortisol in this book. We have also considered how we give hydrocortisone in tablet form to try and mimic as closely as possible the natural circadian rhythm of cortisol. We know that mimicking the circadian rhythm is extremely important as it is the one way that we can ensure that we have firstly, achieved good cortisol replacement as

Congenital Adrenal Hyperplasia. http://dx.doi.org/10.1016/B978-0-12-811483-4.00028-3

well as a proper distribution of cortisol throughout the 24 hour period. Secondly, we know optimal cortisol replacement will normalise 17OHP and androgen production, unless these are being produced by adrenal rest tissue. This helps avoid over and under treatment with the associated side effects which can occur from either extreme. Distribution of cortisol is important. It is as important to see the right amounts of peak cortisol during the day as it is to have periods when levels are naturally low.

When we study the 24 hour hydrocortisone profiles undertaken on oral replacement, we do not achieve the true circadian rhythm of cortisol. If the dosing is correct, then we come very close to it but we still run the risk of over and under treatment through the 24 hour period. This is particularly the case in the early hours of the morning where no matter how hard we try with oral hydrocortisone dosing, it is very difficult to ensure good cover between 04:00 (4 a.m.) and 06:00 (6 a.m.). This is a critical period and one way that we can get the cortisol distribution correct is either to give the last dose of hydrocortisone at 01:00 (1 a.m.) or else to have a way of administering the hydrocortisone at 04:00 (4 a.m.).

We can also see that individual half-life of hydrocortisone and all glucocorticoids is very variable (Fig. 20.10), so the timing of the last dose has to be precisely calculated. Another way in which we have been able to overcome this and to get optimal cortisol replacement distribution, is to use an insulin pump which contains hydrocortisone in place of insulin, which can be set to deliver a continuous amount of hydrocortisone at specific individualised rates over a 24 hour period.

PRINCIPLE OF THE HYDROCORTISONE PUMP

The principle of pump therapy is to vary the amount of cortisol delivered during the 24 hour period. We have to carefully individualise this therapy by taking into account many factors such as the variation in the clearance of hydrocortisone.

There are many combinations of absorption and clearance of glucocorticoids in individuals and the following list gives examples of some of these combinations.

Fast Absorber/Slow Clearance.
Fast Absorber/Fast Clearance.
Slow Absorber/Slow Clearance.
Normal Absorber/Slow Clearance.
Normal Absorber/Fast Clearance.
Very Fast Absorber/Slow Clearance.
Very Slow Absorber/Fast Clearance.

Very Fast Absorber/Very Slow Clearance.
Normal Absorber/Very Fast or Very Slow Clearance.
Very Fast or Very Slow Absorber/Normal Clearance.

The absorption of hydrocortisone when using the pump, is 100% as it gets straight to the vein (Fig. 28.1) so how the individual clears cortisol becomes the most important factor.

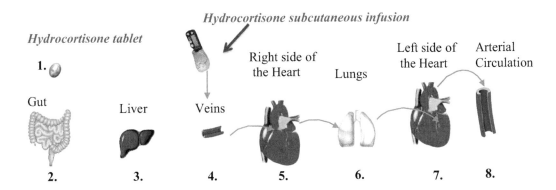

1. Ingestion of oral hydrocortisone tablet.
2. Absorbed in the gut.
3. Carried from the gut to the liver by hepatic portal system.
4. Carried from the liver through the venous (veins) circulation into the right side of the heart.
5. From the right side of the heart carried through the pulmonary arteries to the lungs.
6. From the lungs it is carried back to the left side of the heart.
7. From the left side of the heart it is them pumped out into the aorta.
8. From the aorta it is carried through the arterial circulation.

Figure 28.1 *How the hydrocortisone pump fits into the handling of cortisol by the body.* Note how the pump method bypasses steps 1–3 and the first part of step 4.

Many pumps are available but they all do two things. First, they can deliver a background amount of drug, in this case hydrocortisone throughout the 24 hour period. This is known as the basal hydrocortisone infusion rate.

This background or basal rate can be varied at any time and indeed you can change it every 30 minutes if you wanted to. This is rarely needed in diabetes and even less so in cortisol replacement in CAH.

This is all achieved through a small cannula inserted under the skin into the local fat tissue (Fig. 28.2).

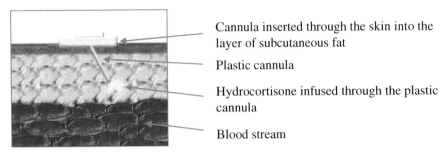

Cannula inserted through the skin into the layer of subcutaneous fat

Plastic cannula

Hydrocortisone infused through the plastic cannula

Blood stream

Figure 28.2 *How the infusion cannula is positioned into the fat under the skin.*

What we have found using the pump, is that we use four to eight different background rates during the 24 hour period to precisely mimic the cortisol profile that you would see in individuals who do not have adrenal problems.

Fig. 28.3 shows an example of a cortisol profile in a young man on a hydrocortisone pump compared to two adult individuals who do not have any adrenal problems.

Unless the individuals are clearly labelled with who is who, it is impossible to tell the person who is receiving hydrocortisone replacement from those who do not have an adrenal problem and producing cortisol normally!

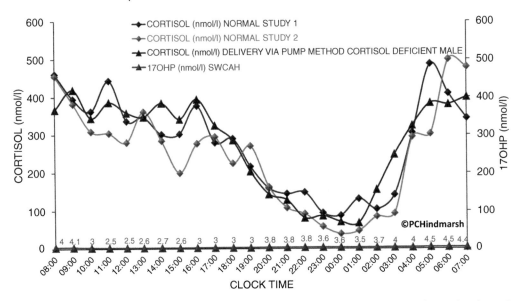

Figure 28.3 *24 hour profile of a young male with SWCAH showing not only optimal cortisol replacement and 17OHP levels as well as cortisol levels superimposed within the normal cortisol production of two males with no adrenal problems.*

The second feature of the pump is that not only can this background rate be varied but it also can be temporarily increased. This is immensely valuable in hydrocortisone replacement, because it means that we can better tailor the dosing of hydrocortisone during episodes when people are unwell. This component to pump therapy, is called the temporary background rate or temporary basal rate and you can increase it by one and a half to twice the normal background that has been programmed in.

This is equivalent to doubling doses of hydrocortisone during periods of stress or illness. We do know, however, that a double dose does not give double the level but we can use another feature of the pump, where you can programme in different basal patterns so that you can have a sickness pattern of say two and a half times the normal daily basal amount.

You need to give extra hydrocortisone before you switch to double or triple dose pattern and this can be done by what is called a bolus which is the third feature. Fig. 28.4 shows how the cortisol takes several hours to buildup if there is no bolus given.

Bolus function

The bolus is similar to giving an emergency injection. On the pump there is a special feature for this and it is really easy to give and only needs three steps. The amount of hydrocortisone which can be given can be quite small (0.025 mg over an hour), or can be a normal dose to cover a stressful event (e.g. 20 mg immediately). It is best not to give too much, as this can damage the infusion site so it is better not to give large doses like 20 mg and instead give several smaller doses such as 5–10 mg. It is also recommended to always carry an emergency injection because you might not have enough in the pump reservoir to cover what you would need.

In Fig. 28.4 a sample was taken at time zero for a premeasurement to see how much cortisol was in the blood. The bolus was administered immediately after this and the pump disconnected, so that we could measure the amount of cortisol that was delivered. There was a level of 364 nmol/l on which the bolus stacked (blue line). The turquoise line shows what would have been achieved if we had started from a zero cortisol level. In illness, the bolus would be given and the pump NOT disconnected, so it would continue to deliver cortisol and the cortisol levels achieved would be much higher. The rates would be doubled or tripled (Fig. 28.6) and the levels of cortisol in the blood would remain high until the pump rates are switched back to normal rate. When using the pump with the rates accurately worked out using the Peter Hindmarsh formula, there will always be cortisol in the blood for cortisol from the bolus to 'stack on' and the increased cortisol levels will still follow the circadian rhythm.

Note: Level 1 user had a level of 364 nmol/l of cortisol at time bolus was given. Pump was disconnected immediately after bolus dose of 25 mg (hydrocortisone) via pump to enable accurate measuring of bolus dose. However, pump would normally continue to deliver at increased rates, so user would have achieved and maintained much higher levels if pump had not been disconnected. Level 2 shows cortisol achieved if there was no cortisol pre bolus.

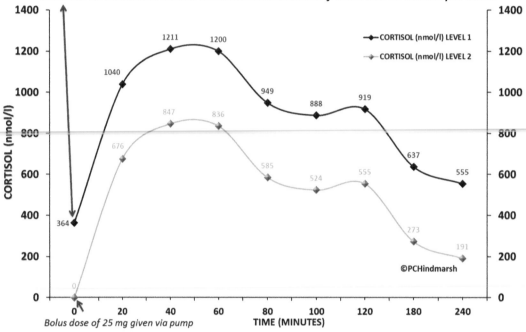

Figure 28.4 *Cortisol levels achieved after a bolus dose of 25 mg was given via the pump.*

Using the pump

Once the dosing is set up and has been checked with a 24 hour profile you do not have to touch the settings unless the dose needs adjusting. The pump automatically delivers the amount it is set to do and this can be adjusted by very small amounts to get the cortisol levels right. For example, there is a natural increase in the ACTH at around 16:00 and even this increase can be factored into the delivery rates.

Patients using the pump find that it gives them much more independence, as they do not have to worry about taking tablets at certain times and it means that they only have to change their site and fill the pump reservoir every 3 days. No waking up to take tablets at weekends and also when ill they know they are well covered in the early hours of the morning.

HISTORY

The pump was developed over 13 years ago for a patient who had a very rapid clearance of hydrocortisone. Formal testing showed a half-life of 40 minutes for hydrocortisone and it was evident he also had rapid clearance of all other glucocorticoids. After many profiles including testing to see if the patient had any aberrant receptors, it was found that he had a problem with the cortisol shuttle conversion of cortisol to cortisone.

Cortisol attained from oral hydrocortisone is converted to non active cortisone by the unidirectional action of the enzyme11-beta hydroxysteroid dehydrogenase type 2 (11β–HSD type 2) (Fig. 20.6). 11β–Hydroxysteroid dehydrogenase type 1 (11β–HSD1) converts the inactive cortisone to cortisol (Fig. 20.6) in the liver. Tests proved that the patient had a problem with 11β–HSD2 and despite large doses of hydrocortisone being taken, inadequate amounts could be measured in the blood implying that 11β–HSD1 was also affected.

It was evident that the patient, who had suffered severe headaches and tiredness from a very young age, had been both under treated and over treated with long periods of the 24 hour period where he had inadequate amounts of cortisol or was totally cortisol deficient. His replacement cortisol was solely judged on his 17OHP levels and it was only when 24 hour profiles were undertaken, it became evident that huge peaks of cortisol were used to bring down the 17OHP. Puberty exacerbated the problem.

To bypass the conversion issue an insulin pump was modified to deliver hydrocortisone subcutaneously. A formula was derived by Professor Peter Hindmarsh to infuse the hydrocortisone in such a way to mimic the circadian rhythm. The rates were calculated to suit his individual metabolism.

Fig. 28.5 shows a profile undertaken before starting the pump method, where the patient took six doses of hydrocortisone a day with a very high total daily dose (over 100 mg per day). As the cortisol was rapidly metabolised to cortisone and little was converted back to cortisol, the overall effect was that the patient was cortisol deficient.

Using high doses made little difference, as it was cleared so quickly by metabolism and the doses used exceeded the saturation of cortisol binding globulin, so was excreted in the urine anyway. Higher doses therefore made no difference to the underlying problem and only made it worse.

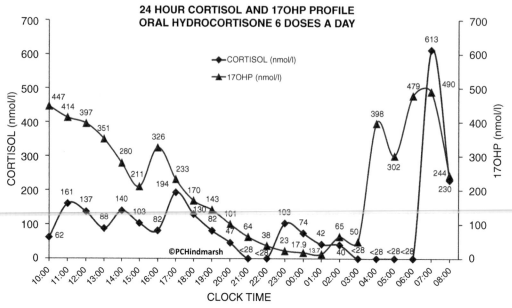

Figure 28.5 *Profile pre pump on high doses of oral hydrocortisone taken 6 times a day.*

CT scan showed that the adrenal glands were enlarged as ACTH levels were very high. An MRI showed a normal sized pituitary gland. IV administration using the formula developed by Professor Hindmarsh over 24 hours, showed good levels of cortisol as the very rapid clearance was accounted for.

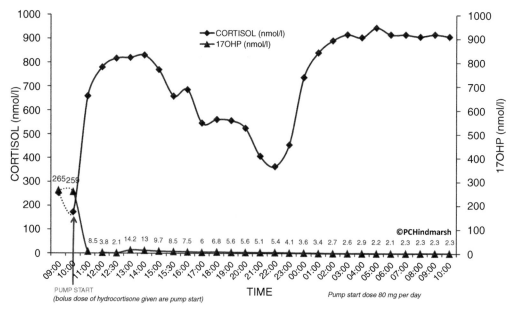

Figure 28.6 *24 hour cortisol profile undertaken at pump start following instigation of hydrocortisone therapy via the pump.*

Fig. 28.6 shows the effect of a continuous infusion of hydrocortisone which was boosted by an IV bolus of hydrocortisone immediately prior to switching on the pump. The bolus is necessary to give the pump infusion a good amount of cortisol in the system to 'stack on' as the cortisol delivered via the pump accumulates slowly.

The pump start dose was calculated at 80 mg per day for this patient due to very rapid clearance and also the enlarged adrenal glands identified on the scan. We can see that the patient needed this amount of cortisol by the 17OHP levels, as they decreased to normal levels.

After several months as the adrenal glands shrank back to normal size, we were able to lower the overall daily dose of infused cortisol by adjusting the amount infused and the rate of infusion. Fig. 28.7 is a profile done 1 month post starting the pump on a reduced infusion rate. The 17OHP helped us to manipulate the rates to deliver lower cortisol levels where needed.

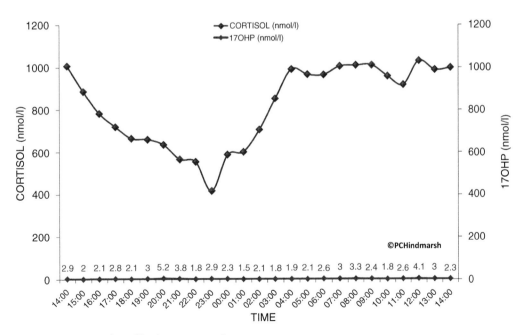

Figure 28.7 *Cortisol profile done 1 month post pump start.*

Not only did the biochemical markers show that this patient was getting towards optimal cortisol levels but his general health improved dramatically. Headaches from low cortisol levels, disappeared and despite the delivery of the high cortisol levels, his weight normalised and remained stable.

Fig. 28.8 is a profile undertaken 18 months post starting the pump. As we can see, 17OHP levels are all within the normal range and cortisol levels are optimal for this patient. There was an unexpected marked increase in growth despite the bone age showing almost complete fusion before the pump start.

All hyperpigmentation disappeared, as well as gut problems caused by the high doses of dexamethasone and prednisolone tried prior to starting the pump. We were able to reduce the rates to deliver 35 mg of hydrocortisone per day which this patient needed due to his fast metabolism of hydrocortisone.

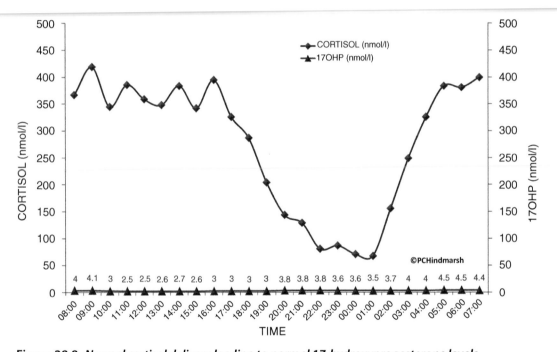

Figure 28.8 *Normal cortisol delivery leading to normal 17-hydroxyprogesterone levels.*

Over the following years we were able to reduce the rates further. CT of the adrenals showed normal size. The patient was able to return to school, go on to University. His quality of life improved dramatically and he now partakes in active and extreme sport, such as surfing, attends the gym and lives a very full active life. His weight is stable and his general health very good.

This improvement in the quality of life for those who use the pump method who have adrenal insufficiency, has been reported by many who use the pump worldwide.

However, what is of utmost importance is to have the rates calculated for the individual and this is done by factoring the individual's clearance rate and half-life of hydrocortisone, weight and height into the Pump Formula.

The delivery formula devised by Professor Peter Hindmarsh is very different to that for oral hydrocortisone. A very small incorrect adjustment in the rates can have a profound effect and unless the rates are calculated for the individual using the formula, the cortisol will not follow the circadian rhythm. In CAH where the adrenal glands are enlarged, higher doses will be needed to start with and then slowly reduced as the glands shrink.

Adjusting rates

As mentioned, a small adjustment to rates of infusion and the timings of the rate changes can not only affect the cumulative cortisol levels but also the distribution.

Fig. 28.9 shows a profile done on a daily dose of 32.6 mg of hydrocortisone infused over the 24 hours.

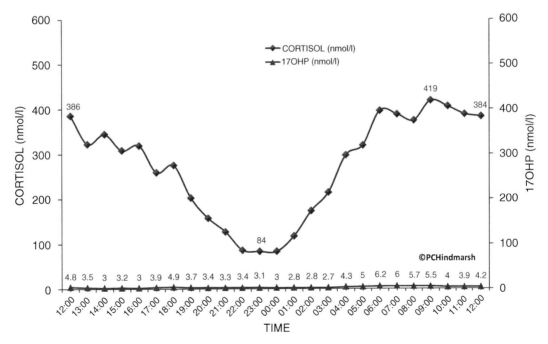

Figure 28.9 *Cortisol and 17OHP levels over a 24 hour period on a total daily dose of 32.6 mg per day.*

A small adjustment in the timing of the rates and amount to 32.8 mg per day was made and Fig. 28.10 shows the difference this small adjustment made to both the cumulative effect of the cortisol, as well as the distribution (pattern of the circadian rhythm) and affect this had on the 17OHP level which shows there is over treatment.

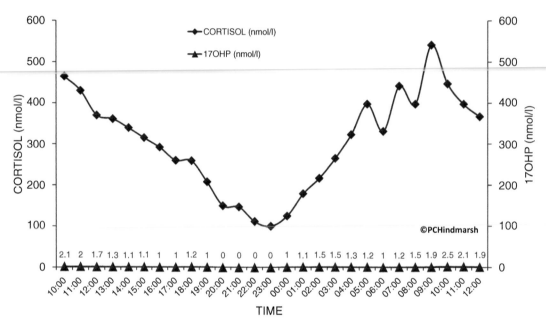

Figure 28.10 *Profile on 32.8 mg of hydrocortisone with slight increase in dose and change of rate caused suppression of 17OHP levels.*

Based on what we had learnt from the previous profiles, we were able to reduce the overall daily infusion rate to 31.9 mg per day (Fig. 28.11). This experimentation with timings and doses, has given us further insight into how cortisol affects 17OHP and how important both the timing and the dose is, as well as how minor alterations in both timing and administration of doses can affect the 17OHP levels.

In fact, what we can achieve can be summarised in Fig. 28.12 where we have taken poor oral hydrocortisone therapy and changed it into a pattern which is indistinguishable from the normal cortisol rhythm in two adult males.

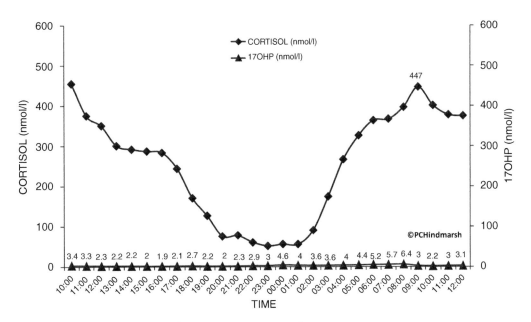

Figure 28.11 *Doses readjusted further to 31.9 mg per day.*

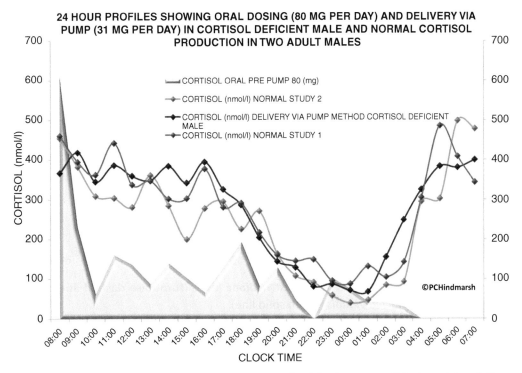

Figure 28.12 *Cortisol circadian rhythm in two normal adults (green and blue) and that delivered by the pump system (purple) compared to the oral route shown as the light blue filled area.*

WHAT HAPPENS TO OTHER HORMONES?

The aforementioned figures show that as the cortisol levels are normalised, in other words we mimic the circadian rhythm, then the 17OHP values follow suit. Once the pituitary ACTH production is regulated properly the increased production of 17OHP is normalised. This change in 17OHP production is also reflected in androstenedione production.

Fig. 28.13 shows androstenedione levels on pump therapy compared to those observed in normal individuals. Note in the case of 17OHP and androstenedione, that normalising cortisol levels does not lead to suppression of 17OHP or androstenedione so pump therapy is not over treating the individual.

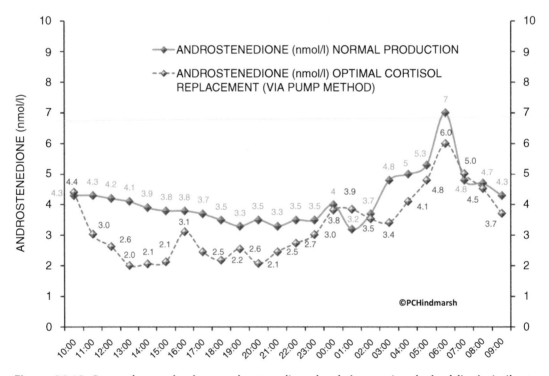

Figure 28.13 *Pump therapy leads to androstenedione levels* (turquoise dashed line) *similar to those observed in normal individuals* (green solid line).

Giving therapy like hydrocortisone raises concerns about how blood glucose might be affected. Fig. 28.14 shows blood glucose measurements over 24 hours on pump therapy and illustrates that blood glucose is not altered by this form of therapy, with values kept within the tight band of 3.5–7.0 mmol/l.

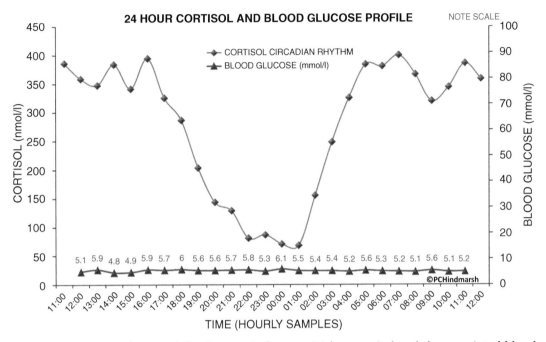

Figure 28.14 *Pump therapy delivering cortisol over a 24 hour period and the associated blood glucose measurements over that time held within a tight zone of 3.5–7.0 mmol/l.*

What is also important to note, is how normalising the cortisol profile impacts on other hormone systems. In particular the hypothalamo-pituitary-testes axis reacts in a very special way.

Fig. 28.15 shows the axis before we got the cortisol right and the adrenal system balanced. LH and FSH are low as is the testosterone.

Notice also, how the LH does not have any bursts of activity in it.

Contrast this with Fig. 28.16 where LH and FSH are higher and LH has bursts of activity. The net effect of this is to raise the testosterone dramatically. This is because cortisol is appearing normally in the blood, normalising adrenal androstenedione production and allowing the hypothalamo-pituitary-testes axis to pulse normally and generate testosterone from the testes.

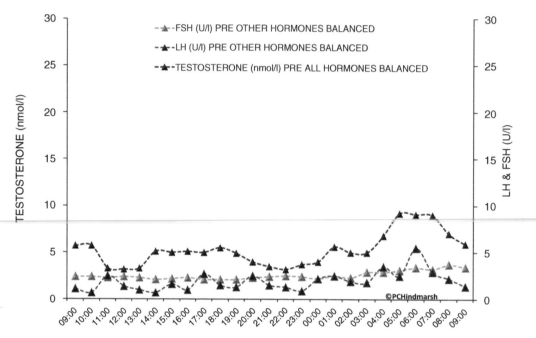

Figure 28.15 *LH (blue), FSH (green) and testosterone (red) prior to pump therapy optimisation with all values low.*

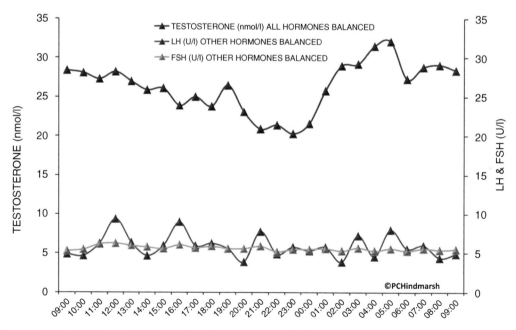

Figure 28.16 *LH (blue), FSH (green) and testosterone (red) after pump therapy optimisation with all values higher than in Fig. 28.15 and pulses in the LH profile.*

WHAT DO WE USE HYDROCORTISONE PUMP THERAPY FOR?

Currently we use hydrocortisone delivered through the pump system in two important situations. Firstly, in those individuals who have a very fast clearance of hydrocortisone from the blood, which is often present in individuals as part of their genetic make up where hydrocortisone is metabolised much more quickly than it is normally. We have seen half-lives reduced to 40 minutes compared to the normal value of 75–80 minutes.

This means hydrocortisone is removed very quickly from the blood stream, which leaves the individual under treated for considerable periods of time. There is often the temptation to get round this, by increasing the dose of hydrocortisone to bring down the 17OHP, but no matter how high you make the peak, it still does not prolong the duration of exposure very much longer as we have seen in previous chapters.

What happens is that doctors chase the situation with higher and higher doses thinking that will give more coverage, but all that is achieved is concomitant over and under treatment.

Secondly, the pump is also very useful for those individuals who have developed gastric problems following exposure to hydrocortisone, or in particular when prednisolone has been used. Individuals can have quite severe stomach problems, ranging from gastritis through to relative immobility of the stomach to contract properly.

The overall effect of this is to reduce how easy it is to absorb hydrocortisone when taken in tablet form. The pump, because it gives the hydrocortisone into the subcutaneous tissues, bypasses the stomach and eliminates this particular problem.

SETTING UP THE PUMP

The pump system delivers hydrocortisone into the subcutaneous tissues. It uses a small plastic cannula that is placed under the skin (Fig. 28.2) and it is through this cannula that the pump delivers the hydrocortisone.

This cannula needs to be changed every 3 days to prevent possible infection occurring at the site of entry. Inserting the cannula is relatively painless and very quick to do, as this all comes in a very user friendly auto inseter disposable device which inserts this fine cannula extremely quickly.

There are a number of places where the cannula can be placed (Fig. 28.17). The cannula should be sited in either the bottom and stomach areas, as there is often not enough fat tissue on the arms and legs.

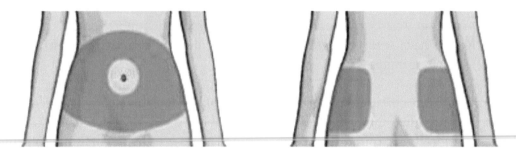

Figure 28.17 *Sites for placing the pump cannula shown in blue.* The best areas are the stomach and bottom. We do not recommend using the arms or legs.

Before starting on the pump it is necessary to know the clearance of hydrocortisone from the blood. This requires a special study to be undertaken, which consists of a dose of hydrocortisone given intravenously, followed by very frequent blood samples at specific intervals to be taken through a different cannula over a period of 2 hours. This is detailed in Chapter 8.

From the results there are a series of calculations which are done to work out the clearance of cortisol from the blood. We can then take the clearance and place it in a set of equations which works out the amount of hydrocortisone that would need to be given to produce a certain level of cortisol in the blood. This takes into account how fast the person removes cortisol from the blood stream. This series of mathematical equations allow us to determine on an hour by hour basis, the amount of hydrocortisone which would be needed to be delivered by the pump to achieve a certain cortisol concentration. This is how the pump delivers exactly what we want, which is the circadian rhythm of cortisol.

Once the clearance has been worked out and the calculations undertaken, then the pump is programmed for the 24 hour period. To be sure of whether fine tuning of the background rates is required, 24 hour profiles are essential to guide doctors to make the correct changes.

What usually happens is that the pump is set up, the formula applied and the background rates programmed. The pump is then attached to the cannula, the dead space cleared by priming the tubing and then the cannula is inserted into the person.

Once running, a 24 hour profile is undertaken to determine whether any further fine tuning or adjustments are necessary to the hydrocortisone delivery.

We use Solu-Cortef for the pump. It comes as a powder you make up into a liquid with sterile water. The Solu-Cortef comes as 100 mg vial so you simply dissolve 100 mg in 1 ml of water, which corresponds to the increments that are in the pump system. This is really important as not only does it make running the pump system easier, but there are also issues with respect to potency of the solution that is made up. This is shown in Fig. 28.18 where a different dilution was used to our standard one resulting in different cortisol delivery.

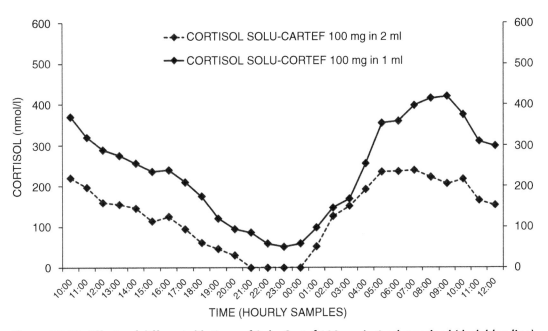

Figure 28.18 *Effects of different dilutions of Solu-Cortef 100 mg in 1 ml standard (dark blue line) and 100 mg in 2 ml (blue dashed line) on the cortisol levels that are produced.*

It is always best to change the set first thing in the morning, so if there are any problems you can identify them and deal with them during the day.

There are a number of safety alarms on the pump. The pump alarms when not delivering and warns when the reservoir is running low. It will not stop alarming until these problems are rectified. The pump also records the delivery of the hydrocortisone so that you can keep check of daily amounts given and parents can check if additional boluses have had to be given at school or nursery. In addition, the pump data can be downloaded using special software to see the total delivery over a period of time.

It is good practice to undertake several profiles when first starting on the pump, especially in CAH, because we take into account the 17OHP levels when profiling. Experience has shown that as the body adjusts to the pump delivery of cortisol, the adrenals reduce to a normal size, androgen levels drop to normal values and often less hydrocortisone is needed. When considering the optimal level of 17OHP on a pump, the normal range is much lower than that when considering oral replacement. Once the rates are set, the pump will require a check profile every 6 months for the first couple of years, but once stable rates are established then an annual profile is sufficient.

Finally, as mentioned, we can bolus on the pump or increase the rates to give extra hydrocortisone. Fig. 28.19 shows this. It also shows, as we have said before, that double or triple doses do not double or triple the blood levels of cortisol. This is because of the effects of the cortisol binding globulin and the pump studies show this very nicely.

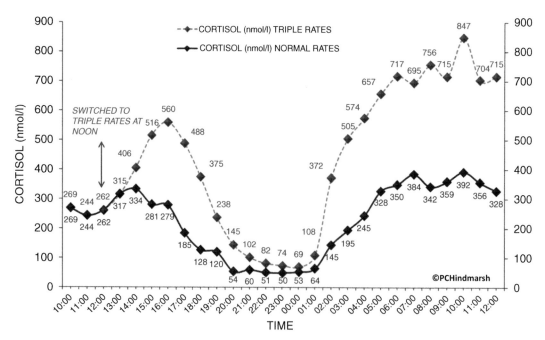

Figure 28.19 *Effect of triple rate (green) compared to standard rate (blue) during pump therapy.*

RESULTS OF PUMP THERAPY

Pump therapy has been extremely effective in delivering a normal cortisol rhythm. Fig. 28.20 shows another example of excellent replacement data in a young girl who required pump therapy, compared to the normal cortisol production of two female individuals which do not have any adrenal problems.

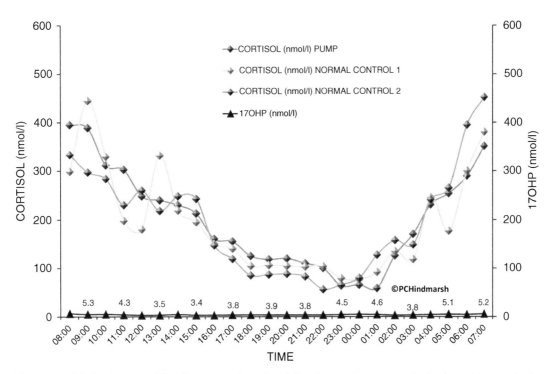

Figure 28.20 *24 hour profile of a young female with salt-wasting congenital adrenal hyperplasia showing a cortisol profile that is indistinguishable from two females with no adrenal problems.*

As with the profiles done in males, the profile is identical to the normal cortisol rhythm. These profiles show again, that the cortisol rhythm does not lead to over treatment because when we measure the 17OHP, it is in the normal range and displays a rhythm with slight fluctuation during the 24 hour period, which means that we have mimicked exactly the feedback system on the pituitary adrenal axis.

We have been able to use this system in one individual for 12 years and several others for over 5 years. The response has been extremely dramatic with a marked reduction in side effects, normalisation of body weight, increased marked unexpected growth in one individual, restoration and normalisation of energy levels and return to normal life in all individuals. In two instances, the individuals were able to return to school with normal good attendance, complete their 'A levels' achieving top grades and go onto University.

Patients noted a marked improvement in their general health and a vast increase in their overall stamina. All now partake actively in sport, such as attending the gym, running, swimming, long distance cycling, skiing and surfing, whereas before using pump therapy, their quality of life was poor.

One patient who initially used Efcortesol (Hydrocortisone Sodium Phosphate) (Fig. 27.1) which is a ready mixed injectable form of hydrocortisone, developed several site abscesses due to a severe allergy to one of the excipients in the preparation and it was noted that others who used this preparation also developed small lumps under the skin. Ultrasound showed pooling of the Efcortesol under the skin due to the high viscosity of the preparation (Fig. 28.21).

Solu-Cortef in the United Kingdom does not cause skin reactions, whereas in the United States and Canada some batches of the ACT-O-VIAL (Fig. 27.1) can cause skin irritation if the pH of the solution is not correct.

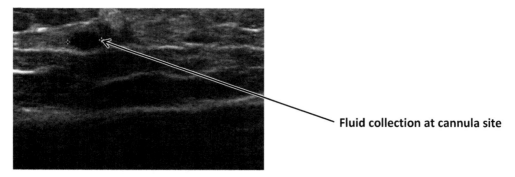

Fluid collection at cannula site

Figure 28.21 *Ultrasound of cannula sites with pooling of hydrocortisone at the infusion site probably related to the viscosity of the hydrocortisone preparation.*

PUMPS AND INSERTERS

There are several types of pumps available. Animas make a waterproof pump which can be worn safely whilst swimming and surfing (Fig. 28.22).

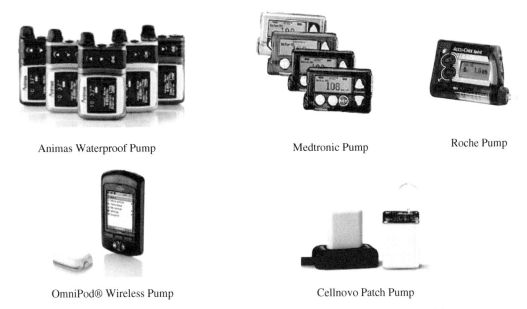

Animas Waterproof Pump   Medtronic Pump   Roche Pump

OmniPod® Wireless Pump   Cellnovo Patch Pump

Figure 28.22 *Examples of some of the different types of pumps that are available.*

There are also a variety of inserters. We recommend the auto inserters; however, it is best to work with a centre which is used to working with diabetes pumps, who will advise you on the best inserter to suit you. Some inserts have 90 degree cannulas which go straight into the skin, whereas some inserts are made with 45 degree cannulas which go into the skin at an angle and are often used by many who do not have enough fat in which to insert the 90 degree cannulas.

The cannulas also come in different lengths, we recommend 6 mm. The tubing also comes in different lengths of 60 and 90 cm. Again, it is best to discuss this with your endocrinologist (Fig. 28.23).

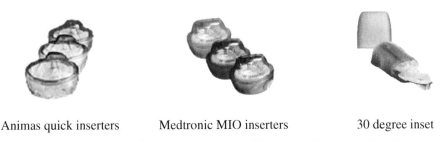

Animas quick inserters   Medtronic MIO inserters   30 degree inset

Figure 28.23 *Examples of some of the different types of inserters that are available.*

Filling the reservoir

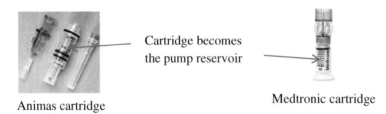

Cartridge becomes
the pump reservoir

Animas cartridge

Medtronic cartridge

Figure 28.24 *Examples of cartridges which once filled with hydrocortisone become the pump's reservoir.*

Different pumps have different types of reservoirs with different filling systems (Fig. 28.24). But essentially, the mix should be 100 mg Solu-Cortef with 1 ml of water for injections. This is made up in the Solu-Cortef vial, then transferred into the reservoir by drawing back out of the Solu-Cortef vial. This is quite easy as the reservoir systems can attach to the bung on the Solu-Cortef vial.

It is important to be taught how to use the pump properly by your endocrine team. To give you a rough idea on how the pump is connected, the following needs to be undertaken. Once the reservoir is full of hydrocortisone, the user needs to flick the reservoir vigorously to move any bubbles to the top and then any bubbles must be carefully pushed out of the reservoir. This is very important as a bubble in the tube means that until it is cleared, hydrocortisone will not be delivered for that time.

Once the bubbles have been removed, the pump will then give instructions on the screen to follow and it will instruct you to rewind the piston that drives the reservoir. Once rewound, the reservoir is inserted into the pump. The pump then instructs you to fill the tubing and the pump is now ready to be primed, which is done manually by holding down the appropriate button on the pump until the drops of hydrocortisone can be seen coming out of the needle. Now you need to remove the paper covering the sticky plaster in the inserter and pull down the bottom of the inserter to prime the needle. Now insert the cannula into the appropriate area as shown in Fig. 28.17.

The final step is to fill the dead space that remains after the needle has been removed. The amount depends on the cannula used, but is about 0.4–0.9 ml.

The pump instructs you to do this and it is an important step, as the dead space volume if not filled, can represent a considerable amount of time when you could be without hydrocortisone.

There is no need to bolus when you change the reservoir. The reservoir and cannula should be changed every 3 days and the area used rotated.

Once you get used to making the change it is very quick to do. Note, it is important to be taught how to do this by your endocrine team.

CONCLUSIONS

Hydrocortisone pump therapy is an extremely good way of mimicking the normal cortisol circadian rhythm and at present is the only way that is available for doctors to achieve this. The system only delivers the necessary amount of cortisol required by the individual, so that periods of over and under treatment are avoided.

The system allows for changes to be easily made in terms of sick days and also allows for bolus doses to be delivered as efficiently as a subcutaneous injection, should they be required.

In the unlikely event of pump failure, which we have not experienced in the years that we have used the pump, the individual can always revert to either emergency injection of hydrocortisone or back to tablets.

Pump therapy, when used for individuals who have a very rapid clearance of hydrocortisone or have gastric problems, is extremely effective. Ultimately, it may be available for all who would like to try this method.

GENERAL INFORMATION

It is important that when considering using the pump method that you seek the expert opinion of an experienced endocrinologist and the following testing must be undertaken.

1. IV cortisol clearance study which needs to be specifically calculated for pump use, with careful consideration to the excess cortisol achieved. Accurate timings of samples are of the utmost importance. We have had instances where several individuals calculating clearance, suggesting the patient is a super fast clearer when in fact the individual has slow clearance.
2. Delivery rates must be carefully calculated using an accredited formula which is different to that for oral calculations.
3. 24 hour profile pre pump and then 24 hours after pump start, for any fine tuning of the cortisol. If the adrenals are enlarged then slow reduction in cortisol basal rates.

4. If the patient has had high 17OHP levels for quite some time on high doses of glucocorticoid, then a CT of the adrenals as well as a CT of the pituitary gland should be undertaken.

5. Social media group treatment and advice is strongly not advised, as small adjustments in pump rates produce significant changes in delivery.

6. Rates should not be altered without the input of your endocrinologist, the pump rates do not need to be altered at any time unless illness occurs.

7. We do not condone the practice of self pump treatment or by anyone who is not an endocrinologist.

FURTHER READING

Bryan, S.M., Honour, J.W., Hindmarsh, P.C., 2009. Management of altered hydrocortisone pharmacokinetics in a boy with congenital adrenal hyperplasia using a continuous subcutaneous hydrocortisone infusion. J. Clin. Endocrinol. Metab. 94, 3477–3480.

Hindmarsh, P.C., 2014. The child with difficult to control congenital adrenal hyperplasia: is there a place for continuous subcutaneous hydrocortisone therapy. Clin. Endocrinol. 81, 15–18.

CHAPTER 29

Stress Dosing for Sick Days, Surgery, Exams and Exercise

GLOSSARY

Adrenalin effects A rise in heart rate and blood pressure, increased movement of the bowels along with feeling of tension and anxiety.

Adrenal insufficiency Term used to cover all causes for deficiency of cortisol. It is not a diagnosis. It is the result of a medical condition that leaves the body unable to produce cortisol or enough cortisol. Adrenal Insufficiency is the key phrase used by ambulance services to get the highest priority call out and alert them to the fact the patient needs a hydrocortisone bolus urgently.

Level 1 Level of action needed when there is sickness without vomiting. Double the normal daily hydrocortisone dose with an extra double morning dose given at 4 a.m. (04:00), (more@4).

Level 2 Level of action needed when there is sickness and vomiting. If vomiting occurs 1 hour after a hydrocortisone dose the medication is likely to have been absorbed and no repeat dose is needed. If vomiting occurs within an hour then the dose should be repeated. If vomiting occurs again then an intramuscular injection of hydrocortisone (doses are 0–1 year, 25 mg; 1–5 years, 50 mg; over 5 years 100 mg) is needed and the person should go straight to hospital.

More@4 During periods of illness a double dose equal to the usual morning dose, to be taken at 4 a.m. (04:00), followed by normal double morning dose to be taken at the usual time. This additional dose is taken to prevent hypoglycaemia occurring in the early hours of the morning.

GENERAL

One of the many questions that parents ask is how to deal with stressful situations. This can range from a child being unwell, visits to the dentist, to higher exams at school and college. We always refer to cortisol as a stress hormone and it is true that in addition to its many roles, higher amounts of cortisol are produced during periods of stress, particularly in association with illness and trauma.

Congenital Adrenal Hyperplasia. http://dx.doi.org/10.1016/B978-0-12-811483-4.00029-5

The stress response is complex and is shown in detail in Fig. 29.1, which shows the brain generating an emotional response through a special part of the brain called the amygdala and also how the hypothalamus responds through cortisol and the pathway that operates through adrenalin production. Adrenalin is a quick response to stress whereas cortisol is a much slower process. However, when we are considering when to replace cortisol in certain situations, we need to consider the implications the increase in cortisol will have in the short term and if repeatedly increased when unnecessary, the long term side effects. The imperative time to double or triple doses is when illness occurs, serious injury, broken limbs, burns, shock and this is because of the changes made in the handling of cortisol when such episodes occur. We will discuss this in further detail during this chapter.

STRESS

What is often sensationalised in the media are reports with headlines such as 'Exams can KILL me', 'Rare disease means student could die if she studies too hard' and 'A young teen with a rare condition that causes her body to shut down fears too much fun will kill her'. These examples refer to the individuals having adrenal insufficiency and have frightened parents and individuals with CAH into feeling they need to increase doses for exams, parties and suchlike.

If your replacement cortisol levels are optimal there is no danger of this happening, in fact, doubling doses before exams can affect the short term memory. Although emotional stress in individuals without adrenal insufficiency will cause a slight natural immediate increase in cortisol, the cortisol level also comes down very quickly and the whole event is over in less than 1 hour. What we are doing in CAH is replacing the cortisol artificially with hydrocortisone and this is a drug which has to be absorbed and has a half-life, so cannot react in the same way. Oral hydrocortisone takes a good 20 minutes to enter the bloodstream and will peak 60–90 minutes later which is well after the event. Overall in this situation the extra hydrocortisone taken will be ineffective. Doubling the dose or even tripling the dose at times when not necessary can cause other unwanted side effects. For example, sudden stress episodes such as a fright or an emotional upset do not need a double dose. This is because this kind of stress is mainly an adrenalin effect.

The important point here is that sudden events and the feelings that they produce are due to adrenalin. The cortisol response is much slower overall than the adrenalin response.

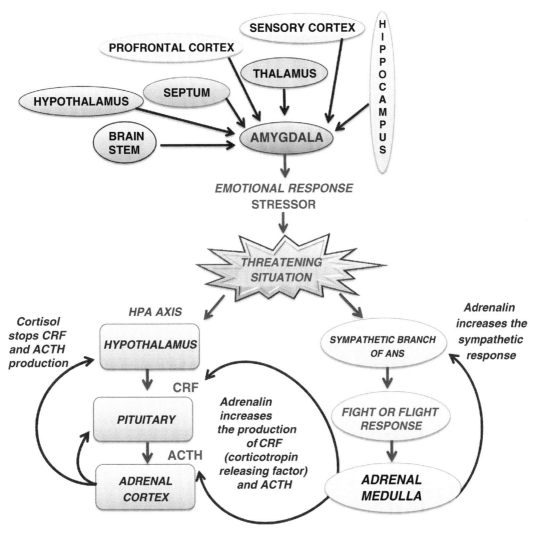

Figure 29.1 *Upper panel shows the emotional response pathway to stress and the lower panel the cortisol and adrenalin pathways for stress responses. Notice that the hypothalamus is in both pathways and is a key player in the overall response.*

For example, if you have a blood test there is an adrenalin response which gives you the rapid heartbeat, cortisol will also increase but for a very brief period of no more than 10 – 20 minutes. The surge then subsides.

Such a brief burst is impossible to mimic with tablets which will take at least an hour to reach a peak which is well after the event has taken place. All that will happen is the person will be exposed to a high amount of cortisol. This may not matter if it is just a one-off event but if the person doubles cortisol regularly for these short frights then they will end up being over exposed to cortisol. As no harm comes from these sudden frights we do not advise to cover them with extra hydrocortisone.

There are particular times where we advise on doubling the dose of hydrocortisone which is mainly during illness and shock.

Doubling the dose or even tripling the dose at other times can cause other unwanted side effects. This is particularly the case in exams where performance in the exam is influenced by the stress, or rather the emotional response to it.

Fig. 29.2 shows that performance is best with a medium degree of anxiety and gets worse if there is too much or even too little anxiety. This is again mainly an adrenalin effect. If you try and deal with this by giving extra hydrocortisone, then you may worsen performance as high doses of glucocorticoids can upset short term memory recall, which is not what you want to do in an exam.

If exams are a problem because of anxiety, then there are ways of dealing with this by either blocking the effect of adrenalin or through coaching methods. Doubling the hydrocortisone dose is not what we would recommend.

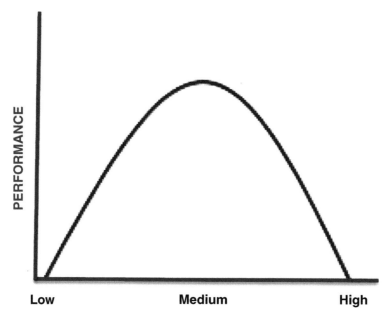

Figure 29.2 *Relationship between performance at a mental task and the level of anxiety either low, medium or high.*

We do recognise however, that there are times during the day when cortisol might be low. This is clear when we undertake 24 hour profiles. If the sudden stress takes place during this period of time, say late evening, then it is probably worth a double dose. In this chapter we will consider the background to this advice and what to do in specific circumstances. We will also look at giving emergency injections of hydrocortisone and how to get help in emergency situations. What we describe is specific for the United Kingdom so may not translate readily to other health care systems.

WHAT HAPPENS DURING ILLNESS, TRAUMA AND SURGERY

During illness especially where there is an associated fever, trauma and surgery, the body responds by increasing the amount of cortisol produced. The amount generated depends on the event but in intensive care and during chest infections, cortisol levels can rise up to 800–1000 nmol/l. Interestingly, when the cortisol is increased, the body does not keep to the circadian rhythm. Rather it tends to move all levels up to these values for the duration of the stress.

Surgery is slightly different in that it is only major surgery such as stomach operations or chest and heart surgery which really cause an increase in cortisol. More minor procedures don't tend to increase cortisol immediately. Cortisol usually tends to rise just after the operation/anaesthetic in those situations. Nonetheless, it is better to err on the side of caution and give extra hydrocortisone before the procedure as well as immediately after.

INCREASED DOSING

Double dose—how much does it actually deliver to the body?

The advice during illness or post surgery is to double the dose of hydrocortisone that is taken daily. This is good advice, but it is important when we are thinking how much we want to achieve in the blood, to realise that there is a limit as to how high you can raise the cortisol level in the blood by increasing the dose.

Increasing a dose, for example from 10 to 30 mg does not lead to a tripling in the blood values as illustrated in Fig. 29.3. In fact, the levels barely double.

The reason for this is because of the various proteins that are in the blood that cortisol binds to, so that they rapidly become saturated and the additional cortisol that is given, is cleared through the kidneys. What we are aiming for in terms of cortisol level during illness is only about 700–800 nmol/l and even in intensive care, levels rarely go over 1000 nmol/l, so doubling the dose is usually enough.

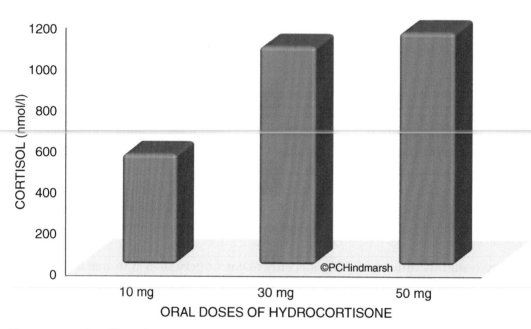

Figure 29.3 *The effect of tripling and quintupling the oral dose of hydrocortisone on the cortisol level achieved in the blood.*

Does a double dose last longer?

Due to the half-life of hydrocortisone, a double dose does not last much longer in the bloodstream at all. In fact, it peaks much higher and excess cortisol is passed out in the urine. We showed this example in Chapter 18 when we were talking about half-life.

Just to reiterate, the half-life is the time taken for 50% of the cortisol in the blood to disappear. This value is on average 80 minutes.

For example, if we have a peak value of 500 nmol/l, then 160 minutes later there would be 125 nmol/l in the blood. If we had a peak of 1000 nmol/l, then 160 minutes later there would be 250 nmol/l. However, 80 minutes after that, the values would be 62.5 and 125 nmol/l respectively.

Both values would be low in a stress situation. The graphs in Fig. 29.4 illustrate this effect for different half-lives of cortisol.

Graph 1 Effect of different half-lives on subsequent cortisol levels

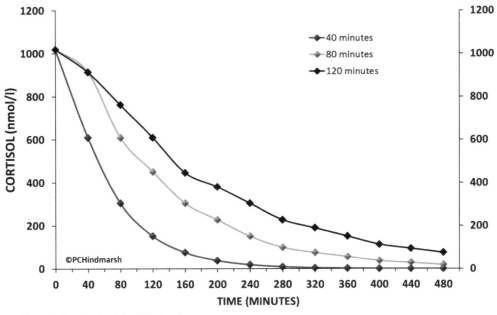

Graph 2 Cortisol half-life clearance

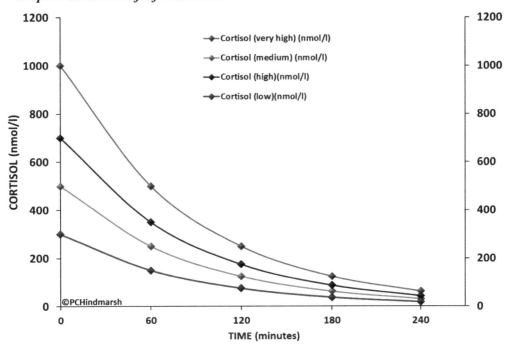

Figure 29.4 *Effect of different half-lives on the amount of cortisol at different stages.* Upper panel (Graph 1: Effect of different half-lives on subsequent cortisol levels) shows the effect of different half-lives of 40 (red), 80 (green) and 120 (blue) minutes starting from a similar peak. The lower panel (Graph 2: Cortisol half-life clearance) shows the same half-life of 60 minutes applied to different peak levels.

The way to deal with this is to give doses more frequently and in a surgery setting or intensive care, this is best achieved by a hydrocortisone intravenous infusion.

MANAGING SICKNESS AT HOME

An unwell child is a worry for any parent and all the more so when they have CAH. The big problem is the development of an adrenal crisis and the components of this are shown in Fig. 29.5. In Fig. 29.5 we have put the features that you might observe in a person with CAH.

Vomiting is the biggest problem because we rely on oral medications to keep the child well. In gastroenteritis which affects absorption from the stomach, there are potential problems that the child has not had the full dose of medication.

ILLNESS

We can classify illness at two levels:

> *Level 1*: There is sickness without vomiting in which case double dosing is needed. In addition, it is important to give an extra dose overnight at 4 a.m. (04:00), during illness.
> *Level 2*: There is sickness and also vomiting.

If vomiting occurs an hour or more after a hydrocortisone dose then the medication is likely to have been absorbed and no repeat dose is needed. However, if vomiting occurs within an hour then the dose should be repeated. If vomiting occurs again, then an intramuscular injection of hydrocortisone is needed and the person should go straight to accident and emergency.

Fig. 29.6 summarises the way illness should be handled.

Taking your child's temperature

A high temperature, i.e. a value more than 38°C, is associated with an infection. The temperature rise results from the immune system attacking the infection and the by-products of these reactions are a series of chemicals that are released into the blood that raise the body temperature.

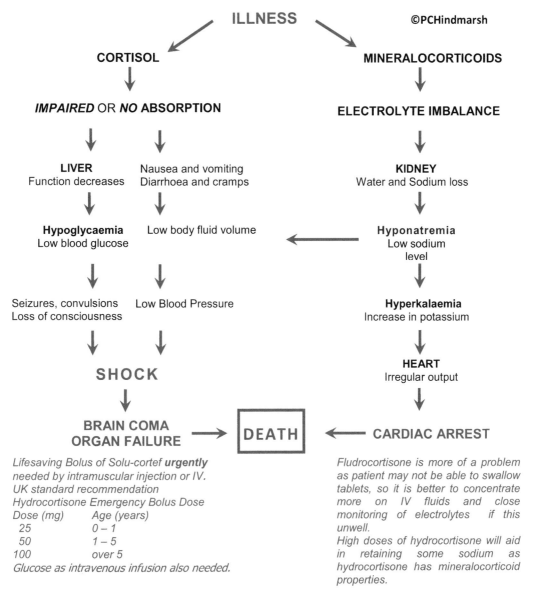

Figure 29.5 *Components of an adrenal crisis which is brought about by loss of both glucocorticoids and mineralocorticoids.*

Interestingly, from the point of view of cortisol, a higher body temperature alters the interaction of cortisol with cortisol binding globulin. This means in local infected tissue, for example, the tonsils, the higher temperature will cause more cortisol to fall off cortisol binding globulin so there will be more in the local tissue to help fight the infection.

WHAT TO DO IN ILLNESS – A QUICK GUIDE

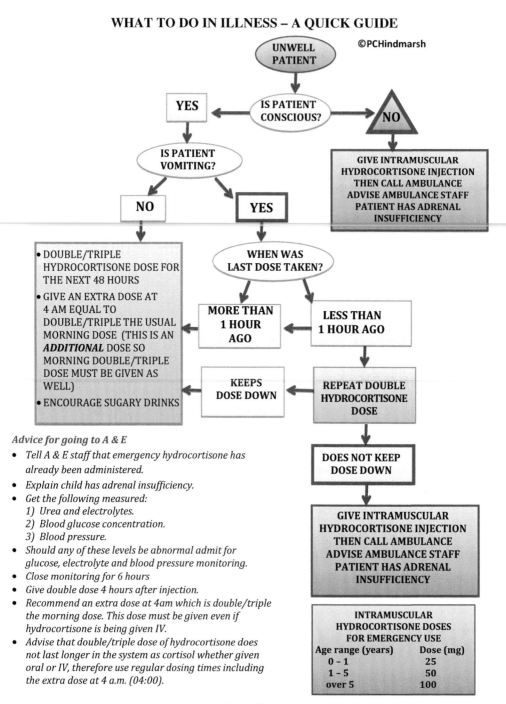

Advice for going to A & E

- *Tell A & E staff that emergency hydrocortisone has already been administered.*
- *Explain child has adrenal insufficiency.*
- *Get the following measured:*
  1) *Urea and electrolytes.*
  2) *Blood glucose concentration.*
  3) *Blood pressure.*
- *Should any of these levels be abnormal admit for glucose, electrolyte and blood pressure monitoring.*
- *Close monitoring for 6 hours*
- *Give double dose 4 hours after injection.*
- *Recommend an extra dose at 4am which is double/triple the morning dose. This dose must be given even if hydrocortisone is being given IV.*
- *Advise that double/triple dose of hydrocortisone does not last longer in the system as cortisol whether given oral or IV, therefore use regular dosing times including the extra dose at 4 a.m. (04:00).*

Figure 29.6 *Flow chart describing what to do with a patient who is unwell, the points at which emergency injection should be given and the patient taken to the emergency department.*

It does mean that in the bloodstream, more cortisol will be free and will be removed more easily which is another reason why we say that doses should be doubled during illness. The graph in Fig. 29.7 shows the fluctuation in body temperature during a 24 hour period.

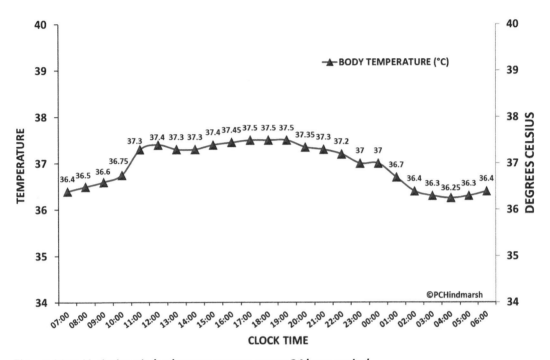

Figure 29.7 *Variations in body temperature over a 24 hour period.*

It is worth quickly comparing Fig. 29.7 and Fig. 29.8. It is almost the inverse of the cortisol rhythm. In fact, there is a lot of evidence to suggest that one of the main determinants of the circadian rhythm is the change in body temperature. This makes sense because if body temperature is low, you would need more energy to keep warm, therefore cortisol production increases, which would increase the glucose levels in the blood to provide energy.

The other important point about Fig. 29.7 is that temperature goes up and down right up to 37.5°C. Normal body temperature varies by person, age, activity and time of day. The average normal body temperature is generally accepted as 37°C but Fig. 29.7 shows the wide range and the fact that values of 37.5°C can be recorded.

What we can be sure of is that a temperature of 38°C and over usually means you have a fever caused by an infection or illness. This is important because slight variations are to be expected and values such as between 37.5 and 37.9°C do not need to be double dosed for, unless the person is actually unwell with other symptoms.

Extra dose at 4 a.m. (04:00) in illness

We have now introduced advice that during illness an *extra double/triple dose* of hydrocortisone be given around 4 a.m. (04:00).

- The dose should be the *same dose* as the *double/triple morning dose*.
- The double/triple morning dose should be given at the usual time, as the 4 a.m. (04:00) dose is an *additional* dose.
- You should give this dose even if you have given a double dose at 1 a.m. (01:00).

The reason why we advise this extra dose should be given at 4 a.m. (04:00) is because at this time in someone who does not have CAH, the circadian rhythm shows us there is usually a lot of cortisol in the system (Fig. 29.8). This cortisol helps keep the blood glucose levels up whilst we are asleep.

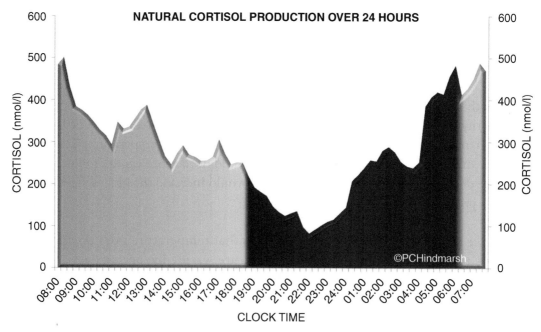

Figure 29.8 *The natural cortisol distribution over 24 hours is known as the circadian rhythm.*

When we are using hydrocortisone to replace cortisol, the evening dose or the last dose taken in that period, will have dropped to a low level by 4 a.m. (04:00) and in illness this can cause hypoglycaemia – low blood glucose levels. Low blood glucose levels can be dangerous and lead to unconsciousness.

What is also very important to remember when taking a tablet the cortisol takes between 1 and 2 hours to peak, so on taking a double dose when ill around 4 a.m. (04:00), will give enough cortisol to cover until the morning dose is due.

Examples 1 and 2 show what happens to cortisol levels when hydrocortisone is taken at specific times to illustrate the cortisol gap which exists in the early hours of the morning.

Example 1

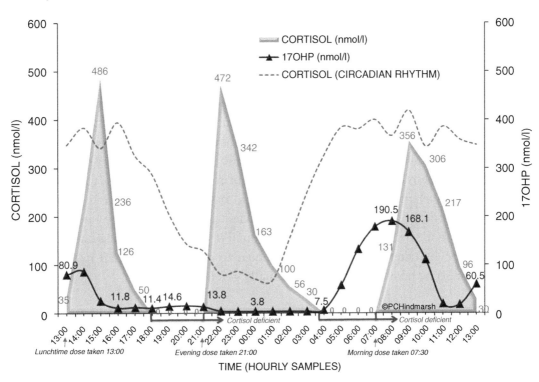

Figure 29.9 *Last evening dose of hydrocortisone taken at 21:00 (9 p.m.).*

The data in the 24 hour profile (Fig. 29.9) is based on a typical three dosing per day schedule, with each dose taken in morning at 07:30, lunchtime at 13:00 and before bed at 21:00. We can see that the doses taken give high peaks of cortisol which does suppress the 17OHP to some extent and if we were basing cortisol replacement on

17OHP levels only using blood spots, the temptation would be to increase the doses. However, when we look at the cortisol, we can clearly see there are multiple periods of the day where there is no measurable cortisol in the blood. The lunchtime dose taken at 13:00 does not last until the bedtime dose which is taken at 21:00, in fact, there is a period of 3 hours (18:00 to 21:00) where there is no cortisol, yet the 17OHP stays at a reasonable level, this is due to the excessive cortisol peak at 14:00.

The evening dose drops to 30 nmol/l from 03:00 and there is no measurable cortisol until the next dose is taken at 07:30. The 17OHP starts to increase not only because the cortisol is very low but because of the natural surge of ACTH which occurs in everyone around this time, to naturally increase cortisol production. In CAH as we know, the adrenal glands do not produce cortisol, so the 17OHP levels increase due to the ACTH feedback system. Interestingly, this patient had an androstenedione level of 5.5 nmol/l at 08:00, 1.38 nmol/l at 10:00 and <1.05 nmol/l at 16:00, 22:00 and midnight, which would indicate over treatment. However, we can clearly see by looking and considering the cortisol level, there are periods of over and under treatment.

In illness even when doubling the doses, the doses would not last much longer, cortisol levels are very low from around 02:00 and by 04:00 there is no traceable cortisol left to measure in the blood. This could lead to dangerously low blood glucose levels. If you look at the blue dashed line which represents the body's own natural production, there is normally a significant amount of cortisol present in the early hours of the morning. At this time of the morning, one of the important roles cortisol plays is to regulate the blood glucose level and in illness the body would naturally produce even higher levels of cortisol in order to ensure that there is sufficient glucose to provide energy, for the increased metabolic demand of fighting infection. This is why we advocate an additional double dose to be taken at 4 a.m. (04:00) equal to double the normal morning dose which must also be taken at the time it is usually given.

Example 2

Fig. 29.10 shows an example a patient who had their last dose at 20:00 (8 p.m.) and we can see they metabolise hydrocortisone at a different rate to the patient in Example 1, as they have good cortisol coverage for most of the day. The morning dose is taken at 06:30 (6.30 am) and when the next dose is taken there is a good amount of cortisol to stack onto the next dose. Pre dose 17OHP blood spots would indicate good replacement and the morning 17OHP level of 40.7 nmol/l would be seen as acceptable, if not a little too high depending on the centre the patient is under, as we know that hydrocortisone only last in the blood as cortisol for approximately 6 hours.

However we can see that the 17OHP is totally suppressed *after* the 20:00 (8 p.m.) bedtime dose which would suggest that this dose is too high and it remains very low until it starts to rise slowly at 4 a.m. (04:00) despite no measurable cortisol in the blood from 02:00 (2 a.m.).

In illness as discussed, even double dosing at 20:00 (8 p.m.) will not make the dose last longer in time, the cortisol will only peak higher. So even with double dose the patient will remain cortisol deficient from around 02:00 (2 a.m.) until the morning dose is taken at 06:30 (6.30am). The patient will also not have eaten as they went to bed at 20:00 (8 p.m.) so without food and any cortisol and if ill the patient will be at risk of hypoglycaemia and adrenal crisis.

In illness a dose double dose of hydrocortisone (equal to double the usual morning dose) needs to be taken at 4 a.m. (04:00) or even earlier and then a double dose taken again at 06:30 (6.30 a.m.).

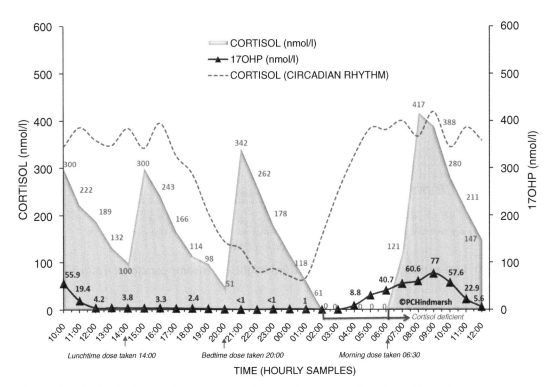

Figure 29.10 *Cortisol levels in someone who metabolises on the slow side with no measurable cortisol in the bloodstream after 02:00 (2 a.m.).*

Despite this patient handling cortisol on the slow side, there are still periods of over and under treatment and they would gain better cortisol levels by taking 4 doses a day which would need to be carefully titrated and timed to suit the way they handle their medication.

Example 3

In the next graph (Fig. 29.11) we can see the patient who has taken the evening dose at the later time of 24:00 (midnight). The profile shows that because the duration of hydrocortisone is 4–6 hours, the cortisol level drops low and there is little around in the early morning and in fact no measurable cortisol from around 05:00 (5 a.m.). This patient has a fast clearance.

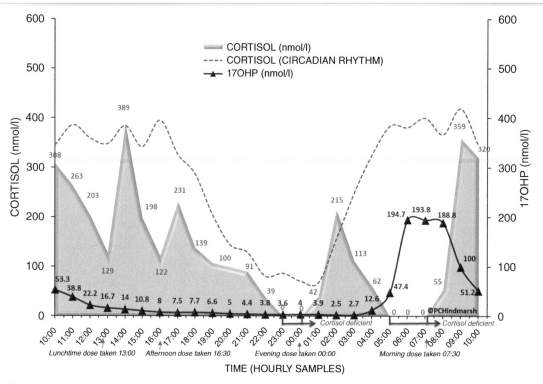

Figure 29.11 *Last evening dose taken at 24:00 (midnight) gives some cortisol at 4 a.m. (04:00) but not much.*

What our profile work has shown is that a double dose should be taken around 4 a.m. (04:00) (equal to double the usual morning dose) in illness, as statistically this is the time when most adrenal crises occur in illness. There have also been several cases reported where young children have woken ill, been put back to bed without a dose being given and have been found comatose in the morning.

WHAT TO DO WITH TRAUMA ACCIDENTS

Many problems with CAH can be handled at home by increasing the dose of hydrocortisone. In general to reiterate, in CAH extra medication is needed when the person becomes unwell or has a serious injury and we do this to prevent a life threatening adrenal crisis from occurring. Our Level 1 and 2 guide shows you what to do for illness. However, what should be done for trauma?

All children have falls, scratches, bumps and bruises and a child will not need any extra hydrocortisone if they recover immediately and carry on what they were doing before their accident.

Intramuscular injection of hydrocortisone is needed immediately for the following:

- Broken limb.
- Bump on the head leading to unconsciousness.
- Burn injury.
- If for any reason the person is found in a condition where they are pale, clammy, drowsy and unresponsive (do not respond as they would normally do).

After administering the hydrocortisone injection, dial 999 (911 in the United States) and ask for an ambulance. What you need to say to them is detailed in the next section. In brief, tell the ambulance control that the person has adrenal insufficiency, that hydrocortisone has been given and they need to be taken to a hospital to be monitored.

It is always safest in these situations to give the IM injection. It will do no harm and it is always better they have the injection as more serious problems may occur if it is not given when needed.

Getting an ambulance

There are several situations where you or your child's carer/nursery/school may need to call an ambulance. Hopefully these will be few and far between. When you ring 999 for an ambulance you need to use these terms as many ambulance services in the United Kingdom are presently following a 'pathways system' and each 999 call is triaged.

The 'pathway' followed for CAH and all other cortisol deficient disorders is 'adrenal insufficiency'. Another key statement is 'on hydrocortisone treatment'.

So in an emergency dial 999 and ask for ambulance service. The call handler will ask for the location which is where the ambulance should be sent.

The call handler will then ask for various details such as name, date of birth and what is wrong – it is most important that you state that the patient has 'adrenal insufficiency and needs an emergency hydrocortisone injection', if one hasn't already been administered. 'Adrenal insufficiency' is the key statement for the ambulance crew who will recognise it, respond accordingly and will act by giving emergency hydrocortisone.

At present, if you have a protocol logged with emergency services this is currently flagged by the patient's address (not by their name) so it is important to make the emergency call handler aware that there is a protocol in place and to give the patient's address if you have it. This is changing, so the name can be registered because ambulance can now track your position if you are using a mobile phone or a landline. This varies from region to region at the time of writing. Your medical team can arrange this for you.

This reinforces the importance of wearing a medic alert with the wording 'adrenal insufficiency' and also carrying an Adrenal Insufficiency Card which should have the home address details on.

When to call an ambulance

Just as a reminder you should call an ambulance when:

1. You have given an emergency injection and there has been no response.
2. If your child is involved in an accident.
3. There is loss of consciousness.
4. Your child is vomiting and cannot keep medicines down.
5. If your child is very unwell and you do not have an injection kit or unable to give the injection.

When the ambulance arrives give a copy of your emergency letter prepared by your medical team or Adrenal Insufficiency Card to the ambulance crew.

On the way to hospital, the ambulance crew will alert accident and emergency that you are on your way, but it is good idea to ring your medical team as well to tell them what has happened as they will be able to liaise with accident and emergency and assist with what needs to happen next.

Please note the medical team will only look for a medical alert, they are not authorised and do not have the time to check mobile phones, go through bags or check for stickers on car windows. Having a notification sticker on the car window could lead to confusion as the person with the condition may not be in the car. It is extremely important to wear a medic alert ID bracelet or necklace as this is what the paramedics are trained to look for and act upon.

In accident and emergency

When you get to accident and emergency the team will be ready for you if you arrive via an ambulance. If you arrive by other means then the triage system will deal with you and for children this has to be within 15 minutes after arrival.

It is extremely important that you are seen by a doctor immediately after triage and you should tell them that your child has 'adrenal insufficiency' because of congenital adrenal hyperplasia. It is important to show them the Adrenal Insufficiency/Steroid Card as this has details of what to do in this situation.

The important steps are:

1. Insert an intravenous cannula so that salt replacement and glucose can be given.
2. Get urgent blood tests ordered. These include:
   a. Basic metabolic panel including sodium, potassium, chloride and bicarbonate, urea, glucose, creatinine and calcium.
   b. Cortisol.
   c. Check capillary blood glucose level and perform any other appropriate tests (e.g. urine culture).
3. Start treatment.
   This should consist of an intravenous or intramuscular injection of hydrocortisone if not already given by the parent or paramedic.
   Just to recap the doses are:

Age range (years)	Dose (mg)
0 – 1	25
1 – 5	50
Over 5	100

4. Start intravenous fluids.
   This gets a bit technical but we have included this as it might be helpful for accident and emergency teams. The key points are:
   a. Commence IV fluids infusion of 0.45% sodium chloride, 5% glucose at maintenance rate (extra if patient is dehydrated). Add potassium depending on electrolyte balance.
   b. Commence hydrocortisone infusion in 50 ml 0.9% sodium chloride via syringe pump.
   c. Monitor for at least 12 hours before discharge.
   d. If blood glucose is <2.5 mmol/l give bolus of 2 ml/kg of 10% glucose.
   e. If patient is drowsy, hypotensive and peripherally shut down with poor capillary return, give 1 ml/kg of 3% saline.

Following the aforementioned recommendations will mean fluid and salt balance are properly corrected and blood glucose is kept in the normal range. The tests will also pick up any cause for the patient becoming unwell which might need additional treatment, such as a chest infection.

SURGERY IN PATIENTS RECEIVING GLUCOCORTICOIDS

Hopefully most of the time people with CAH do not need surgery. There are times when surgery is needed and this is done in a planned way known as an elective procedure. The other type of surgery is emergency surgery, for example, appendicitis. The ways in which we advise glucocorticoid cover for these two types of surgery differ slightly but the basic principle is the same – more glucocorticoid is needed. For all surgical procedures including tests such as MRI scanning we use hydrocortisone as the preferred glucocorticoid.

Elective surgery

Here are some useful points to remember for planning elective surgery. This is what doctors will be thinking when they are organising surgery, so it is really a good idea to know what they are planning so that you can make sure it really does happen.

1. The doctor in charge, usually the surgeon, should always let the anaesthetist know beforehand so they can plan for the operation, getting intravenous hydrocortisone available, for example.
2. It is best if you are placed first on the surgical list in the morning. This is not always possible because lists are arranged in terms of complexity and whether the case is infective or non infective but the principle should be where possible, CAH patient first. You should take your normal evening dose of hydrocortisone. The ward staff should start monitoring your blood glucose concentrations from 06.00 (6 a.m.) and hourly thereafter until you get to the operating theatre. These blood glucose checks will be continued at 2 hourly intervals after the operation until you resume taking food and drink normally. At the same time a dextrose with saline (sugar with salt mixture) intravenous drip should be commenced and maintained until tolerating oral fluids.
3. If you are on an afternoon list then take your usual morning dose of hydrocortisone and fludrocortisone.
4. You will be given an intravenous dose of hydrocortisone (2 mg/kg body weight) (Fig. 29.12) when you get to the operating theatre. Extra bolus injections will be given if the operation is expected to exceed 4 hours. Alternatively, for prolonged procedures and when post operative recovery is likely to be slow, hydrocortisone infusion using a pump will be set up.

Minor surgery

Minor Surgery can be defined as a procedure that lasts less than 90 minutes in total such as dental work needing a general anaesthetic.

At induction: Hydrocortisone IV 2 mg/kg and repeated if procedure exceeds 4 hours.

Post op: Can use repeat IV regimen of hydrocortisone (2 mg/kg) in lieu of routine medication until tolerating oral fluids. Then return to oral therapy which must include that day's fludrocortisone dose.

Always make sure that you are only written up for post op bolus when you are able to take oral medications.

Note that after short procedures such as an MRI or CT scan, an increased need for cortisol is required after the scan if it is under taken under anaesthesia or sedation, so take double morning dose straight after the scan and then continue the rest of day on usual therapy.

Major surgery

Major Surgery can be defined as a procedure which lasts more than 90 minutes for example chest or stomach operation.

At induction: Hydrocortisone IV 2 mg/kg.

During op: Repeat IV hydrocortisone on 4 hourly basis or use a hydrocortisone infusion.

Post op: Can use repeat IV regimen of hydrocortisone. Alternatively, when post operative recovery is likely to be slow a hydrocortisone infusion is better. Continue IV administration until tolerating fluids. Then return to **oral therapy at twice normal dose for 24 hours**.* Then return to normal requirements. As soon as on oral therapy reintroduce fludrocortisone dose.

*Post operative dosing schedule will be determined by the extent of the surgical procedure and should be conducted in liaison with your endocrine team.

Fluids: 100 ml/kg/day if weight < 10 kg
80 ml/kg/day if weight 10–30 kg
60 ml/kg/day if weight > 30 kg

If salt-wasting congenital adrenal hyperplasia use 5% glucose with 0.45% sodium chloride.

For other cases use 4% glucose with 0.18% sodium chloride.

Hydrocortisone infusion

Infusion rate to achieve the average serum cortisol concentration achieved on PICU during sepsis of 1000 nmol/l (0.36 mg/ml) is shown in Fig. 29.12.

Situation	Cortisol clearance (ml/24 hours)	Infusion Rate (mg/24 hours)
Prepubertal: <10 kg	74	25
10-20 kg	147	50
>20 kg	294	100
Pubertal	430	155
Postpubertal	290	105

Infusion Rate (mg/24 hours) = clearance (ml/24 hours) × steady state cortisol concentration (mg/ml)

Figure 29.12 *Hydrocortisone infusion schedule.*

Emergency surgery

If you need to have emergency surgery, then you will almost certainly have a drip so all your hydrocortisone will be given intravenously as a bolus or infusion, just as in major surgery.

Things can happen quickly in these situations so it is very important the staff know that you have to take hydrocortisone. This is why it is so important to carry with you your Adrenal Insufficiency Card and to wear a 'medic alert' bracelet with the words 'adrenal insufficiency' stamped on it. Remember, you may not be conscious when all this is going on so you do need some way to tell people about your or your child's condition.

Dental surgery

By dental surgery we mean fillings and root canal work that can be undertaken with a local anaesthetic. If a general anaesthetic is needed then the minor surgery routine aforementioned will need to be followed. Extra hydrocortisone is not needed for a routine dental appointment even though you might be stressed about visiting the dentist!

For dental work requiring a local anaesthetic, give double the dose of hydrocortisone on the day of the procedure. Start with doubling the morning dose if the work is in the morning, or the lunchtime dose if in the afternoon. You should continue with double the dose for 24 hours after the procedure particularly if it is painful such as root canal work or removal of wisdom teeth.

EXAMS

School and university examinations can be very stressful but usually most of the feelings we have are related to adrenalin rather than cortisol. That said, you probably do need slightly more cortisol to get through them especially if profile work shows that you have dips late morning or late afternoon.

What we would suggest is if the exam is in the morning then you have the usual morning dose of hydrocortisone when you get up. Then, if you normally have a dose at lunchtime, you should take half that dose at 10:00 (10 a.m.) to keep you going during the exam and of course have your normal lunchtime dose. This will prevent any cortisol dip late morning.

If the exam is in the afternoon then take the normal lunchtime dose as usual. You should then take a further dose at 15:00 (3 p.m.). The dose should be equivalent to half the normal lunchtime dose and this will keep you going in the late afternoon. If you have morning and afternoon exams then you will take half the lunchtime dose at 10:00 (10 a.m.), then the normal lunchtime dose and a further dose of half the lunchtime dose at 15:00 (3 p.m.). It is always a good idea to check that you can take your extra hydrocortisone into the exam room.

VACCINATIONS

All childhood vaccinations are recommended for children with CAH. There are rules about giving some vaccines to people receiving glucocorticoids. These rules are for those receiving high doses of glucocorticoids for inflammatory conditions and do not apply to the replacement doses which we use in CAH.

The way a person reacts to a vaccination varies. If there is a rise in temperature then double dosing with hydrocortisone should be started and the 'Sick Day Rules' outlined previously followed. If you are unsure about how the person is reacting to the vaccine then it is always best to get medical advice either from your endocrine team, your general practice or accident and emergency.

GETTING YOUR FAMILY DOCTOR INVOLVED

Family doctors are very good at dealing with common problems. However, they are unlikely to know a lot about CAH. In an average practice they may only come across one case every 10 years or so, if that!!

That said, there is a lot that they can do and what we have done is create a guide to help you, which you can also share with them. What the family doctor can do is to make sure that all the normal things that occur in childhood such as immunisation, happen. There is no reason why a child with CAH should not have all their immunisations.

What needs to be done is the responsibility for care to be clearly defined between the hospital and the family doctor so everybody knows what is expected of them. This is particularly important during illness when rapid review by the family doctor can prevent an admission to hospital.

Hospital responsibilities

Hospitals take charge of monitoring the condition and in particular:

- height and weight,
- blood pressure monitoring,
- medication dose changes,
- arrangement of specialist hospital appointments and
- annual review assessments and 24 hour profiles.

It is important this information is supplied regularly to the family doctor to keep them up to date.

General health

This can be provided as is usual for any child, by the family doctor. This includes the full range of immunisations and developmental checks.

Emergency care

There are several aspects that family doctor can help with:

1. Arranging and ensuring the continuation of "Open Access" with the local paediatric team to avoid unnecessary delays in accident and emergency.
2. Have a copy of the emergency letter for all health care professionals at hand along with a copy of the hospital emergency guidelines plan.
3. Allow priority appointments when unwell.
4. Ensure that practice nurses and out of hours services are aware of the emergency protocol and are familiar with importance of increasing steroids when ill, as well as the correct dose of hydrocortisone which should be administered IM.
5. That the patient's condition is flagged on the practice GP system, so locum doctors, practice nurses are alerted the patient has adrenal insufficiency.
6. Reinforce the need to wear medic alerts with the wording 'adrenal insufficiency'.

ILLNESS—DOSING GUIDE

ISSUE/CIRCUMSTANCE	AMOUNT OF EXTRA HYDROCORTISONE NEEDED	COMMENTS
Raised Temperature >38°C	Double dose	Extra double dose at 4 a.m. (04:00) equal to double morning dose. See GP for diagnosis of cause of raised temperature
Raised Temperature >39°C	Triple dose	Extra triple dose at 4 a.m. (04:00) equal to triple morning dose. See GP for diagnosis of cause of raised temperature
Broken bone	IM injection (see dose schedule)	Give IM injection (appropriate dose) call for ambulance
Unconscious	IM injection (see dose schedule)	Give IM injection (appropriate dose) call for ambulance
Serious burns	IM injection (see dose schedule)	Give IM injection (appropriate dose) call for ambulance
Severe scalding	IM injection (see dose schedule)	Give IM injection (appropriate dose) call for ambulance
Minor burns	Double dose	Extra double dose at 4 a.m. (04:00) equal to double morning dose. See GP or A & E for assessment of burn area
Head injury where loss of consciousness	IM injection (see schedule)	Give IM injection (appropriate dose) call for ambulance
Serious injury	IM injection (see schedule)	Give IM injection (appropriate dose) call for ambulance
Minor injury (grazes and bruises)	None needed	
Surgery with General Anaesthetic	Bolus pre surgery and bolus post-surgery	See surgery guidelines
Minor Surgery with Local Anaesthetic	Depending on surgery extra dose 30 minute pre-surgery	This will ensure there is adequate cortisol at time of procedure
Dental Work with General Anaesthetic	Bolus pre surgery and bolus post-surgery	See surgery guidelines. Must always be carried out in hospital not in dentist chair
Dental Work with Local Anaesthetic	Depending on surgery extra dose 30 minute pre-surgery	This will ensure there is adequate cortisol at time of procedure
Common cold with no temperature	None needed	Add in 4 a.m. (04:00) dose
Vaccinations	None needed unless a fever develops	If fever develops include more at 4 a.m. (04:00)

STRESS—DOSING GUIDE

OCCASION	AMOUNT OF EXTRA HYDROCORTISONE NEEDED	COMMENTS
Exams	Not recommended	See exam section if you have cortisol dips on your profile late morning or late afternoon
Birthday parties	None needed	
Shock from bereavement	Not really needed but no harm to take small extra dose	
Sport	None needed	Some people may need extra if exercise is done before next dose is due ©PCHindmarsh

Figure 29.13 *Summary guide of what to do with hydrocortisone dosing in various situations.*

Drug interactions

This is important to consider especially with hydrocortisone, so it is always good to remind the family doctor that you are on hydrocortisone so they can check for drug interactions. You can always check with our table in Chapter 20 (Fig. 20.15).

The main interaction to watch out for is with the oral contraceptive pill. This is associated with a need to alter the hydrocortisone dosing (Fig. 20.9).

CONCLUSIONS

We have covered a lot in this Chapter so in Fig. 29.13 we have put a summary of what needs to be done in the various situations.

FURTHER READING

Hahner, S., Burger-Stritt, S., Allolio, B., 2013. Subcutaneous hydrocortisone administration for emergency use in adrenal insufficiency. Eur. J. Endocrinol. 169, 147–154.

Hsu, C.Y., Rivkees, S.A., 2005. Chapter 9 Stress Dosing. In: Hsu, C.Y., Rivkees, S.A. (Eds.), Congenital Adrenal Hyperplasia: A Parents' Guide. AuthorHouse, Indianna.

Weise, M., Drinkard, B., Mehlinger, S.L., et al., 2004. Stress dose of hydrocortisone is not beneficial in patients with classic congenital adrenal hyperplasia undergoing short term, high-intensity exercise. J. Clin. Endocrinol. Metab. 89, 3679–3684.

CHAPTER 30

Practical Information Emergency Kit and School Information

GLOSSARY

Adrenal insufficiency Term used to cover all causes for deficiency of cortisol. It is not a diagnosis. It is the result of a medical condition that leaves the body unable to produce cortisol or enough cortisol. Adrenal Insufficiency is the key phrase used by ambulance services to get the highest priority call out and alert them to the fact the patient needs a hydrocortisone bolus urgently.

Emergency kit A steroid/adrenal insufficiency card, copy of emergency letter and an emergency kit which consists of cotton wool ball, alcohol wipe if available or alternatively hand sanitiser, syringe and needle. AmpSnap (plastic top to help snap open glass ampoules safely) ampoules of hydrocortisone for injection either; Hydrocortisone Sodium Phosphate (100 mg in 1 ml) or Solu-Cortef 100 mg in 2 ml, tube of Glucogel.

Medic alert Essential identifier of condition. Needs to be engraved with term 'adrenal insufficiency' as this is the only item that ambulance crews will search the person for and the words will trigger their emergency pathway.

MEDIC ALERT

Adrenal insufficiency is used as a descriptive term, this is *not a diagnosis*. However, adrenal insufficiency is the most appropriate wording to be used on medic alerts as it is the recognised terminology used by the ambulance services in their pathway system. The pathway alerts the emergency service that an injection of hydrocortisone is needed urgently.

It is highly recommended that everyone who has CAH, wears a medic alert at all times and the wording on the medic alert is 'Adrenal Insufficiency'. If the medic alert is inscribed with congenital adrenal hyperplasia there is a strong probability that emergency staff will not recognise the condition and may not appreciate that emergency hydrocortisone is needed.

Congenital Adrenal Hyperplasia. http://dx.doi.org/10.1016/B978-0-12-811483-4.00030-1

Babies and toddlers will soon get used to wearing one and the chain can be shortened and links can be added back on, as your child grows. Although parents feel they are always with their child, something may happen which might leave you unable to communicate with the emergency services. Paramedics who are usually on the scene first, as well as all other emergency staff involved in urgent care, are all trained to look for medic alerts! If your child (or you) is not wearing a one, emergency staff would not be aware that lifesaving injection of hydrocortisone is needed urgently and a life could be lost as a result. Other wording maybe added such as 'Steroid Dependent' but it is important to use 'Adrenal Insufficiency', as the latter highlights the individual has a medical condition where the adrenal glands do not function properly (Fig. 30.1).

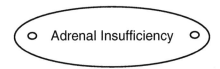

Figure 30.1 *Medic alert should be inscribed with the words Adrenal Insufficiency and be worn at all times.*

EMERGENCY KIT

All patients should carry a steroid/adrenal insufficiency card and an emergency kit which consists of the following:

Cotton wool ball.

Alcohol wipe if available or alternatively hand sanitiser.

Syringe and needle.

AmpSnap (plastic top to help snap open glass ampoules safely).

Ampoules of hydrocortisone for injection either:

- Hydrocortisone Sodium Phosphate (previously known as Efcortesol) (100 mg in 1 ml)

  or

- Solu-Cortef 100 mg in 2 ml. Solu-Cortef comes in powder form with 1 vial of sterile water (2 ml to mix), see insert on how to mix.

Tube of Glucogel (used to be known as HypoStop).

Glucogel should be only used when the patient is showing signs of low blood sugar levels. Glucogel should be used AFTER the hydrocortisone injection has been given. Gradually squirt the Glucogel into the side of the mouth, between the gums and the cheek. Alternatively, squirt the Glucogel onto your fingertip and apply it between the gums and cheek. Up to one third of a 25 g tube may be needed. Massage into the cheek to allow the gel to be absorbed, which should raise blood sugar levels within 10 minutes.

Keep the entire emergency pack together in a safe place where children cannot reach it. Keep it at room temperature, out of direct sunlight or heat. The injection ampoules do not need to be kept in the fridge.

It is also very helpful to keep a copy of an emergency letter with all relevant information and up to date phone numbers which will be helpful to the emergency services (Fig. 30.2). An example of an emergency letter can be seen in Fig. 30.3.

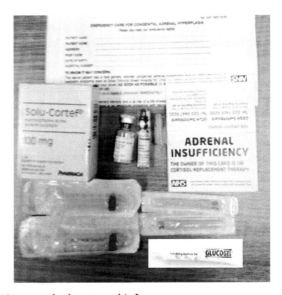

Figure 30.2 *Important items to be kept as a kit for emergency use.*

EMERGENCY INJECTION

It is important that your endocrine team teaches you how to draw up and administer an emergency injection. We recommend that you keep a note and diarise the expiry date of the vials of hydrocortisone you have, allowing enough time to request a repeat prescription so you are never left without a supply. Emergency injections are really important and we have covered when they should be done and how much should be given.

EMERGENCY CARE FOR CONGENITAL ADRENAL HYPERPLASIA

PATIENT NAME   ....

PATIENT HOME   ....

ADDRESS   ....

POST CODE   ....

DATE OF BIRTH   ....

HOSPITAL NUMBER ....

TO WHOM IT MAY CONCERN:

The above patient has a rare genetic disorder congenital adrenal hyperplasia and is under the care of our team at .... Please contact the Endocrinology team **AS SOON AS POSSIBLE** on .... and ask to be put through to the Paediatric Endocrine Registrar on call.

~~He/she must been seen by a medical physician IMMEDIATELY.~~ Time in a waiting room or triage situation is INAPPROPRIATE.

The patient is on replacement steroids and is at risk of a life threatening adrenal crisis if not treated quickly. A crisis will occur when there is an electrolyte imbalance with febrile illness, fluid depletion from vomiting and diarrhoea, burns, serious illness and injury. Signs of an impending crisis can include weakness, dizziness, floppiness, failure to respond, nausea and vomiting, hypotension, hypoglycaemia, pallor, and clammy sweating.

1. INSERT IV CANNULA

2. URGENT BLOOD TESTS REQUIRED

- Basic metabolic panel including: urea and electrolytes, glucose and calcium.
- Cortisol and 17OHP to get idea of current status.
- Check capillary blood glucose level (BM Stix) and perform any other appropriate tests (e.g. urine culture).

3. TREATMENT

STAT: Solu-Cortef injection IV or IM, if NOT already given by the parent or paramedic

Doses are as follows:

Age range (years)	Dose (mg)
0 – 1	25
1 – 5	50
Over 5	**100**

4. IV FLUIDS:

1. Commence IV fluids Infusion of 0.45% sodium chloride, 5% glucose at maintenance rate (extra if patient is dehydrated). Add potassium depending on electrolyte balance.
2. Commence hydrocortisone infusion in 50 ml 0.9% sodium chloride via syringe pump.
3. Monitor for at least twelve hours before discharge.
4. **IMPORTANT** If blood glucose is <2.5 mmol/l give bolus of 2 ml/kg of 10% glucose.
5. If patient is drowsy, hypotensive and peripherally shut down with poor capillary return give: 20 ml/kg of 0.9% sodium chloride stat.

IF IN ANY DOUBT ABOUT THIS PATIENT'S MANAGEMENT, PLEASE CONTACT ....

Figure 30.3 *Example of an emergency letter.*

NEEDLE INFORMATION

Another point which also needs to be considered is what size needle should be used to administer the injection.

Choosing the correct needle is important because we don't want one which is too short, otherwise the injection will not only go into fat tissue, it will hurt. It will also not be absorbed as well. The gauge of the needle is important as we don't want the needle to be too fine. The gauge is how wide or narrow the needle tube is. If it is too narrow it will make giving the injection difficult. This is especially the case when using Hydrocortisone Sodium Phosphate the readymade hydrocortisone solution, as it is quite thick so you need to use a wider bore needle. Although it may sound odd, longer needles hurt less and cause less of a local reaction. It is important to never reuse the needle and also to dispose of it safely once used.

The length of the needle for all ages from infants to adults is 1 inches or 2.5 cm. The gauge varies so that for children less than 12 months of age, a gauge 25 needle can be used. This is coloured orange. This is probably a bit too small for Hydrocortisone Sodium Phosphate use, so it is better to use a gauge 23 or blue needle. For children and young people the blue gauge 23 works well but again if using Hydrocortisone Sodium Phosphate it is better to use a green gauge 21.

If we look at the emergency dosing guide, we can add our recommended needle gauge to it (Fig. 30.4).

Age (years)	Hydrocortisone dose (mg)	Needle Gauge and Colour	
		Solu-Cortef	Hydrocortisone Sodium Phosphate (Efcortesol)
0–1	25	25	23
1–5	50	23	21
Over 5	100	23	21

Figure 30.4 *General guide of which gauge needle to use.*

All these numbers can be rather hard to understand so Fig. 30.5 illustrates what the needles look like and is for illustrative purposes only. These will vary depending on what your team has available.

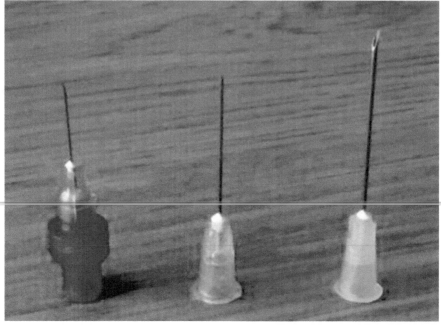

| 25 Gauge | 23 Gauge | 21 Gauge |

Figure 30.5 *Picture of what the different needles look like.*

INFORMATION FOR SCHOOL AND NURSERY CARE

Schools and nurseries/day care also need to know exactly what to do, as they will need to give doses during the day and also double doses if the child has an accident or becomes unwell.

They are not obliged to give the emergency injections but many will if shown how to. Below is an outline school/nursery plan for the administration of hydrocortisone and a plan to handle illness and trauma at school/nursery.

It is important to ensure the school has the contact numbers for both parents/carers and that the school is informed of any changes, or if the parent will not be contactable. If this is the case, then another contact must be given.

Children do not like to be excluded from normal activities and there is no reason why any child with CAH cannot be included on school trips and activities. It is important to ensure that medication is taken along as well as the emergency kit. The staff must understand if a dose needs to be taken, it needs to be given on time and what needs to happen if the child becomes unwell. Also ensure that the child has a drink available so they are able to take their tablet!

Here is an example of the information that should be supplied to a school or nursery.

MEDICAL MANAGEMENT PLAN FOR SCHOOLS OR NURSERY CARE

Steroids School Supply

Type of steroid:	hydrocortisone
Dose of steroid to be administered at school:	….mg
Time of administration:	….h

ILLNESS AT SCHOOL OR NURSERY

In CAH, extra medication is needed when the student or child becomes unwell or has a serious injury to prevent a life threatening adrenal crisis occurring. All children have falls, scratches, bumps and bruises and a child will not need any extra hydrocortisone if they recover immediately and carry on what they were doing before their accident.

Always notify parents/guardian or emergency contact of any illness or injury.

SERIOUS INJURIES

Intramuscular injection of hydrocortisone is needed immediately for the following:
- Broken limb.
- Bump on the head leading to unconsciousness.
- Burn injury.
- If for any reason the student or child is found in a condition where they are pale, clammy, drowsy and unresponsive (do not respond as they would normally do).

After administering the hydrocortisone injection, dial 999 ask for an ambulance.

Advise ambulance control that the student has Adrenal Insufficiency and the student or child must be taken to hospital to be monitored.

Even if the student or child did not necessarily need the IM hydrocortisone injection, it will do no harm and it is always better they have the injection as more serious problems may occur if it is not given when needed.

GENERAL ILLNESSES

If a student or child becomes unwell at school or nursery they will need extra medication if she/he has:

- High temperature that is 38°C or above (degrees centigrade).
- If the student or child faints.
- Stomach upset that is severe enough to prevent normal school or nursery activities.

A double dose of hydrocortisone should be given, whether the dose is due or not.

VOMITING

It takes about an hour for the oral hydrocortisone to be absorbed so if the student or child has vomited up the administered steroid at lunchtime:

- Repeat oral dose but double the amount.
- Contact parent.
- If the second dose is vomited then give intramuscular hydrocortisone.
- Call ambulance on 999 and the student or child should be taken by ambulance to the nearest Accident and Emergency department.

Sometimes a student or child might start to vomit before the medication is due. In this situation the parents should be contacted immediately and seek medical advice. Carefully monitor the student's/child's level of consciousness, if they become drowsy give an intramuscular hydrocortisone and call an ambulance.

It is important that you meet with the school or nursery staff before each new term starts and give the school/nursery a good supply of the tablets needed, allowing extra to be given for emergencies. Most schools or nursery staff will help with administering tablets and many pupils use a watch alarm to remind them to go to the office to take their tablets. Although they may feel singled out, if this practice starts at a very young age, it soon becomes routine and many children take medication for different reasons throughout the day at school. It is important that tablets are taken and taken on time.

There have been some campaigns where parents are urged not to send sick children to school or nursery due to the risk that is put on children who have adrenal insufficiency. Unfortunately, the most contagious stage is often before symptoms appear and there is just as much risk in picking up these viruses from other family members, or when out and about.

CHAPTER 31

Other Treatments for Congenital Adrenal Hyperplasia—Prednisolone, Dexamethasone and Adrenalectomy

GLOSSARY

Adrenalectomy Surgical removal of the adrenal glands.

Dexamethasone Synthetic glucocorticoid made by modifying prednisolone by adding in a fluorine atom.

Duration of action The time over which a drug or hormone produces a biological effect (i.e. the inflammatory effects of hydrocortisone last for approximately 8–12 hours, which is longer than the drug is in the system).

Enteric coated A special coating applied to a tablet to prevent the tablet being broken down by stomach acid.

Glucocorticoids Group of steroid hormones (glucose + cortex + steroid) which regulate glucose metabolism and suppress inflammation.

Half-life The time taken for the level of a drug or hormone in the blood, to fall by half the value.

Hydrocortisone Synthetic form of cortisol.

Prednisolone Synthetic glucocorticoid made by modifying cortisol with a double carbon bond.

GENERAL

Prednisolone and dexamethasone were developed not as glucocorticoid replacement therapies, but for their anti-inflammatory and immune suppressive actions. This is important because the biological effect which is anti-inflammatory lasts approximately 36–54 hours for dexamethasone, so for anti-inflammatory effects, dexamethasone only needs to be given once per day. This is what they are licenced for and not for adrenal replacement therapy. Giving these medications more frequently for replacement therapy will lead to short and long term side effects. Dexamethasone was a derivative of 9-alpha fludrocortisone and the potency of both of these steroids comes from the introduction of the fluorine atom. Prednisolone very closely resembles dexamethasone structurally, but lacks the fluorine (Fig. 31.1).

Congenital Adrenal Hyperplasia. http://dx.doi.org/10.1016/B978-0-12-811483-4.00031-3

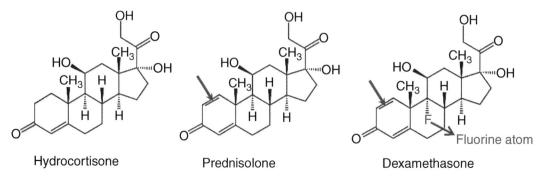

Hydrocortisone   Prednisolone   Dexamethasone

Figure 31.1 *The chemical structures of hydrocortisone, prednisolone and dexamethasone.* Prednisolone differs from hydrocortisone by the presence of a double carbon bond (red arrow) and dexamethasone differs from prednisolone by the introduction of a fluorine atom (red F).

Prednisolone and dexamethasone have different properties in terms of duration of action and growth suppressing effects compared to hydrocortisone (Fig. 31.2).

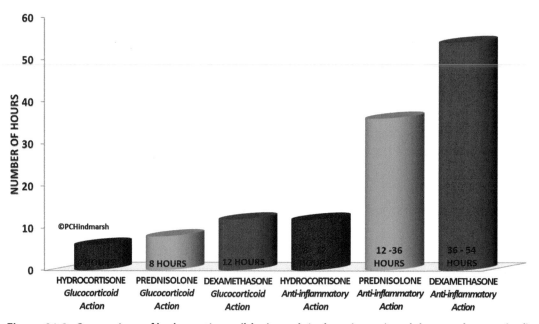

Figure 31.2 *Comparison of hydrocortisone (blue), prednisolone (green) and dexamethasone (red) in terms of glucocorticoid and anti-inflammatory action.*

PREDNISONE AND PREDNISOLONE

Prednisone is derived from altering cortisol (Fig. 31.1). Prednisone is a synthetic glucocorticoid that is used for its anti-inflammatory properties and its duration of action as an anti-inflammatory agent is 12–36 hours. Prednisone is metabolised to its active form prednisolone in the liver (Fig. 31.3) and the relationship between the biological effects of cortisol and prednisolone is shown in Fig. 31.4.

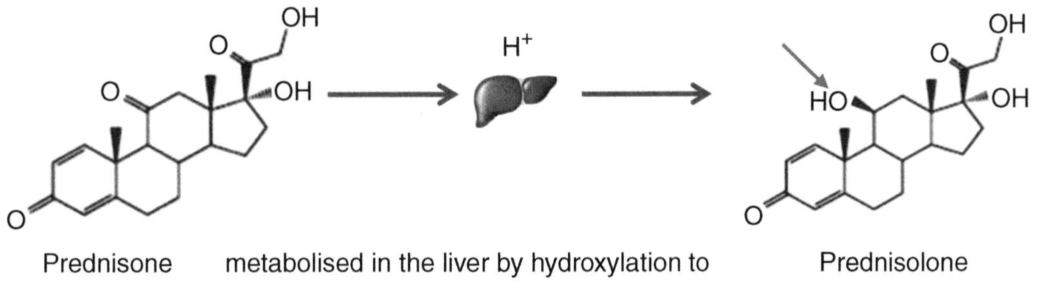

Prednisone   metabolised in the liver by hydroxylation to   Prednisolone

Figure 31.3 *Prednisone is the precursor of prednisolone and is converted in the liver to prednisolone.*

Prednisone acts like hydrocortisone and will suppress ACTH production and endogenous glucocorticoids. Prednisone has a slight mineralocorticoid activity, retaining sodium and water in the kidney which can lead to hypertension. Prednisone can stimulate secretion of acid in the stomach and it also has a direct effect on the lining of the stomach. This can lead to the development of stomach ulcers which leads to stomach pain, especially associated with food intake and on rare occasions bleeding from the ulcer site.

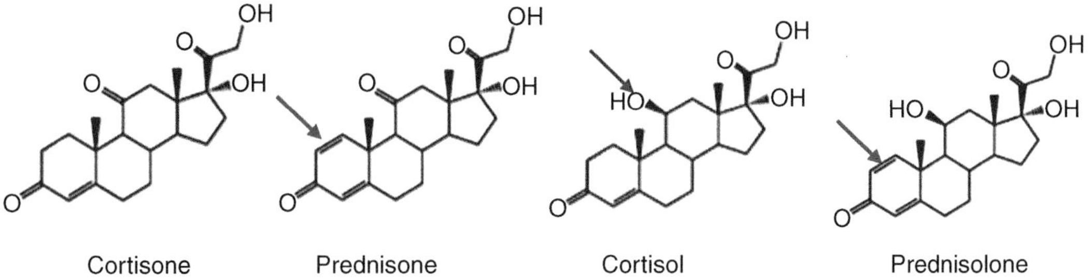

Cortisone   Prednisone   Cortisol   Prednisolone

Figure 31.4 *Similarities and differences between cortisone, cortisol and prednisone and prednisolone. Cortisone was altered by adding a carbon double bond (red arrow) in the A ring to form prednisone. Cortisone has a hydrogen atom attached to form cortisol (blue arrow) cortisol was altered to form prednisolone by adding a carbon double bond (red arrow).*

The pharmacology profile of prednisolone is shown in Fig. 31.5. Prednisolone is readily absorbed by the gastrointestinal tract in its metabolically active form and the peak plasma concentration is reached some 1–2 hours after oral administration. It has a half-life in the blood of 180 minutes and the duration of action is longer than hydrocortisone. The initial absorption of prednisolone, but not its overall bioavailability, is affected by food. Prednisolone cannot be measured accurately in the blood because there are no routine assays available. It will cross react in the cortisol assay. When prednisolone was measured, the blood profile is as shown in Fig. 31.6. Prednisolone is bound to plasma proteins, although less so than hydrocortisone.

Prednisolone will last in the blood for about 8 hours which means it has to be given at least 3 times per day.

To avoid some of the stomach side effects, there is an enteric-coated preparation available which means that prednisolone is not released until the tablet gets into the small bowel. The profile differs however (Fig. 31.6), with a delayed peak 5 hours after ingestion and a lower overall peak value. Due to this delay it is not recommended as a form of cortisol replacement.

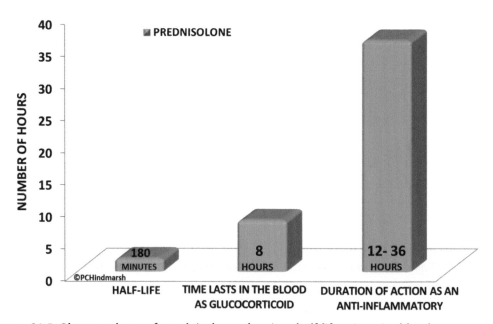

Figure 31.5 *Pharmacology of prednisolone showing half-life, time in blood stream as a glucocorticoid and duration of action as an anti-inflammatory glucocorticoid.*

The potency of prednisolone is much greater in terms of growth suppression. This limits its use in paediatric practice and it has proven very difficult to use prednisolone in a way that does not inhibit growth. In addition, prednisolone appears to be associated with significant alterations in mood, particularly depression, in about 5% of those that take it. Osteoporosis is also more common in patients who take prednisolone, as it blocks the stimulation of the cells that buildup bone in the skeleton in response to vitamin D. Calcium and vitamin D supplements are advised when prednisolone is used long term. Prednisolone is more likely to produce side effects of weight gain, fat gain and diabetes than hydrocortisone. As it is so potent, the adrenal glands in normal individuals will shut down very quickly when the daily dose exceeded 7.5–10 mg per day for anything more than 14 days and recovery can be slow especially when repeated doses are used.

Although prednisolone is usually prescribed to be taken twice daily when used in replacement therapy for CAH, unless you have a slow clearance rate, dosing twice a day would most certainly lead to periods of under replacement and in fact periods of glucocorticoid deficiency. It would be more suited to a three times per day dosing schedule. Prednisolone, like prednisone, has slight mineralocorticoid activity. As with hydrocortisone tablets, prednisolone tablets have a number of fillers: lactose, maize starch, stearic acid, purified talc and magnesium stearate.

Prednisolone formulations

Prednisolone comes in different formulations. An enteric coated version is available, which means that the special coating prevents break down in the stomach and reduces the chances of the drug irritating the stomach lining and causing gastritis. This alters the way that the prednisolone gets into the blood stream as is shown in Fig. 31.6.

DEXAMETHASONE

Dexamethasone has received some popularity recently because it could be given as a once a day drug, although it should be taken twice a day when used for the replacement of cortisol. The main problem with dexamethasone is that in the current way it is made, it has an extremely flat profile. This means whilst it could easily be titrated to match the troughs of the circadian rhythm, at other times of the day the individual is under treated. Equally, if one tried to match the peaks then there would be times of the day when over treatment would result. The features of dexamethasone are shown in Fig. 31.7.

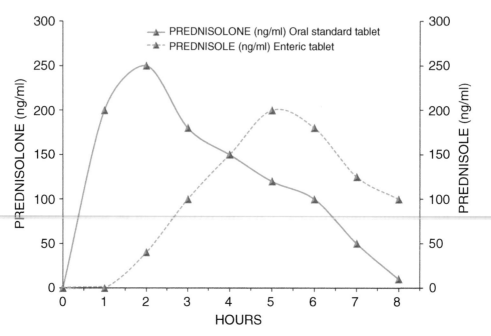

Figure 31.6 *Effect of enteric coating of prednisolone on the appearance in the blood stream. Note the delay in achieving a peak concentration. (Data taken with permission from Adair et al., 1992. Br. J. Clin. Pharm. 33, 495–499).*

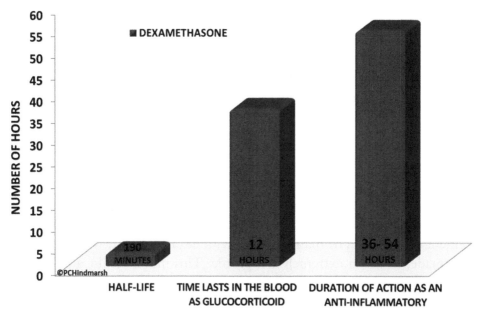

Figure 31.7 *Pharmacology of dexamethasone showing half-life, time in blood stream as a glucocorticoid and duration of action as an anti-inflammatory glucocorticoid.*

There is a liquid preparation of dexamethasone available in the United States that seemed to work in children, but has been associated with increased weight gain in many individuals. Until further studies are forthcoming dexamethasone is not used as the first line of treatment in CAH. The liquid preparation, like the tablet, would still need to be given twice daily to ensure good glucocorticoid cover.

Dexamethasone, like prednisolone, has marked effects on growth. One milligram of dexamethasone is equivalent to 80 mg of hydrocortisone in terms of growth suppression! So if you were replacing 10 mg of hydrocortisone with dexamethasone, the equivalent dose would need to be 0.125 mg. For prednisolone in comparison, the equivalence factor is 4 (2.5 mg prednisolone equates to 10 mg hydrocortisone). Dexamethasone is readily absorbed after oral administration achieving a steady level in the blood after 1 hour. Binding to plasma proteins is less than for hydrocortisone and prednisolone. The biological half-life of dexamethasone is approximately 190 minutes which is almost twice as long as hydrocortisone. The duration of action is even longer, lasting approximately 36–54 hours, so there is the potential for overlapping effects on a twice daily dosing schedule hence the high incidence of side effects with dexamethasone. Elimination occurs via liver metabolism and renal excretion and it is not altered by the enzyme 11-hydroxysteroid dehydrogenase type 2, unlike hydrocortisone. The bioavailability is 90% similar to prednisolone and hydrocortisone.

CONTRA-INDICATIONS AND DRUG INTERACTIONS OF PREDNISOLONE AND DEXAMETHASONE

The contraindications and drug interactions for prednisolone and dexamethasone are similar to those for hydrocortisone (Chapter 20). Birth control pills alter prednisolone metabolism.

ADRENALECTOMY

Adrenalectomy has been suggested as a method to remove uncontrolled androgen production. This procedure entails the surgical removal of both adrenal glands. The rationale for adrenalectomy is that it removes the source of adrenal androgen and means that less glucocorticoid is required for replacement. The latter could be a factor in situations where there is weight gain. It is said the glucocorticoid replacement required for Addison's Disease is less than that needed for CAH, hence less would be needed if the adrenal glands are removed. Actually, this is not correct as once cortisol replacement is titrated to the individual's needs, then the dose would be similar because the androgen production normalises. Adrenalectomy has been helpful in some cases of infertility associated with high androgen production and for correcting the high blood pressure associated with 11–hydroxylase deficiency (see Chapter 4). It would have been interesting in these cases to study the cortisol replacement before adrenalectomy.

There are a number of additional problems that ensue following adrenalectomy.

General outcomes have been poor with a high risk of adrenal crises reported. Adrenaline production is lost so the individual is more at risk of hypoglycaemia as they have lost this important blood glucose raising hormone. Not only does the loss of adrenaline occur if cortisol is not replaced optimally, ACTH will increase and in turn drive androgen production from any adrenal rests, which can occur in the gonads, so that all the symptoms of excess adrenal androgens will reoccur. This increase in ACTH requires optimal cortisol replacement and distribution to be undertaken, otherwise the high ACTH level will lead to hyperpigmentation along with all the symptoms which occur with an increase in androgens.

It is commonly suggested that the reason for 'difficult to control CAH' is poor compliance. What we do not know in these cases, is if the cortisol replacement was closely examined and measured, with consideration paid to the individual clearance and the distribution of cortisol derived from their dosing schedule.

Cortisol, as well as 17OHP, ACTH and androgen levels, should be measured using 24 hour profiles before undertaking the removal of both adrenal glands. If cortisol replacement is not correct before adrenalectomy, then it is unlikely to improve following the procedure. This seems to be the outcome reported in the literature. We have cases, where with pump therapy, a total daily dose of 80 mg of hydrocortisone was initially needed to shrink the adrenal glands and then the dose was slowly titrated down, as the adrenal glands shrank, to 26 mg per day. A similar situation has been observed with oral therapy.

CONCLUSIONS

Prednisolone and dexamethasone look on face value as good ways to replace cortisol, but they were not designed for cortisol replacement. They are designed as anti-inflammatories and immunosuppressants. They cannot be measured easily in the blood and should not be used as first line cortisol replacement therapy. Adrenalectomy should be the last resort in treating androgen excess, optimal cortisol distribution should be carefully considered by a 24 hour profile, medication adjusted accordingly with further profiling reducing the dose at appropriate intervals as the adrenal glands shrink, prior to any surgery being performed.

FURTHER READING

Loew, D., Schuster, O., Graul, E., 1986. Dose-dependent pharmacokinetics of dexamethasone. Eur. J. Clin. Pharmacol. 30, 225–230.

Pickup, M.E., 1979. Clinical pharmacokinetics of prednisone and prednisolone. Clin. Pharmacokinet. 4, 111–128.

Van Wyk, J.J., Ritzen, E.M., 2003. The role of bilateral adrenalectomy in the treatment of congenital adrenal hyperplasia. J. Clin. Endocrinol. Metab. 88, 2993–2998.

CHAPTER 32

Fludrocortisone
9 Alpha-Fludrocortisone

GLOSSARY

Fludrocortisone Cortisol modified with fluorine atom which prolongs action on the mineralocorticoid receptor which retains salt and water.

Glucocorticoids Group of steroid hormones (glucose + cortex + steroid) which regulate glucose metabolism and suppress inflammation.

Haematocrit An indirect measure of the circulating blood volume (a ratio of total red blood cell volume and the total blood volume. As total red blood cell volume does not change much haematocrit reflects changes in total blood volume). When high this implies dehydration, when low water overload.

Hyponatraemia A low sodium level (less than 130 mmol/l).

Mineralocorticoid Hormones which regulate the balance of electrolytes such as sodium and potassium. A member of the steroid family which increases sodium uptake from the kidney and large bowel.

Prednisolone Synthetic glucocorticoid made by modifying cortisol with a double carbon bond.

Renin Protein made by the kidney that instructs the liver to make angiotensin which in turn is involved in making aldosterone (salt retaining hormone) in the adrenal glands.

WHAT IS FLUDROCORTISONE?

Fludrocortisone is a synthetic corticosteroid based on cortisol. You will remember that when we looked at the structure of dexamethasone it had been modified slightly and a fluorine atom had been introduced. This introduction of a fluorine atom always prolongs the duration of action of a steroid. Fludrocortisone is cortisol with a fluorine atom introduced into the ring structure at position 9. That is why it has the name '9 alpha–fludro' as it describes the fluorine added at position 9 in the alpha orientation. The effect of this is to prolong the action of cortisol so its duration of action begins to look more like that of dexamethasone (Fig. 32.1).

Fludrocortisone is rapidly and completely absorbed after oral administration rather like hydrocortisone. The blood level reaches a peak between 4 and 8 hours. Fludrocortisone

Congenital Adrenal Hyperplasia. http://dx.doi.org/10.1016/B978-0-12-811483-4.00032-5

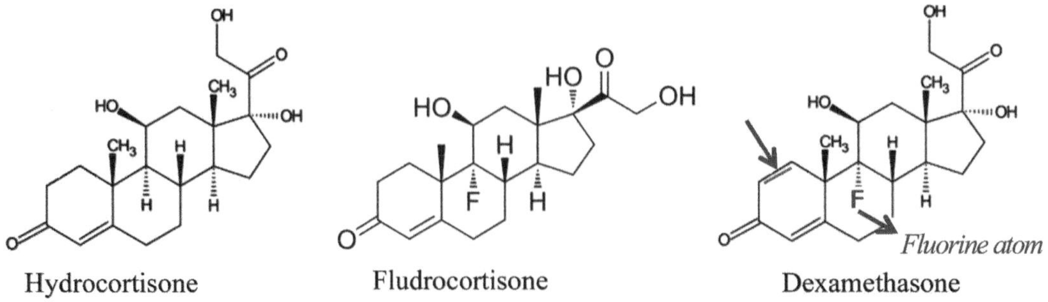

Figure 32.1 *Chemical structures of hydrocortisone on the left, fludrocortisone in the middle and dexamethasone on the right. Note the similar position of the fluorine atom in dexamethasone and fludrocortisone.*

is attached in the blood to various proteins which act as a pool for the drug and evens out the way in which it is distributed throughout the 24 hours.

HOW DOES FLUDROCORTISONE RETAIN SALT WHEN IT IS LIKE CORTISOL?

The change to the duration of action of cortisol not only makes its action longer, but also the introduction of the fluorine means that the modified cortisol is no longer easily broken down by the special enzyme 11β-hydroxysteroid dehydrogenase type 2 (see Chapter 20). 11β-Hydroxysteroid dehydrogenase type 2 has a specific effect of converting cortisol which is the active glucocorticoid to cortisone which is biologically inactive. By introducing the fluorine atom the chemists effectively made fludrocortisone resistant to breakdown by 11β-hydroxysteroid dehydrogenase type 2. The levels of 11β-hydroxysteroid dehydrogenase type 2 are very high around the aldosterone (salt retaining hormone) receptor in the kidney. This prevents cortisol from binding to the aldosterone receptor. Fludrocortisone, however, can bind to the aldosterone receptor and will retain salt. This clever manipulation of the chemical structure of cortisol by the introduction of the fluorine atom, allows for a prolonged duration of action and the opportunity to avoid conversion to cortisone and hence ability to access and bind to the aldosterone receptor in the kidney.

IF FLUDROCORTISONE HAS A PROLONGED CORTISOL LIKE ACTION, CAN IT BE USED INSTEAD OF HYDROCORTISONE?

The short answer to this question is no. The reason is that the profile of dexamethasone, or for that matter fludrocortisone, is rather flat in the blood and does not display the circadian rhythm we want for cortisol. What we don't want are people exposed continually to high concentrations of glucocorticoid because we know they can develop problems with handling sugar, become obese and develop osteoporosis if that is the case.

As a result, it would not be advisable to have fludrocortisone as our sole source of glucocorticoid. We use fludrocortisone for its salt retaining properties, but in our calculations we also have to remember that it will have a dexamethasone like action, so this needs to be factored into the total daily dose of glucocorticoid a person receives.

FLUDROCORTISONE AND SALT BALANCE

Fludrocortisone helps retain sodium in the kidney and also in the large bowel. The amount of sodium that can be retained per day by the kidney and for that matter re-absorbed through the gut, is limited to the total amount of sodium that is taken in. We normally take in about 2 millimoles (mmol) per kilogram body weight of salt per day. If you become salt depleted, then unless you increase the amount of salt in the diet, you will never make up the deficiency because there is only a certain amount of salt fludrocortisone can retain per day, namely the normal daily intake. What some individuals do is to increase the amount of fludrocortisone but as we've said, doing this will not make any difference to the amount of salt which is retained because it is relatively fixed in the diet. What it will do, is have a glucocorticoid effect, so it may actually make things worse as the individual becomes overexposed to glucocorticoids.

So when planning fludrocortisone replacement, it is important that consideration is given to the total daily salt intake and sometimes after a salt losing crisis, salt supplements are required. If you also travel to a very hot country such as near the equator, then it is possible that salt supplementation will be required because of the increased salt loss in sweat.

Current brands of fludrocortisone do not require storage in a fridge unlike their predecessors.

WHAT IS THE DOSE OF FLUDROCORTISONE THAT IS NEEDED?

As with hydrocortisone, the dose of fludrocortisone is worked out initially in terms of the size of the body. However, the amount required varies with age. In the newborn period the dose is 150 $\mu g/m^2$ body surface area/day whereas in childhood it is 100 $\mu g/m^2$ body surface area/day. The reason for this is newborn baby's kidneys are not as responsive to aldosterone as later in childhood. More aldosterone is needed. In addition, in CAH, the increased adrenal androgens that are present at diagnosis have an anti fludrocortisone effect which again means that more fludrocortisone is required. In late adolescence and adulthood, even less may be required, except during the last 10 weeks of pregnancy when an increase in the adult dose is often needed as the high levels of progesterone counteract mineralocorticoid action.

So the usual plan is to start with doses as mentioned earlier. It probably does not matter if the fludrocortisone is given once or twice daily, so most people opt for once per day. Fine tuning of the dose is then required and we consider that now.

HOW DO WE MONITOR FLUDROCORTISONE REPLACEMENT?

Fludrocortisone replacement can be evaluated clinically. Symptoms and signs to look out for include salt cravings and/or light headedness, as well as whether there is any body swelling that might indicate water overload. However, this approach only detects marked under or over replacement, so it is better to use biochemical measures to determine how good the replacement is.

There are several in which we can look at fludrocortisone replacement.

1. Measuring the amount of sodium in the blood. This is quite a useful measure after a salt–wasting crisis, but it does not give us a good overview of the total body sodium. Measuring total body sodium is much more complicated and what we prefer to do is to measure the plasma sodium, coupled with an estimate of the plasma renin activity. You will remember from Chapter 1 (renin–angiotensin system), that renin is produced by the kidney in response to a lowering of sodium in the body. Renin then acts via angiotensin to produce aldosterone from the adrenal glands. In CAH of course, the individual cannot make any aldosterone so what we are doing is replacing it with fludrocortisone. If we have the fludrocortisone correct and by that we mean that it is acting on the kidney to retain sodium, then the plasma renin activity once the body sodium has been restored, will stay within the normal range.

   We do know, however, that not getting the blood sodium correct leads to long term problems. Firstly, the total blood volume will be low and symptoms of this may be headaches or dizziness, particularly when standing up quickly. Secondly, in the long term low sodium levels (less than 135 mmol/l) lead to osteoporosis. In fact, because the salt content of bone is so high, low sodium over long periods of time has a greater effect on osteoporosis than almost any other known factor. Thirdly, sodium is present in many other tissues of the body including cartilage and ligaments. The sodium in cartilage and in the discs of the spine is important as it takes with it, water. This makes the cartilage and discs very strong and capable of resisting huge stress forces when we walk, run and jump. It is not clear what the effect of low sodium does in these situations, but it probably means the bones and joints are less able to stand the wear and tear of normal activity.

In addition to measuring the sodium, we can also measure potassium. These two tend to go in opposite directions if we have not got the fludrocortisone dose right. If the dose is too low, the person will lose sodium in the urine and the blood potassium will rise. High and for that matter low potassium levels, can lead the heart to beat irregularly and if too high, stop beating altogether. If the dose is too high the sodium will be at the upper end of the normal range, but will not go over 145 mmol/l as the body will always compensate by retaining water, which will have the effect of increasing blood pressure. However, a high sodium will be accompanied by a low potassium which as we have said, is not good for the function of the heart.

2. Measuring plasma renin activity can be difficult. We tend to do it in two ways. Initially, in the resting position after lying down for a period of 2–3 hours and then after standing for 2–3 hours. This gives us important information because plasma renin activity tends to increase slightly in the standing position, to cope with the changes in blood volume, resulting from the upright position. In CAH what we are really interested in, is if there is adequate fludrocortisone being taken, to keep both the resting and the standing plasma renin activities within the normal range. If the standing plasma renin activity were higher than the normal range, then this might indicate we are under replacing with fludrocortisone and the blood volume is low. Sometimes patients can tell this because they become rather dizzy when standing up quickly from the sitting position. This is called postural hypotension (low blood pressure on standing upright). You can also pick this up if you measure blood pressure in the lying and standing positions. Normally blood pressure will drop slightly on standing upright but by no more than 10 mmHg.

3. The next way we test whether we have got the fludrocortisone dose correct in the longer term, is to measure blood pressure. As fludrocortisone retains sodium, water will also be retained with it. This increase in the retention of water in the body leads to an increase in blood pressure. As long as the plasma renin activity is within the normal range, then blood pressure will also be within the normal range for height. However, we do like to check on this and to make sure there is no movement into the upper half of the normal range. If that were to happen, this might indicate that in the long term we are giving too

much fludrocortisone. Blood pressure changes with age and size in children, so we use charts like the one shown in Fig. 32.2 to determine how the measured blood pressure relates to the normal standards.

Just as a high blood pressure (hypertension) can be a problem, low blood pressure (hypotension) can indicate that we are under dosing with fludrocortisone. Again, this might manifest itself in the blood pressures we record when you are lying down and then standing up. This probably reflects reduction in the blood volume and would explain why people become dizzy when standing up quickly.

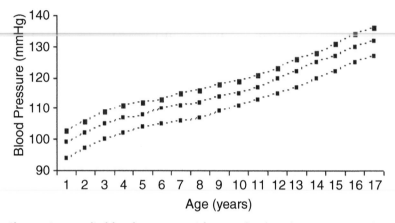

Figure 32.2 *Change in systolic blood pressure with age.* *The three lines represent the average blood pressure (bottom line), the next line shows the levels described for high blood pressure and the blue line is the levels above which the blood pressure is described as hypertension. Centiles constructed from the 4th Paediatric Hypertension Task Force dataset with kind permission.*

4. The final way to assess fludrocortisone replacement is to measure the haematocrit. The haematocrit (a ratio of total red blood cell volume and the total blood volume. As total red blood cell volume does not change much haematocrit reflects changes in total blood volume), gives a guide to how the circulating blood volume is maintained. If the haematocrit is raised, this suggests that the circulating blood volume is reduced and in CAH often means more fludrocortisone is needed. Haematocrit is really useful for fine tuning as it can show changes before they manifest in terms of blood pressure or plasma renin activity.

Another way we can check on the blood volume is to measure the urea level in the blood. Urea levels which are low, may reflect too much water in the circulation, whereas a high urea level might imply dehydration or a low blood volume. Unfortunately, urea is also influenced by other factors such as body nitrogen turnover so it is not as specific as the other measures we have talked about.

SIDE EFFECTS, CONTRAINDICATIONS AND DRUG INTERACTIONS

As fludrocortisone is a derivative of cortisol, the side effects, drug interactions and contraindications are exactly the same as those we have described in the hydrocortisone section. If you would like to review these they are in Chapter 20. The most important difference from hydrocortisone is the effect on blood pressure, which we have talked about earlier.

In addition, there are some specific drugs that need to be considered. Diuretics and drugs that affect blood pressure and electrolytes, might interact with fludrocortisone and may require dose adjustments. Liquorice and grapefruit juice, potentiate the mineralocorticoid effect of hydrocortisone by reducing the conversion of cortisol to cortisone, so may enhance the overall effect of fludrocortisone and should be avoided.

DO I NEED TO DOUBLE DOSE WITH FLUDROCORTISONE WHEN UNWELL

This is a good question. *The answer is NO.*

The reason extra dosing is not needed is that you will only create more problems by doing this. If you take extra fludrocortisone, it will retain slightly more sodium and therefore water, which will expand the blood volume and may even lead to high blood pressure. Although this might be thought of as a good idea, the major problem is that fludrocortisone will retain sodium and lose potassium. Potassium loss leads to low blood potassium levels, which are really dangerous as this leads to heart rate problems and can lead if they get too low, to the heart stopping working.

The right treatment if unwell, is to double the hydrocortisone dose and also ensure a good intake of fluids such as sports drinks which contain extra sodium and glucose. If you have an adrenal crisis and the sodium is low, then intravenous fluids are the way to rectify the problem, as the total body sodium will have fallen and no matter how much fludrocortisone is given, it will not raise the sodium. The only way to do that is to give more sodium in the fluids.

Summary

1. Fludrocortisone is a very powerful steroid which has both mineralocorticoid (salt retaining) (Fig. 32.3) and glucocorticoid properties. Due to its potency it is used and measured in micrograms.

2. Fludrocortisone is used to replace the missing hormone aldosterone which plays a vital role in maintaining the correct balance of electrolytes. Aldosterone causes the cells in the body to retain sodium (salt) and in turn this keeps the potassium levels correct. The sodium in turn retains water which is important for good blood circulation.

3. Hyponatremia is a condition which occurs if the sodium levels are too low (less than 130 mmol/l) and if this happens the potassium levels will rise. Hyponatraemia occurs when someone has vomiting and diarrhoea, or omits the fludrocortisone medication. Hyponatremia is serious and needs treatment as it can lead to seizures, low blood pressure, coma and death. A high potassium level is known as hyperkalemia and is often associated with hyponatraemia. This can cause the heart to beat irregularly which is known as an arrhythmia. This can cause the heart to stop and cause sudden death.

4. Fludrocortisone retains sodium, but for it to work properly you have to have adequate amounts of salt.

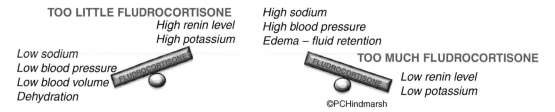

Figure 32.3 *The fludrocortisone seesaw. Too little or too much fludrocortisone leads to problems with blood volume and blood pressure. Careful measurement of blood pressure and plasma renin activity are required to get replacement correct.*

CONCLUSIONS

Fludrocortisone is a synthetic modification of cortisol which allows it to retain sodium. Careful dosing is required as the dose does change with age. The aim of therapy is to maintain a normal plasma renin activity and blood pressure, at the same time ensuring under treatment does not lead to troubling effects such as headaches and dizzy spells.

FURTHER READING

Sterns, R.H., 2015. Disorders of plasma sodium—causes, consequences, and correction. N. Engl. J. Med. 372, 55–65.

Upala, S., Sanguankeo, A., 2016. Association between hyponatremia, osteoporosis and fracture: a systematic review and meta-analysis. J. Clin. Endocrinol. Metab. 101, 1880–1886.

CHAPTER 33

Travel and Time Zones

GLOSSARY

Clock changes or daylight saving As the clocks are adjusted at 01:00 (1 a.m.), take your evening dose at the usual time. Adjust the clock time according to the season either back or forward before you go to bed and then take your morning dose at the usual time which will accommodate the adjustment in time.

Dioralyte Oral rehydration solution that has the right balance of salts for treating dehydration due to vomiting and diarrhoea.

Fludrocortisone Cortisol modified with fluorine atom which prolongs action on the mineralocorticoid receptor which retains salt and water.

Medic alert Essential identifier of condition. Needs to be engraved with term 'adrenal insufficiency' as this is the only item that ambulance crews will search the person for and the words will trigger their emergency pathway.

More@4 During periods of illness a double dose equal to the usual morning dose, to be taken at 4 a.m. (04:00), followed by normal double morning dose to be taken at the usual time. This additional dose is taken to prevent hypoglycaemia occurring in the early hours of the morning.

GENERAL

Holidays abroad should be great fun. Generally, all goes well and with some forward planning most situations can be dealt with. This chapter suggests some ways to plan ahead and what to do should problems occur. It all depends of course, on your destination, so it is always a good idea to discuss your plans with your consultant at an early stage.

You might also need advice on additional vaccinations or tablets. You can usually get this from your GP. Some surgeries run a specialised 'Travel Clinic'.

THINGS TO REMEMBER WHEN YOU TRAVEL

- You/your child should wear your or his/her medic alert bracelet or equivalent at all times.

Congenital Adrenal Hyperplasia. http://dx.doi.org/10.1016/B978-0-12-811483-4.00033-7
431

- Ensure you have a copy of your/your child's emergency letter and it is always a good idea to get it translated into the local language.
- Take your/your child's steroid or treatment card with you and make sure it is up to date.
- Carry your/your child's supply of tablets and hydrocortisone for emergency use (make sure it is in date) in your hand luggage. It is always a good idea to get a customs letter from your consultant to explain this and the fact that you are carrying other medications.
- Ensure you have enough supplies of everything for the length of your holiday. Then double the amount, as getting medicines abroad can sometimes be difficult and the formulations are not always the same.
- For travel to the United States make sure that all your/your child's medications are carried in the packaging that was issued by your pharmacist. They need to show the name of the drug and that they were dispensed by the pharmacist. Most pharmacies place their label on the drug package which is all that is needed. Do not carry loose medications.
- Ensure you have your/your child's hospital contact number in your phone.

FLUDROCORTISONE

For patients who take fludrocortisone, it is perfectly safe to keep fludrocortisone tablets out of a fridge for a 2 week holiday, as only your backup supply needs to be kept cool. Taking them in and out of the fridge for short periods will do no harm; however, current brands of fludrocortisone do not require storage in a fridge unlike their predecessors. If you are going to a really hot country where the temperature will be above 35°C, it is a good idea to take extra salt with you or make sure that snacks are savoury foods such as crisps.

IMPORTANT INFORMATION

If you are flying, all medication needs to be carried in your hand luggage for accessibility during the flight. If it goes in the baggage in the hold and the baggage goes on its own holiday, you could be left short! Also the hold on an aircraft gets very cold, so the intense cold might alter how the medication works.

You will need a letter from your endocrinologist to enable you to carry your emergency kit through customs (Fig. 33.1). The letter should give flight details and which medications you are carrying.

To whom it may concern

Name of patient:

Date of Birth:

Medical Condition: Congenital Adrenal Hyperplasia (*Adrenal Insufficiency*)

Hospital Number:

_____ has the above medical condition and receives treatment with hydrocortisone and fludrocortisone. This is lifesaving medication as are the emergency injections of hydrocortisone that he/she carries (his/her parents carry for him/her).   He/She needs to have this medication with them in the cabin of the plane and not in the luggage in the hold to avoid freeze damage to the medications.

_____ will also need to carry syringes and needles for emergency intramuscular injection.

They will be flying to _____ (flight details).

I trust this letter will facilitate his/her safe passage through customs. Should there be any problems please contact _____ on the telephone number _____.

Figure 33.1 *Example of a letter for customs.*

DEALING WITH DIARRHOEA

Diarrhoea is the major problem because of the fluid loss. This is the same whether the child has CAH or not. If it is associated with vomiting, then you are best to get medical help quickly as you cannot be sure that any of the medication has either stayed down or been absorbed.

Key points are as follows:

- Diarrhoea is a particular problem due to the fluid losses.
- Oral rehydration solutions such as Dioralyte should be used.
- Make sure your child is passing urine regularly.
- Seek medical advice early especially:
  - If there is a fever.
  - Blood in the diarrhoea.
  - Your child becomes confused.

- The diarrhoea does not stop after 24 hours.
- There is associated vomiting.
- Do not use antidiarrhoeal drugs.

In some countries it is wise to use only bottled water for drinking, even when cleaning teeth and avoid ice in drinks.

ON HOLIDAY

Most people do not get ill on holiday or become involved in accidents; however, in the event those problems arise, then these problems need to be dealt with in the same way as they would be at home (see Chapter 29).

However, always remember:

- If you think that your child is ill, double or treble the hydrocortisone dose.
- If there is associated vomiting intramuscular hydrocortisone should be administered.
- If you have used the intramuscular injection of hydrocortisone, take your child to the nearest Accident and Emergency department as soon as possible and tell the doctors of the condition and that emergency hydrocortisone has already been given.
- The doctors need to check, with blood tests, for salt balance and blood glucose, so don't leave until this has been done.
- In any situation of doubt insist that your child is admitted for glucose, electrolyte and blood pressure monitoring.
- Give an additional double dose of hydrocortisone at 4 a.m. (04:00). This *extra* dose should be equal to double the usual morning dose, which must also be a double dose and given at the usual time the morning dose is given.

TIME ZONES

Increasing air travel means that many patients receiving hydrocortisone treatment have to face changes to their dosing schedule.

For travel within Europe this is not a problem, but longer journey times may need some adjustment to the timings of doses (Fig. 33.2).

No change to fludrocortisone is required as it is taken on a once a day basis and this should be continued. For those travelling to hot climates, an increase in salt intake may be required.

AFRICA   (Including South Africa)

Journey to and from Africa

No change required as within a 1–3 hour time shift.

EUROPE

Journey to and from Europe

No change required as within a 1–3 hour time shift.

FAR EAST, AUSTRALIA OR NEW ZEALAND

Journey to and from Far East, Australia or New Zealand

No significant changes as dose schedule is already 8 hourly.

Simply take tablets as normal until arrival, then switch to local time and dose as normal at usual times.

MIDDLE EAST OR INDIA

*Journey **to** Middle East or India*

> ➢ Evening dose as usual.
> ➢ Half morning dose on arrival.
> ➢ Normal dose schedule from the morning of arrival day.

*Journey **from** Middle East or India*

> ➢ Repeat evening dose on boarding plane.
> ➢ Usual morning dose on arrival in United Kingdom
> ➢ Second dose late afternoon.
> ➢ Normal evening dose.
> ➢ Normal dose schedule the following day.

UNITED STATES OF AMERICA

*Journey **to** USA*

> ➢ Morning dose as usual.

> ➢ Half morning dose on arrival.

> ➢ Evening dose before going to bed.

> ➢ Normal dose schedule the following day.

*Journey **from** USA*

> ➢ Evening dose as usual.

> ➢ Normal dose schedule the following day.

Figure 33.2 *Dosing times for different time zone travel.*

HYDROCORTISONE MEDICATION CHANGES DURING TRAVEL

Clock changes or daylight saving

Many countries have set times in the year when clocks are put forward or back by an hour to extend the periods of daylight during winter mornings. The exact dates chosen for these changes vary between countries. The evening dose should always be taken as late as possible, but as hydrocortisone lasts approximately 6 hours, the following adjustment should be implemented:

Clocks forward:

When the clocks go forward you lose an hour.

By example, if you take a tablet at midnight and your next dose is at 06:00, when the clocks change, the 06:00 will become 07:00. To overcome this, adjust your clocks before you go to bed and take your tablet at midnight as usual and then at the clock adjusted time of 06:00.

Clocks back:

When the clocks go back, you gain an hour.

By example, if you take a tablet at midnight and the next dose at 06:00, when the clocks change, 06:00 will become 05:00. To overcome this, adjust your clocks before you go to bed and take your tablet at midnight as usual and then at the clock adjusted time of 06:00.

For the other doses during the day no changes to the timing of the doses are required.

CHAPTER 34

Thinking Through Blood Results–A Quiz

GLOSSARY

Hydrocortisone Synthetic form of cortisol.

Over stacking The phenomenon which happens if the timing of doses is incorrect. Occurs where the dose is taken to too early and builds onto the cortisol remaining from the previous dose, leading to higher cortisol levels than would have been expected from the dose given.

Stacking The addition of a dose upon another dose within a certain time frame, usually the time the drug is in the circulation.

Useful stacking Cortisol is added when cortisol drops to a desired level, which not only prevents levels dropping too low but also allows a smaller amount to be added to give the optimal peak.

GENERAL

As we have gone through this book we have looked at how to replace cortisol with hydrocortisone. In Section Two, we looked at things that can go wrong in CAH and in Section Three, what we are trying to do with our treatment to prevent potential problems from occurring.

We saw in Section Two, that we have many options to try and put right the problems that arise. However, this is often a bit too late in the day and it is better not to let things get into a sorry state in the first instance.

Central to this, has been the observation that the hormone that is missing in CAH is cortisol and we are replacing what is missing with cortisol in the form of hydrocortisone, so what we should measure to know where we are, is cortisol. We have demonstrated that if the cortisol replacement is optimal and by that we mean it mimics the circadian rhythm, then all the other components such as 17-hydroxyprogesterone (17OHP) and androstenedione will fall into line.

It is important that we concentrate on cortisol replacement, because all the problems that crop up in Section Two and all the side effects that we looked at in Section Three, arise purely and simply from either over or under exposure to hydrocortisone. In other words, they are the symptoms and signs of cortisol excess or deficiency.

In this chapter, we are going to review what information we get from blood tests and the decisions these results help us make. We are going to do this as a piece of revision and along the way there will be a few questions for you to think about!

SINGLE BLOOD TESTS AND BLOOD SPOTS FOR 17-HYDROXYPROGESTERONE

Now firstly, imagine that you are in a clinic and that you have had a blood test, or perhaps it was a blood spot measurement for 17OHP. Here it is plotted for you in Fig. 34.1 and the result is from a sample taken at 09:00.

What questions or further information might you need to interpret this value? Jot down your thoughts and then have a look at Fig. 34.1 on what we think might be needed.

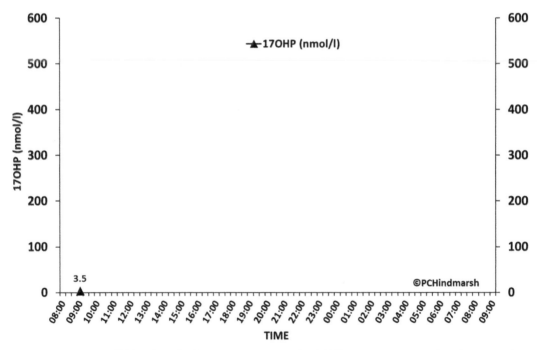

Figure 34.1 *One-off blood 17-hydroxyprogesterone (17OHP) measurement taken in outpatient clinic.*

If your response to the question was "Well, I am a bit stuck as not sure what it is telling me but it looks good," then you are partly in agreement with us! We are struggling too!

The value at 3.5 nmol/l is within the normal range. However we do not know:

- How it relates to the hydrocortisone treatment schedule. Was the blood sample taken before or after the morning dose? If before, that might mean the evening dosing is too much. If it is just after the morning dose, then yes the dose is right but the 17OHP might come down even lower, in which case the morning dose may be too much.
- Could the 17OHP have been high overnight and just come down because the morning dose was taken earlier and has kicked in?
- What will happen next? In other words what is the rest of the day like? Do we need information during the rest of the day to tell us what we should be doing? For example, if we are going to alter the morning dose surely we want to know what the knock on effect would be during the morning! Might the patient end up cortisol deficient and symptomatic late morning?

Well alright, what if we put in another measurement that people often use to assess the adequacy of cortisol replacement, namely, androstenedione. Here it is in Fig. 34.2.

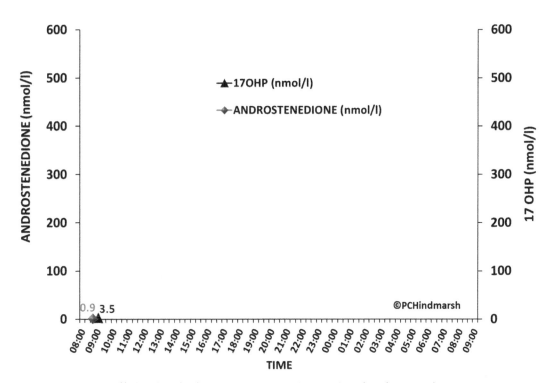

Figure 34.2 *One-off blood 17-hydroxyprogesterone (17OHP) and androstenedione measurements taken at 09:00 before clinic.*

When assessing CAH, 17OHP and androstenedione are the usual measurements which are used to assess 'control' in most centres worldwide.

Adding in ACTH does not help that much more, as we can see in Fig. 34.3, where we now have a single measurement of 17OHP level, androstenedione and ACTH.

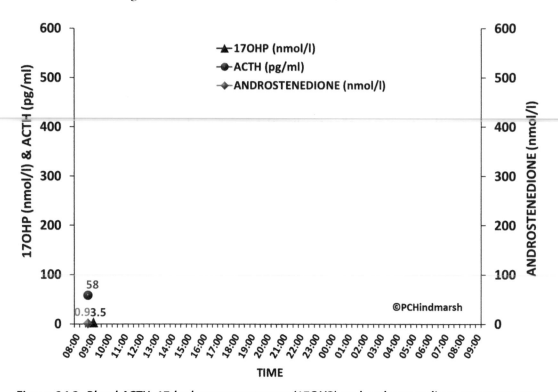

Figure 34.3 *Blood ACTH, 17-hydroxyprogesterone (17OHP) and androstenedione measurements taken at 09:00 before clinic.*

Excellent 'control' is suggested, but there is no indication of what time the morning tablet was taken, or how much cortisol there is in the blood.

Would pre dose 17OHP blood spots taken over the 24 hour period give us more of an idea, as we would know what time doses were taken? The results are plotted in Fig. 34.4. Again, good replacement with hydrocortisone might be the conclusion, although some may feel that the 09:00 17OHP level of 3.5 nmol/l could be a bit low so may suggest a decrease in the evening dose.

So, what if we were able to do home cortisol blood spots (which is not possible), in addition to the 17OHP blood spots done before each dose is taken during a 24 hour period. The results are shown in Fig. 34.4? If we had the cortisol as well, what would they show us? Look at Fig. 34.5.

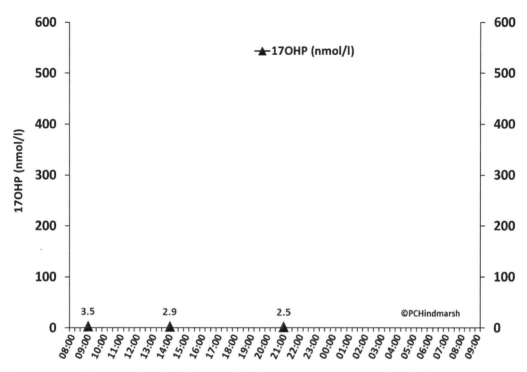

Figure 34.4 *A bit more detail with extra blood spot measurements of 17-hydroxyprogesterone (17OHP) taken pre dose.*

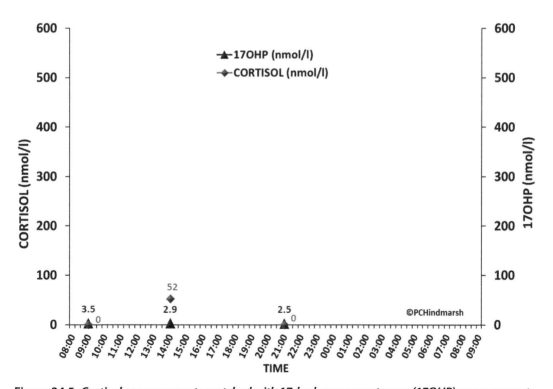

Figure 34.5 *Cortisol measurements matched with 17-hydroxyprogesterone (17OHP) measurements.*

Well, looking at the data in Fig. 34.5, there is no cortisol in the morning (09:00), we can expect that because we know that hydrocortisone would not last, if the previous dose had been taken the night before. It is still tempting to reduce the evening dose of hydrocortisone as the 17OHP is low (3.5 nmol/l).

The pre lunchtime dose results (14:00) appear really good. The 17OHP (2.9 nmol/l) is low but the cortisol is really low (52 nmol/l), however, the next dose is due. When we come to the evening dose, the 17OHP is still good (2.5 nmol/l) but there is no cortisol to be measured. This could mean that we need to increase the dose at 14:00.

So that is as far as we can get. Now the patient is seen in the clinic and the following observations are made:

BMI kg/m²	HYDROCORTISONE mg/m²/day	FLUDROCORTISONE µg/m²/day)	PLASMA RENIN ACTIVITY (nmol/l)
38.8	19.9	124.1	3.74

That Body Mass Index (BMI) is very high. Goodness, what is this patient eating – you are what you eat!

Growth is doing well, highish hydrocortisone dose, but because this is a 'large' person, they need it and they probably have a fast clearance (Fig. 34.6).

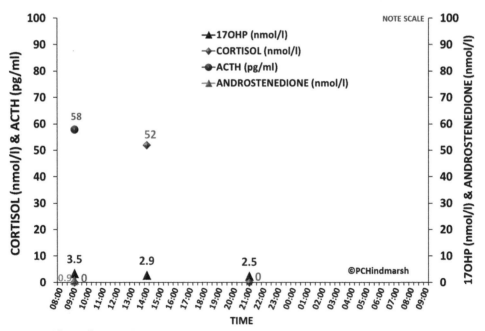

Figure 34.6 *Altogether now!*

Considering all the data that could be collected by blood spots, one-off blood sample and the measurement of the cortisol at the same time, where have we got to? Not many patients have cortisol measured as the focus has been on 17OHP. But we are not replacing 17OHP, we are replacing cortisol!

So in effect, what is really being looked at to judge the overall replacement is the 17OHP as this is usually the only level that is measured, especially with 17OHP blood spots, which are done at home. Even when we look at 17OHP over a 24 hour period, we are not much the wiser in respect of what to do with our hydrocortisone dosing (Fig. 34.7).

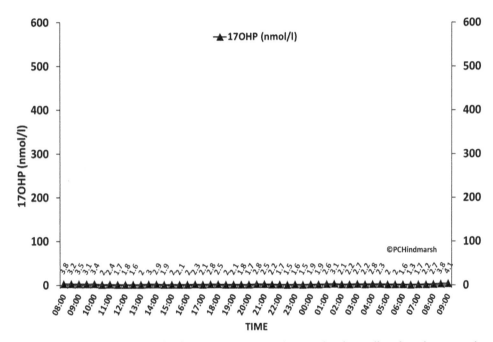

Figure 34.7 *Job done! Blood 17-hydroxyprogesterone (17OHP) values all within the normal range so all must be well.*

What we also know is that this patient has a slightly fast cortisol clearance. The fasting glucose is normal, but there is a lot of insulin produced to keep it normal and the leptin is high, indicating a high fat mass. None of this is good as this suggests we are running into metabolic problems.

HALF-LIFE (minutes)	FASTING GLUCOSE (mmol/L)	INSULIN (Mu/L)	LEPTIN (ng/ml)	CBG (µg/ml)
63.1	3.5	18.2	71.6	42.5

From this data we assume there is good cortisol replacement judged on the 17OHP. However, it appears there is also obesity and metabolic problems which could lead to the development of diabetes.

This all points to cortisol excess so what does the 24 hour cortisol profile look like?

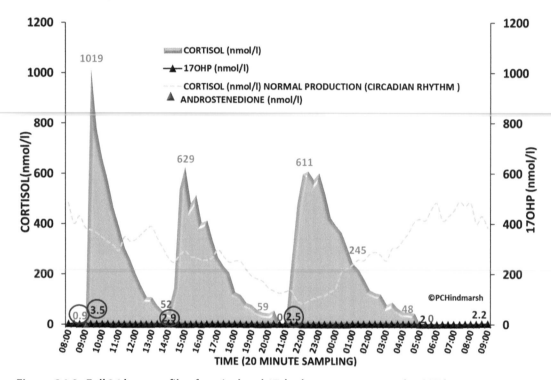

Figure 34.8 *Full 24 hour profile of cortisol and 17-hydroxyprogesterone (17OHP).*

Now in Fig. 34.8 we can see what is going on and where we will have to make changes.

1. The patient has no cortisol in the system from 04:00 until 09:00, yet there is no significant rise in the 17OHP at this time.
2. The morning dose is giving a peak of 1019 nmol/l, with a high peak of 629 nmol/l from the lunchtime dose and the evening dose peaking at 611 nmol/l.

So this patient is obese through *over* dosing with hydrocortisone. Many may not accept this because they are judging the treatment solely on the three 17OHP levels which are circled in red, or the one taken at 09:00, along with the androstenedione level, if measured. None of these could possibly depict the cortisol values.

What this full profile does show, is androstenedione is low and the cortisol exposure very excessive; however, 17OHP production is not completely blunted, which gives us valuable information, as this 17OHP is probably not from the adrenal glands but from the ovaries.

The cortisol levels show us that there is very obvious over treatment when we consider the very high peaks. There are periods of under treatment which are also very obvious as we can see that for 5 hours from 04:00 to 09:00 and an hour from 20:00 to 21:00, where the patient is totally without measurable cortisol, totalling 6 hours of the 24 hours.

These periods of over and under treatment are not obvious when only 17OHP is measured and will lead to both short term and long term side effects. Studies on male patients with CAH, report that a high number of males develop adrenal rests. It has been remarked that some males have developed adrenal rests despite good 'control'. However, this may well be because their cortisol levels have not been assessed over the 24 hours and their cortisol replacement assessed solely on 17OHP and androstenedione levels.

ANOTHER EXAMPLE

Here is another example for you to work through. We will start again with 17OHP blood spots and buildup from there.

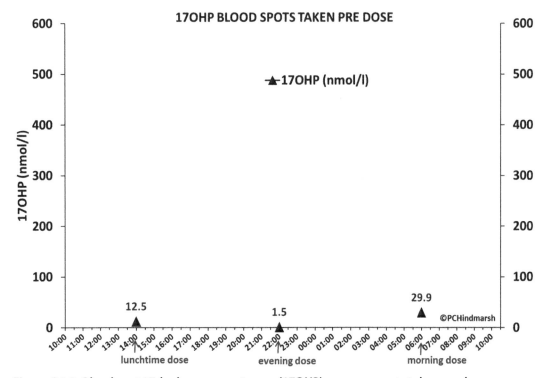

Figure 34.9 *Blood spot 17-hydroxyprogesterone (17OHP) measurements taken pre dose.*

In Fig. 34.9 we can see the information which is most commonly used for assessing cortisol replacement in CAH. There is considerable variation in what doctors think the morning 17OHP pre dose level should be and this can range from 5 to 100 nmol/l. We can be relatively certain that there is no cortisol remaining from the dose taken the previous night, as we know hydrocortisone lasts 6 hours at most.

Looking at the data in Fig. 34.9 the level of 29.9 nmol/l may be deemed acceptable, over treated or under treated. In other words, the adjustment of the evening dose will depend on the centre you are under. As this level is measured pre dose and we know that hydrocortisone only lasts for at most 6 hours, the cortisol level will be either zero or extremely low and will depend on the individual's metabolising of the medication.

Most centres aim to keep the 17OHP, which is measured using modern assays, to below 5 nmol/l in the morning and below 10 nmol/l over the rest of the day. The afternoon pre dose level of 12.5 nmol/l indicates that an increase in the morning dose is needed as the 17OHP is slightly high, in other words, not being 'controlled'.

The pre evening 17OHP level of 1.5 nmol/l is a little on the low side.

So what to do?

Morning dose: considering the lunchtime 17OHP of 12.5 nmol/l is raised, the morning dose is increased to bring this down.

Evening dose: the morning 17OHP level of 29.9 nmol/l is probably fine, we know that there is no cortisol around as it will have run out from the evening dose, so we will leave it.

Lunchtime dose: evening 17OHP level of 1.5 nmol/l is fairly good, so no changes to the afternoon dose.

So what if we were to adjust the doses when looking at all the 17OHP levels over the 24 hours, as remember this is the way almost all centres assess dosing schedules, based solely on the 17OHP levels? In Fig. 34.10 we can see the 17OHP levels over the 24 hours.

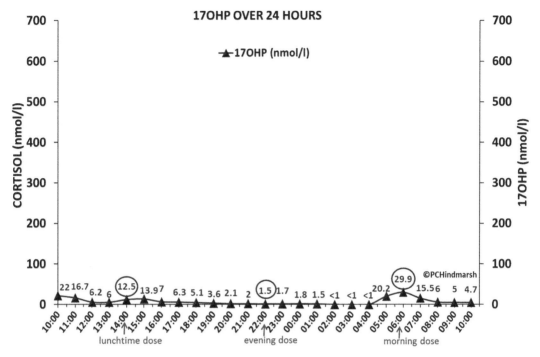

Figure 34.10 *17-Hydroxyprogesterone (17OHP) measured over the 24 hour period.*

What further information does looking at a full 17-hydroxyprogesterone profile over 24 hours give?

Firstly, we can see at the beginning of the profile as the cannula was inserted at 10:00, 17OHP was 22 nmol/l which is significantly higher than at the same time the next day where it measures 4.7 nmol/l. Although 17OHP levels could vary from day to day, this rise is almost 5 times higher and runs true to what we have seen in our patients who use pump therapy, where we know that the cortisol delivery is the same every day. If this was a one-off blood sample in clinic at 10:00, we would see this rise in 17OHP from the blood test and consider changes to the dosing schedule.

Next, we can see that the 14:00 17OHP result is higher than the optimal level for that time of the day and it takes some time for 17OHP to fall to where we want it, so if we increase the morning dose this, in theory should bring down the 17OHP level.

The evening pre dose level is 1.5 nmol/l and although 17OHP is not measurable for several hours, as we are increasing the morning dose, we could slightly decrease the evening dose as the patient does have weight issues. Any increase in 17OHP as a result, would be dampened by the increase in the morning dose, which would lower the slightly elevated pre dose afternoon 17OHP level. So, we will decrease the dose.

If this is the way replacement cortisol dosing is currently assessed in CAH, judged solely using the 17OHP levels, are we right?

Well let's add the cortisol and see if we have it right.

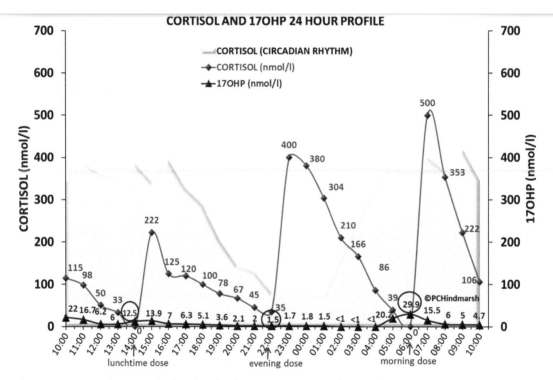

Figure 34.11 *24 hour cortisol and 17-hydroxyprogesterone (17OHP).*

Acting on the 17OHP only (Fig. 34.10), the following changes were made to the dosing schedule. Consider these changes now in the light of what the cortisol levels are during the 24 hour period (Fig. 34.11).

1. The morning dose was increased to bring down the afternoon 17OHP level. (We can see that this may not have been a good idea because the morning cortisol level is already high at 500 nmol/l).

2. The afternoon dose was not altered.
(This is probably correct).

3. The evening dose based on the blood spots (Fig. 34.9), no changes made. (This would have been incorrect as when we look at the cortisol peak, this is too high. This is evident when we look at the 17OHP level as there is no measurable 17OHP from 02:00 to 04:00. Remember, the dosing is based solely on 17OHP measurements and as none of the 17OHP levels are excessively high, we can assume that the androgens levels are within acceptable range).

4. Although tempted to leave this dose as it was, looking at all the 17OHP levels we decided to lower the evening dose as the 17OHP at 22:00 was 1.5 nmol/l. This was already low and estimating that a dose would be taken at this point, 17OHP would become over suppressed by the high cortisol level at 400 nmol/l, which occurs at a time when cortisol is naturally low. So we decrease this dose.

The patient then had another 24 hour profile on the new dosing schedule.

We now look at what happened with these changes in place.

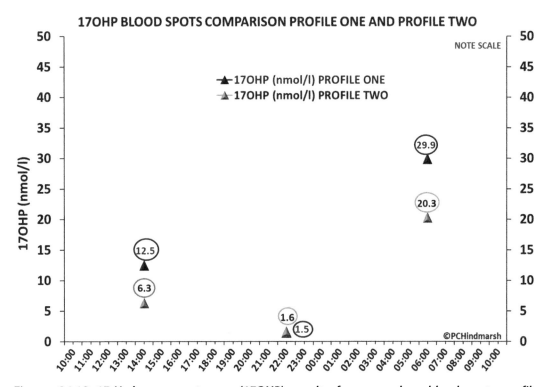

Figure 34.12 *17-Hydroxyprogesterone (17OHP) results from pre dose blood spots profile undertaken before (Profile 1) and after (Profile 2) the dose changes.*

In Fig. 34.12 we can see the changes to the pre dose 17OHP levels in Profile 1, before the dose adjustment and the effect these changes have made in Profile 2. Remember, we increased the morning dose which has brought down the 12.5 nmol/l to 6.3 nmol/l. We decreased the evening dose and actually this has lowered the morning 17OHP level from 29.9 to 20.3 nmol/l, so in fact we can be extremely pleased with these 17OHP results.

Let's compare all the 17OHP results (Fig. 34.13).

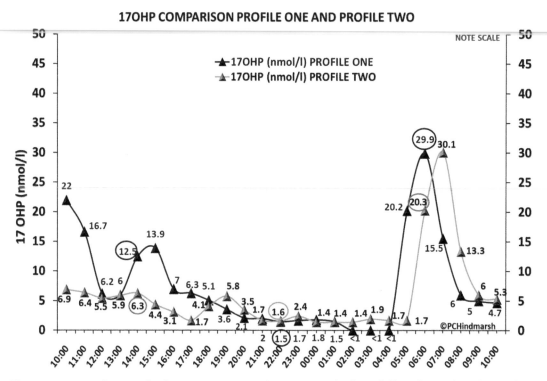

Figure 34.13 *24 hour 17-hydroxyprogesterone (17OHP) results from full profile undertaken before (Profile 1) and after (Profile 2) the dose changes.*

In Profile 2, to overcome the response to pain, the cannula was inserted 2 hours before the profile was started. Overall, we can see that throughout the day the 17OHP levels are 'well controlled' and surely this confirms we made the right adjustments! Well did we?

We need to remember and consider the following facts:

• It is the missing hormone cortisol which is being replaced.

- Raised 17OHP levels are driven by elevated ACTH production from the pituitary gland, as a result of a lack in cortisol production.
- The 17OHP level is affected by the amount of replacement glucocorticoid which is taken.
- There is a delay to this effect.
- There can be no cortisol in the body for several hours, but 17OHP levels can be within normal range, or in fact no 17OHP can be measured in the blood.
- High doses of glucocorticoid can totally switch off 17OHP production.
- 17OHP production can be temporarily elevated from the pain of the blood sampling, insertion of a cannula or blood spot sample.
- A raised 17OHP level may not be indicative of a lack of cortisol, but elevated due to 17OHP production from adrenal rests or polycystic ovaries.
- 17OHP is a steroid hormone in the glucocorticoid pathway and not an androgen.
- The accepted optimal 17OHP level in replacement therapy varies considerably between centres, this can range from >100 nmol/l for the pre dose morning level, down to 5 nmol/l.

Let's have a look at the cortisol replacement.

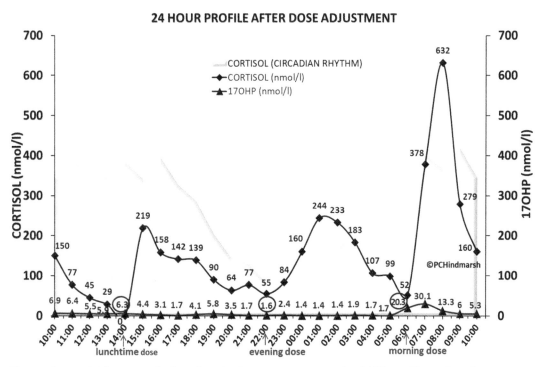

Figure 34.14 *24 hour cortisol and 17-hydroxyprogesterone (17OHP) profile undertaken on new dosing schedule.*

When we look at the cortisol replacement (Fig. 34.14) we can see that we are not doing too well with this. The morning cortisol peak is too high and this will lead to side effects. We can also see that the patient is still low on cortisol from 11:00 with no cortisol left pre dose. To get a detailed look at what the increase has done to the cortisol levels, we now compare cortisol levels from both dosing schedules (Fig. 34.15).

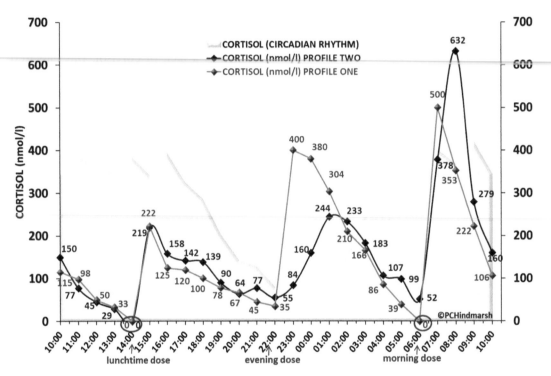

Figure 34.15 *24 hour cortisol and 17-hydroxyprogesterone (17OHP) profile undertaken before (Profile 1) and after (Profile 2) the dose changes.*

Studying the cortisol replacement values, we can see that from midmorning the cortisol levels drop very low, normal production levels should be in the hundreds. This is not surprising as the morning dose was taken at 06:00, the next dose is taken at 14:00, 8 hours after the morning dose which lasts around 6 hours.

The second profile, even with the higher dose in the morning, the cortisol does not last any longer in the blood and there is a period where there is still no cortisol. This period of inadequate cortisol is termed as under replacement and will lead to low energy, headaches, dizziness and all the other associated signs of low cortisol. What is also very evident, is the very high peak from the dose increase and this over replacement will lead to both short and long term side effects, especially weight gain.

The evening dose even though lower, lasts longer, a phenomenon we have seen occur in many of the profiles we have undertaken.

So, if we were treating the 17OHP as opposed to using it as a guide as to how cortisol is actually influencing 17OHP levels, we would be doing well. BUT as our principal objective in CAH is to replace missing cortisol, we can see that cortisol replacement is suboptimal. Many suffer low energy levels, mood swings, headaches, problems which are usually resolved when the cortisol replacement is adjusted and fine tuned. Even if the patient did not suffer short term side effects, these periods of over and under treatment over many years may very well be responsible for the poor health and quality of life which CAH adult studies have highlighted.

This patient actually needs four doses of hydrocortisone a day, with careful attention to timing of medication. This would ensure that optimal 'stacking' would occur to avoid cortisol levels dropping too low and smaller doses given at the appropriate time to stack the correct amount onto the cortisol left in the system, avoiding excessive levels of cortisol.

Summary

What is evident from these profiles is the following:

1. You cannot accurately assess the amount of cortisol in the blood by simply looking at the 17OHP levels.
2. Increased doses do not last longer, they dampen down 17OHP production as we can see in Profile 1 where the high evening dose totally suppressed 17OHP for several hours.
3. The patient needs a better distribution of cortisol which could be achieved by taking four doses a day, with careful attention to the timing of when to 'stack' the dose, so there are no periods of inadequate cortisol replacement or indeed 'over stacking'.
4. As the aim of therapy is to sustain life by replacing cortisol, it is important to ensure replacement is optimal, by looking at both the cortisol achieved from the hydrocortisone and the effect it has on 17OHP which should be used as a check.

What we need to think about when dealing with CAH:

Are we treating the 17OHP levels or are we replacing cortisol which in turn stops the ACTH drive and subsequently lowers the 17OHP levels? These data support the latter approach.

CONCLUSIONS

These short clinical exercises tell us how complex the replacement of hydrocortisone can be. In assessing replacement therapy, we need to consider what the aims of therapy are, which is to replace cortisol as close to the circadian rhythm as is possible without over or under treating. We know that statistics tell us we need detailed measurements and that comes from profiles. These case studies show this perfectly.

CHAPTER 35

Discussing the Emotional Aspects of Living With Congenital Adrenal Hyperplasia

GLOSSARY

Adolescence Period of time from 13 to 25 years during which puberty takes place and the person becomes more of an individual learning to be independent of parents.

Developmental stages The evolution of complex thought and consequences which starts from very simple concrete thinking to abstract thought.

Disclosing The process of giving information about a diagnosis and what it means in a staged manner using terms which are appropriate for the age and understanding of the patient.

GENERAL

Many parents wonder how best to tell their child about CAH. Like many chronic conditions parents often do not know when it is the right time to do this. The short answer to that question is that there is probably no right time, it is more a question of seeking opportunities. For example, sitting down and working through the whole steroid pathway is unlikely to generate interest in many individuals, even doctors! One way to think about this is to consider the various developmental stages which a child goes through and then to tailor the information accordingly. In this chapter we will consider parents of a child with CAH which has been diagnosed at birth. In the first few years as the child develops, the parent is largely involved in the normal child development steps such as learning to walk, talk and recognise objects. This is also a difficult time in terms of CAH, because parents have to be extra vigilant to detect early signs of infection when responsive intervention with increasing doses of hydrocortisone is going to be required.

EARLY YEARS AGES 0–5 YEARS

Between the ages 0 and 5 years there is a considerable change in the child, the doubling of height and weight (see height and weight charts in Chapter 6). Motor skill development is immense with the acquisition of skills to use crayons and pencils, to attain balance and to undertake coordinated activities such as catching. Expressive language also develops with the basics of adult language in place by the age of 5 years. Associated with this, children start using symbols and think about what is happening at any particular moment in time. Logical thinking is not really established at this age so what CAH might mean for the future is hard for them to grasp. This means that any talk has to be simply about the now. This can be looked at and discussed with the child. The parent might say that you need to take tablets to help you feel better and keep you healthy. This is a good way to start thinking about CAH. It appeals to the child because it is about something which happens to them in the here and now and is also very concrete in that they can then recognise the need to take the medicine and there is a very simple short term consequence in that they feel better and do not become unwell. This is good because they do have experience of being well or unwell, so this whole phrase helps tie things together very neatly in a way which is understandable. In another way, approaching the discussion with the child this way can be used to make the child feel quite special, that they have this extra thing, medicines, that others do not have. This puts a slightly more positive approach to the condition in that rather than just being singled out as being different, the child is also special.

Even at this very early stage, it is important for the family to recognise the impact that the condition has on other siblings. There is in CAH, the need to take medicines regularly and it is important that other siblings are not excluded by the child with CAH receiving more attention. This is understandable on both sides as parents are naturally worried about their child with CAH becoming unwell, so are more on the lookout for signs and symptoms pointing to a developing illness. Whilst there is probably not much that can be done to reduce the level of anxiety regarding their child, it is good for parents to recognise this and perhaps between them divide their attentions so that the other siblings do get special events as well.

Research has shown that siblings of children with chronic conditions have a higher risk of emotional and behavioural problems. The sibling may feel uncared for, unimportant, angry with the child with CAH and at the same time, guilty. Siblings may adopt different roles and become the supporter for the child with CAH, or take on a low profile so as not to cause problems or act out to gain attention. This needs careful work with medical teams. It is a normal response, so if you find it is happening then ask your doctor to get you support and help. There is nothing wrong in asking. It is not a sign of weakness nor shame. These are important and powerful emotions and often it is better to talk things over like this with someone outside the family who can offer a different perspective.

Whilst all this is going on parents have to work through their own emotions after the diagnosis of CAH. There are three main components to this process. *Shock*, which lasts, from the moment of diagnosis and lasts for 3–4 weeks. This often involves feelings of, no it is not real the docs must have got it wrong. This is a period of time of high anxiety often with upset sleeping and eating patterns, all superimposed on dealing with a new baby. This period of time needs a lot of support from family, friends and doctors.

Confrontation, this takes place from arrival at home with the new baby because this is where the parents now face reality. We have our baby which is great and the baby has CAH which we have to deal with to keep the baby safe and well. Again, support is needed as this is very stressful as it comes on top of the shock period.

Finally, there is *recovery*. This phase usually takes about 12 months. Things are seen in perspective. A more positive outlook develops. It is really important that parents get to this stage otherwise they can end up in a situation of endlessly mourning the loss of their 'normal' child.

CHILDHOOD AGES 6–12 YEARS

From 6 to 12 years of age physical growth slows. Over this time period children develop the ability to think logically and in abstract terms. By 9 years of age they can tell stories as well as expressing their own opinions. It is during this period that children can start to feel 'different' from their peers. This is particularly so at school where they need to have their hydrocortisone dose at lunchtime, or during activities when they have to take along their emergency injection kit. At this stage the question often arises 'why me?'. 'Why am I different and why do I have to take these medicines?'

The 'why me?' can be rather alarming for parents. They may resurrect their own feelings, particularly of guilt, that they have 'given the child the condition' or bring back the feelings that they had at diagnosis. It is important therefore, to be totally open in any discussion with the child. Often it can be helpful to say that many people have something wrong with them and when you were being made, one part, the adrenal glands, went wrong.

When introducing the idea of something going wrong, it is always good to follow on with reassurance all will be well as doctors have found a medicine that puts it all right. It is particularly important at this age, because although the abstract part of their thinking is developing rapidly, there is still a lot of concrete thinking going on and this requires a reassurance statement to be followed. We do know as adults that CAH is not as simple as just giving the medicine. There are a lot of things that have to be done as well, such as checking levels and looking out for complications. Those facets of care are important, but as far as the child is concerned, they reflect events which are going to happen a long time in the future and as such, do not necessarily impact on their way of thinking just at this particular age. There are certainly concepts which are important, but can be deferred in terms of discussion until later in adolescence. At this stage, curiosity will often lead the child to ask about how long they need to take medicines for. As we said, because of this stage they can think ahead a little, so you can say for life and they will accept this.

Sometimes a child will want more detail of the condition, although at 10 years of age this is less likely. If you are going to explain the condition you are better to do it in small chunks and do not do the whole steroid pathway in one go! We always like to work out what the child likes doing best. So if they are into cars, then you can make up a story along the lines of a motorway journey where the road to cortisol is blocked at Junction 21 and the diversion takes you off the motorway into androgen land instead. Then you can say that the medicine that you take creates a slip road to help you get by a different route to cortisol without having to go to androgen land. Using what your child is interested in, is a good way of using that interest and channelling the information so it fits more with what they can comprehend most easily.

Looking out for opportunities to bring up the subject of CAH is far better than trying to create set times and scripts to talk it through. School curricula include a lot of biology these days, so it is always worth keeping an ear open as to what the child is learning at school. Even genes are taught about at school, so this can give an opportunity to talk about when genes go wrong. If you need to refresh your memory on that, Chapters 2–4 will help.

ADOLESCENCE

Adolescence is a period of physical, psychological and social change. It is a period of time of the emerging adult personality and independence. This will be a difficult time as the young person seeks to be independent, but at the same time they might not be fully mature. It can be best summarised by a book title 'Get Out of My Life, but First Could You Drive Me and Cheryl to the Mall'! During this period of development there is a gradual appreciation and realisation of causation. In other words, something you might do today might have an impact in the future. That future might be weeks, months or years ahead. The realisation of causation and the fact that what you do today might have an impact on something tomorrow, develops slowly during adolescence and isn't fully in place until about 16–18 years of age. Even then, it probably requires further testing in the world until it fully becomes mature around about 20 years of age. This lack of appreciation of causation which is a natural developmental step, is why smoking cessation programmes in adolescence usually fail. It is not that the message smoking is bad for you and can lead to lung cancer which is the problem. It is simply the fact that the idea of causation and the time frames involved have not fully set themselves in the mind of the individual. At this point the adolescent regards themselves as immortal! Nothing can harm them which probably also explains why there is an element of increased risk taking at this particular age. Gradually, as the person progresses through the teenage years, importance of cause and effect becomes well established and risk taking and lack of long term appreciation, dwindle.

One of the issues which can raise itself at this stage is to be in control. The young person may want to be in control, for example, taking their tablets but social activities, for example sports and lunchtime may mean medicines are forgotten. This is rarely wilful and more a 'I forgot because there was so much going on' event. The standoff arguments which can arise at home are unhelpful. Rather, gentle persuasion and questions such as 'what might you do to remind yourself' are better approaches. The idea is to promote responsibility which is what they want, but in a way which is safe and achievable. The 'you must' approach is counterproductive; people, as always, are more likely to do something if it is their own idea, even if it isn't!

Again, discussions during adolescence have to be opportunistic. Face to face meetings to discuss CAH are not likely to be very productive. Rather, it is seeking opportunities as they arise. In addition, planting the seeds for longer term health is most likely to bear fruit in the mid to later teenage years. Again, this reflects the idea of cause and effect. Certainly, around 14–16 years of age any adolescent will want to know more about a particular condition and it is at this stage more detailed discussions can take place.

One area we have not covered here is the issue of surgery in girls. This is complex and one that needs to be worked through with the medical team. The topic could take up a whole book and we are not placed to talk about the practicalities. That is for surgeons. From our point of view it is best to be transparent about the decisions that were made and the implications of those decisions. This can be done along the lines of the parent acting in the child's best interest. When facing these discussions it is a good idea to rehearse them with the medical team. Psychology input into how best to present information can be immensely helpful for families. It is important, in all this to respect the child as an individual and also to recognise their right to privacy regarding their medical condition. This is extremely important with CAH and its association with DSD. Social media, is not the place to discuss children's issues and using photos of them makes it easy to be identified. Teenagers, in particular, do not want to be seen to be different and often do not want people to know they have a medical condition. Careless disclosure of their condition could possibly lead to future negative repercussions, e.g. bullying, lack of confidence, employment prospects. They are individuals and their medical condition is first and foremost theirs.

INTERACTION OF CONGENITAL ADRENAL HYPERPLASIA WITH NORMAL DEVELOPMENT

One of the difficulties parents often face in understanding behaviour in their children, is how much the condition itself and/or its treatment is the cause of the behaviour, compared to what might be expected normally. Certainly, it is helpful to have other siblings to compare developmental changes with, particularly if the siblings are older. We know that when glucocorticoids such as hydrocortisone, but particularly prednisolone and dexamethasone are given in doses that are higher than required, then side effects can arise especially with mood and behavioural changes. In addition, if insufficient hydrocortisone is given, adrenal androgens will come to the fore which in themselves although weak, can lead to behavioural changes as well. Separating what might be attributable to the condition which is being treated versus natural development is quite hard. It is in these situations that 24 hour profiles play a very important role. If we have cortisol replacement correct, which brings all the other hormones such as the adrenal androgens into the normal range, then we can be assured that any changes in behaviour are more likely to be due to normal development and not related to CAH. It is only when we know CAH is well managed with hydrocortisone replacement, that we can be assured whatever we advise about behaviour is based on normal development and not on CAH itself.

CONCLUSIONS

The way to tell a child or young person about their condition is quite difficult. Rather than having set periods of time when this should happen, parents should use opportunities in the child's life to introduce an explanation about the condition. This will vary depending on the age of the child and as the child progresses through nursery and primary school, this will largely be talked about it in more general terms and gradually focused on areas as opportunities arise. During adolescence, engagement with the young person may be more difficult but there will be times when questions will arise. The skill of parenting is to spot these particular times and then to use them to raise the topic which is understandable to the individual.

FURTHER READING

Hopson, B., Scally, M., Stafford, K., 1992. Transitions: The Challenge of Change. Lifeskills Personal Development Series. Lifeskills Communication, London.

Wolf, A.E., 2002. Get Out of My Life, but First Could You Drive Me & Cheryl to the Mall: A Parent's Guide to the New Teenager. Farrar Strauss Giroux, New York.

APPENDIX 1

Converting System International (SI) Blood Measures Into North American Values or Conventional Units

In this book we have used the units of measurement that are used in Europe called the System International (SI). If you are from North America or some other part of the world where this system is not commonly used, then blood results are presented in different units, often referred to as conventional units. To help you understand the graphs better, you can convert the SI measures to the conventional or North American measures using the following table.

Measure	SI units	Conversion	North American units
Cortisol	nmol/l	÷27.6	mcg/dl
17-Hydroxyprogesterone	nmol/l	÷0.03	ng/dl
Androstenedione	nmol/l	÷0.035	ng/dl
Testosterone	nmol/l	÷0.035	ng/dl
ACTH	pg/ml	No difference	pg/ml
LH	U/l	No difference	U/l
FSH	U/l	No difference	U/l
Estradiol	pmol/l	÷3.67	pg/ml
Blood glucose	mmol/l	×18	mg/dl
Growth hormone	mcg/l	No difference	ng/ml

ACTH, Adrenocorticotropic hormone; FSH, follicle-stimulating hormone; LH, luteinising hormone.

Congenital Adrenal Hyperplasia. http://dx.doi.org/10.1016/B978-0-12-811483-4.00036-2

APPENDIX 2

List of Abbreviations

COMMON ABBREVIATIONS	
A4	Androstenedione
ACTH	Adrenocorticotropic Hormone
BG	Blood glucose
CBG	Cortisol binding globulin
CRH	Corticotropin releasing hormone
CYP11B1	11-Hydroxylase
CYP21	21-Hydroxylase
DHEA	Dehydroepiandrosterone
E2	Estradiol
FSH	Follicle-stimulating hormone
GH	Growth hormone
GnRH	Gonadotropin releasing hormone
HCG	Human chorionic gonadotropin
HPA	Hypothalamo-pituitary-adrenal axis
LH	Luteinising hormone
LOCAH	Late-onset congenital adrenal hyperplasia
NCCAH	Non-classical congenital adrenal hyperplasia (also termed LOCAH)
17OHP	17-Hydroxyprogesterone
PRA	Plasma renin activity
SVCAH	Simple virilising congenital adrenal hyperplasia
SWCAH	Salt-wasting congenital adrenal hyperplasia

nmol/l	Nanomoles per litre
mmol/l	Millimoles per litre
pmol/l	Picomoles per litre
pg/ml	Picograms per millilitre
U/l	Units per litre

Congenital Adrenal Hyperplasia. http://dx.doi.org/10.1016/B978-0-12-811483-4.00048-9

INDEX

Printed and bound by CPI Group (UK) Ltd, Croydon, CR0 4YY

03/10/2024

01040318-0006